What People Are Saying About
Own Your Health . .

"I recommend this book to all pe⟨...⟩ ⟨...⟩ navigate the confusing world of alternative medic⟨...⟩ ⟨...⟩s that work. Whether you intend to use alternative ⟨...⟩ ⟨...⟩egrate them with conventional medicine, the infor⟨...⟩ ⟨...⟩ *Health* can guide you to making the right decisions."

—Andrew Weil, M.D.
author, *8 Weeks to Optimum Health*

"*Own Your Health* is truly a landmark book in integrative medicine. It combines moving, personal stories with the latest scientific research in alternative medicine. Most importantly, Dr. Brian Berman is one of the few international authorities with the depth of both clinical and research experience to accomplish this task. With this practical guide, he and Ms. Weisman have elegantly articulated the potency of individual empowerment and informed choice as the cornerstone of health and healing."

—Kenneth R. Pelletier, Ph.D., M.D. (hc)
clinical professor of medicine, University of Arizona and University of
Maryland Schools of Medicine; former director, NIH Complementary and
Alternative Medicine Program at Stanford School of Medicine; author, *The Best
Alternative Medicine: What Works, What Does Not*

"*Own Your Health* is an impressive combination of the inspirational, the factual and the potential for integrative medicine. By telling the stories of patients who became 'medical pioneers,' determined to discover how to choose the best medical treatments from both worlds of medicine, this book is a welcome breakthrough and valuable tool for all patients and their doctors."

—H. Eugene Lindsey Jr., M.D.
cardiologist, internist and chairman of the board,
Harvard Vanguard Medical Associates

"A responsible book for getting the best out of medicine. Inspiring yet grounded in science, *Own Your Health* is for everyone."

—Wayne B. Jonas, M.D.
director, Samueli Institute; former director,
Office of Alternative Medicine, National Institutes of Health;
coeditor, *Essentials of Complementary and Alternative Medicine*

"*Own Your Health* is a book with several important messages. For patients, it is an exciting, beautifully written and well-informed guide to alternative medical strategies. In particular, it offers direct firsthand experiences of several of these treatment options, with a careful discussion of the contribution each approach made possible. As a teacher of medicine I also found the volume important. Many of the comments are of great significance in a medical world increasingly incarcerated by technology, and in which the individual contribution of the physician as healer is being neglected. Finally, it is essential for all physicians to be made aware of the other therapeutic routes available outside their normal professional experience—and this book eloquently describes many of the additional advantages of a clinical practice which integrates these."

—**David Morris, M.A. (Cantab.)**
member, Royal College of Physicians,
associate professor of medicine, reproductive
endocrinology, McGill University, Montreal, Quebec

OWN YOUR
HEALTH

Choosing the Best from
Alternative & Conventional Medicine

EXPERTS TO GUIDE YOU, RESEARCH TO
INFORM YOU, STORIES TO INSPIRE YOU

ROANNE WEISMAN WITH BRIAN BERMAN, M.D.

Nov. 14, 2003 Jewish Book Fair speaker

Health Communications, Inc.
Deerfield Beach, Florida

www.hcibooks.com

Library of Congress Cataloging-in-Publication Data

Weisman, Roanne
     Own your health : choosing the best from alternative & conventional
 medicine : experts to guide you, research to inform you, stories to inspire you /
 Roanne Weisman, with Brian Berman.
        p. cm.
     ISBN 0-7573-0011-1 (tp)
     1. Health.   2. Alternative medicine.   3. Medicine, Popular.   I. Berman, Brian.
 II. Title.

 RA776.5 .W456 2003
 613—dc21

                                                                    2002038713

©2003 Roanne Weisman
ISBN 0-7573-0011-1

All rights reserved. Printed in the United States of America. No part of this publication may
be reproduced, stored in a retrieval system or transmitted in any form or by any means, electronic, mechanical, photocopying, recording or otherwise, without the written permission
of the publisher.

HCI, its Logos and Marks are trademarks of Health Communications, Inc.

Publisher: Health Communications, Inc.
                3201 S.W. 15th Street
                Deerfield Beach, FL 33442-8190

Cover design by Lawna Patterson Oldfield
Inside book design by Dawn Von Strolley Grove
Author photo by Robin Z. Boger

To Michael,
who has been a vital force in my life for twenty-five years.
And to our children, Benjamin and Elizabeth,
each one a miraculous blessing.

CONTENTS

ACKNOWLEDGMENTS

It took more than a year to write this book, but I have been thinking about health and illness for much longer than that. Thoughts alone do not create a book, however. Peter Vegso and Tom Sand, of HCI, had the vision and the imagination to crystallize the structure of this book and to help make it a reality, and I thank them both. Tom's enthusiasm and curiosity were contagious, as was his unwavering belief that I could use both my background as a science/medical writer and my own experiences to produce a book that would be useful to those who are facing serious medical problems, recovering from illness or trying to create lifestyles that promote longevity and good health.

I will always be grateful to Tom for inspiring me to reach deeper within myself as a writer to discover new truths.

I am also grateful to Brian Berman, M.D., director of the Complementary Medicine Program at the University of Maryland. Besides my family, I only have one "day job": I write. He has at least three: In addition to being an authority in the field of integrative medicine (combining conventional and complementary treatment), he is a caring physician, a respected scientist and a talented teacher, lecturing in this country and abroad. Despite his busy schedule and the fact that we live in different cities, he was always available to advise me on the structure and content of this book. He helped ensure that we covered the most important topics, and directed me to fascinating physicians and researchers who are experts in their fields. In addition, he contributed valuable expertise on using integrative medicine in the treatment of pain and cancer, as well as advice on ways to "own your health" by combining complementary and conventional medicine. And throughout the writing process, his guidance and thoughtful review of the manuscript helped ensure a balance between humanity and science.

The Voices in These Pages

As I look through almost every page of this book, I can hear again the voices behind the names: Some belong to the courageous patients who shared their stories of struggle; some belong to the physicians, scientists and practitioners who described their passion to heal. Others are less visible, but no less important: those who read the manuscript, talked with me about health and illness and provided solid editorial consultation. This book would not exist without these people. I give them my deepest gratitude.

Eugene Lindsey, M.D., a healing physician—and a gifted writer as well—who has been my doctor for twenty-five years, whose gracious generosity of spirit helped make this book possible, and whose wisdom and openness helped me to own my own health.

Christine Belleris, HCI editorial director, whose perceptive advice helped to shape both structure and content.

Carla Lane, a good friend and a science and medical editor on a relentless quest for clarity and accuracy.

Erica Orloff, who contributed not only her editorial skills but also her own courageous story of healing.

Alexa Fleckenstein, M.D., who played so many important roles: expert, constant encourager and tireless reader of the entire manuscript. Her comments and editorial suggestions were invaluable, as is her friendship.

Deborah Adams and Eurydice Hirsey, D.C., both extraordinary practitioners who help me find my own healing power. I thank them for their passionate belief in this book and for sharing both their time and their stories.

Ester Shapiro, Ph.D., for her wisdom about the nature of healing.

Julie Gleason, who helped me discover my strength.

Deborah Levinson, a bottomless fount of Macintosh wisdom, who seems to know everything and can explain it perfectly.

Ann MacDonald, a friend and writer of extraordinary talent who is always generous with ideas and advice.

HCI staff members, including: Kim Weiss, director of public relations; Randee Feldman and Kelly Johnson Maragini in the marketing department; Allison Janse and Kathy Grant in editorial; Larissa Hise Henoch, director of the art department, and her staff, Lawna Patterson Oldfield, Anthony Clausi and Dawn Von Strolley Grove; and copyeditor Nancy Burke.

William ("Mac") Beckner, of the Complementary Medicine Program at the University of Maryland, for his vast, comprehensive knowledge of research and resources in the field and for his helpfulness in making it available to me.

Jill Kneerim and Patricia Nelson, Esq., for their wise counsel.

The members of a very special writers' group: Alexa Fleckenstein, Carol Michael, Eleanor Rosellini, Kathryn Silver and Diana Tsomides.

Emile Lievore and Fabiano Roque for keeping the essential details of life smoothly operating.

In addition to those already mentioned, I thank so many experts who took the time to talk to me and share research studies, articles and information, including:

Practitioners Martin Anderson; Ghanshyam Singh Birla; Doreen Friedman; Xiao Ming Cheng; Paul Fraser; Christine Harris; Susan Himmelman, M.S.; Fern Ross Israel; Andrea Lindsay, LI.C.S.W.; Sarena Morello, M.S.; Carol Nelson; Chandan Rugenius; Betty Solbjor; Enza Stabilé; Cindy Stewart; Adele Strauss; Ayelet Weiselfish; Erika Wilton; Shu Xian Yang, M.D.

Integrative medicine physicians and researchers Rachel Brooks, M.D.; Barrie R. Cassileth, Ph.D.; Ted Chapman, M.D.; Andreas Constantinou, Ph.D.; Phuli Cohan, M.D.; James A. Duke, Ph.D.; James S. Gordon, M.D.; Jennifer Jacobs, M.D., M.P.H.; Wayne Jonas, M.D.; Ted J. Kaptchuk, O.M.D.; David E. Krebs, Ph.D., P.T.; D. Vasant Lad, B.A.M.S., M.Sc.; Frederic Luskin, Ph.D.; Gail Mahady, Ph.D.; Victoria Maizes, M.D.; John D. Mark, M.D.; Margaret Naeser,

Ph.D.; Pamela Peeke, M.D., M.P.H.; Kenneth R. Pelletier, Ph.D., M.D., (hc); Thomas Perls, M.D., M.P.H.; Srinivasa N. Raja, M.D.; Glenn Rothfeld, M.D., MAc; Virender Sodhi, M.D.; Marty Sullivan, M.D., (and with special thanks to Karen Gray in his office); Jill M. Tall, Ph.D.; Laura Wood, R.N.; Andrew Weil, M.D.; and Grace Ziem, M.D., M.P.H.

Physicians and scientists Joseph M. Alexander, Ph.D.; Dario Fauza, M.D.; Rudolf Jaenisch, M.D.; Aaron Rapoport, M.D.; Harold Rosen, M.D.; Michael Rosenblatt, M.D.; Clifford Woolf, M.D.; and the surgical and research team at Massachusetts General Hospital Transplantation Biology Research Center, directed by David H. Sachs, M.D., and including Nina Tolkoff-Rubin, M.D., Thomas Spitzer, M.D. and transplant surgeons A. Benedict Cosimi, M.D. and Francis Delmonico, M.D.

People of courage who overcame tremendous challenges and had the generosity to share their stories: Julie Aredondo, Miriam "Mimi" Berger, Jinny Chapin, Elinor Cohen, Deborah Dunham, BJ Goodwin, Marjorie Heffernan, Barbara Kivowitz, Marin, Janet Madden McCourt, Maureen and Walter Mercer, Jacqueline Miller, Geeta Sharma, M.D., M.P.H., Mike Siddall, Mark Soler, Marcelle Tennenbaum, Benjamin Lee Weisman (who is my son, and who continues to teach me how to create a life of joy even in the midst of physical challenges), Lillian and Paul Weisz, and finally, "Anna Olivera," "Ellen Johnson" and "Charlotte Harrington" (you know who you are).

Three reference and textbooks became my "bibles" during the research phase of this book:

The Best Alternative Medicine, What Works? What Does Not? by Kenneth R. Pelletier, Ph.D., M.D., (hc) of the University of Maryland and the University of Arizona Schools of Medicine.

The Desktop Guide to Complementary and Alternative Medicine, by Edzard Ernst, M.D., Ph.D., F.R.C.P., of the University of Exeter, U.K.

Essentials of Complementary and Alternative Medicine, by Wayne Jonas, M.D., director of the Samueli Institute for Informational Biology and an associate professor in the Department of Family Medicine at the Uniformed Services University of Health Sciences in Bethesda, MD.

Both Dr. Pelletier and Dr. Jonas, who work in the United States, generously granted me lengthy interviews, and their views appear in the text, as well as quotes from their books. Geography made it difficult for me to interview Dr. Ernst, but his comprehensive review of research on complementary and alternative medicine informs almost every chapter in this book. Dr. Pelletier's book, which is useful both for professionals and the general public, combines the history, philosophy and practice of most complementary/alternative practices with a thorough review and analysis of the research literature. Dr. Jonas's book, one of the first textbooks for physicians on the subject, brings together experts in such diverse fields as Ayurveda, Chinese medicine, spirituality, Tibetan medicine and homeopathy to explain each practice, including its history and relevant research evidence.

Throughout my own recovery and the subsequent writing of this book, my family and friends showered me with the gifts of love, support and encouragement. My gratitude and love to my parents Elinor and Seymour Cohen, my sister Carol Cohen, Lora Weisman, Matthew Weisman, Dan and Barbara Weisman, Mark Soler and Andrea Weisman, Sharon Polk Sadownik, Laura Lubestsky and Carl Sussman, Julietta Appleton, Susan Luther, Rosemarie Sansone, Ellen Glazer, Ellen Beth Lande and Detlev Sudcrow, Shelley and Dick Brown, Anne Callahan, Nancy Adams, Mark Schwartz and Adrienne Knudsen.

There are research studies in this book that found significant health benefits from connections with others in a community. But I did not need research to understand the significance of the astonishing outpouring of support from our friends and neighbors. During my own medical crisis, elaborate, full-course dinners began to arrive on an almost-daily basis (so much food that we had to put a second refrigerator in the basement), along with household and childcare help and a flood of warm, life-affirming feelings. How could I not get better?

And finally, to three of the most important people in my life: my husband and children, whose love sustained me during the hard times and who continue to fill my days with joy.

When the book was at its most consuming, my son, Benjamin, became a transportation manager, doing grocery shopping, driving his sister, her friends and the dog, and making countless trips to the store for still more paper and supplies. And Elizabeth surprised us: We always knew that she has a gift for nurturing and healing, but in the past year we also discovered a hidden talent for gourmet cooking! To Ben and Elizabeth: You make everything worthwhile.

And to Michael, who in the past twenty-five years has given meaning to the words, "in sickness and in health." Your love has sustained me and your constant support and encouragement made both my recovery and this book possible. Thank you for being in my life.

Roanne Weisman

I am deeply grateful to Roanne Weisman for taking the initiative derived from her own journey to health to write and research this book. It was her clear vision—that what she did others could do also—that drove this book forward. Knowing that people need information, knowledge and confidence, she was tireless and thorough in her search for the right sources that will help other people feel they can take control of their own health. I would like to also thank the many people who were willing to share their stories in order to inspire and inform others, and my many colleagues and friends who were open and willing to be interviewed for the book. Finally, I am especially grateful to my wife, Sue, for her support and encouragement to keep searching for the "best in both worlds."

Brian Berman, M.D.

FOREWORD

This is a book about healing journeys. It is not just a "how to" book, but an inspiration derived from the deeply moving stories of individual people, both patients and practitioners, who have grasped the challenge of illness and sought a meaningful way of achieving and owning health. In large part the book is an exploration of an approach to medicine that is broad and inclusive of many healing traditions. This vision of medicine embraces all of the wonders of modern medicine and the huge strides it has made in overcoming life-threatening diseases and acute trauma, but it also embraces the rich diversity of life itself by including approaches from other cultures and schools of thought. Perhaps most importantly though, it is an approach that attempts to right what has been called "the leaning Tower of Pisa of modern medicine." For all of the advances and great technological breakthroughs in health care over the last century, medicine has fractured the person it aims to cure into parts, even infinitesimal parts. In its focus either on the germ that causes the disease, the system or organ of the body that has been attacked, or the gene that predisposes a person to be susceptible to that germ, modern medicine has come to neglect the patient as a whole being with emotions, thoughts, beliefs, and cultural and environmental influences—all of which can also contribute to making that person sick, and . . . well and healthy again. Ultimately, this book is a celebration of the desire of people to re-humanize medicine, to reclaim a role in their own healing, and to be educated about and have access to choices in treatment.

My own journey to find a new way of healing began with the stories told to me by my own patients. It also began out of the frustration I felt when, as a young, fully trained and qualified doctor, I listened to these stories and felt the only thing I had to offer was a prescription pad or a surgical procedure. Like most aspiring doctors I had started out in medical school with all the altruistic ideals of alleviating human suffering and bettering the lot of my fellow man. Fortunately, my experience as a medical student only whetted my passion. Out of a desire to experience cultures other than my own in the United States, I had chosen to go to medical school in Ireland, and there I was embraced by a way of life that at that time was less technologically advanced than in the United States but was rich in unhurried time for personal interaction and storytelling.

Tagging along on the ward rounds of some of Dublin's hospitals, I saw the value of this emphasis in some of the clinicians who were my mentors and teachers. These caring individuals taught me that medicine was much more than the test results we were interpreting or the diseases and drugs we were try-ing to match up. Each patient had a story to tell, and the doctors were there to listen. I realized at the time that I was privileged to be witnessing true masters practicing the art of medicine, and though I took these gems with me when I went on to my residency training in the United States, disillusionment began to creep in.

Residency is a grueling experience with long hours, yet little time to give to each patient because of a hectic and overloaded schedule, and a great deal of information to learn and incorporate. By the time I finished my three years of training in family practice I was respectful of the tremendous achievements of medicine, but I was also exhausted and frustrated, ready to quit a profession that I felt had lost its heart.

On the one hand, I was aware that we have made huge advances in diagnos-tic testing and in understanding how the body functions down to the molecular and genetic levels as well as in improving public health and the management of acute trauma. On the other hand, however, I felt medicine had become a slave to technology, economics and the large machine of the pharmaceutical business. What was more, chronic diseases continued to baffle us, and in all truth, we had little to offer to alleviate symptoms, let alone cure. If anything, our powerful drugs were at best only giving us a false sense of accomplishment that we were "doing something" and at worst were allowing us to get people in and out of our offices quickly, not to mention causing problems of their own, so-called "side effects." There had to be a different way of practicing medicine, I thought, one that was more fulfilling and effective than this.

From these beginnings I went on to dedicate much of my career to learning about other medical traditions and approaches. Many of these therapies fall under what we call in Western countries "alternative" or "complementary" medicine. I began to integrate these techniques into my medical practice and, as I did so, felt a greater sense of satisfaction with what I had to offer my patients. In learning about systems of medicine, such as traditional Chinese medicine and homeopathy, I gained new insights into illness and healing patterns and how to consult with my patients. At one level I felt my practice was enriched because I now had more tools added to my medical black bag, but at another level I realized I was being challenged to reevaluate my thinking and my role as a doctor.

First of all, these approaches did not fit neatly into the scientific paradigm of my conventional training. They talked of concepts such as *qi* and *vital force* and used diluted medicines or techniques such as acupuncture, which were almost impossible to comprehend. What was this idea they shared of a life force that if blocked could cause illness and if stimulated could restore health? It is a concept that continues to fascinate me and one that I hope my own research and that of other medical scientists or even physicists will begin to decipher. Perhaps we will gain new insights that are as groundbreaking as the discovery of the nervous system! However, at this point in time, life force is not too far-fetched when we think of it in terms of the healing response, or the natural ability of the body to cure itself. Put differently then, the focus of these therapeutic approaches is on activating the body, the individual, to self-heal. And this is the important emphasis.

In incorporating these approaches into my practice, I realized I would lose their essence if I saw them only as other potential magic bullets. When it came down to it, whether using conventional techniques or alternative approaches, my role as a doctor was to be a partner with the person who will do the healing—my patient. The word doctor comes from the Latin *docere*, to teach, and as I altered and broadened my practice, I realized it was more important for my patients to feel in control of their own self-coping than rely on my treatment.

In *Own Your Health* the stories you will read are about people who have come to a similar realization as my own about a new approach to medicine and healing. The stories weave together themes of human suffering and dignity, and they uplift and as a whole paint a picture of the possibilities contained in the mysteries of life and the potential contained within each one of us. Sometimes it takes the experience of adversity, such as sickness, for us to realize we need to open our horizons as well as reclaim our own power. For me as a newly trained doctor I had felt gravely wounded and had to embark on a journey that led me to question many of my ingrained beliefs and turn away from some of my medical indoctrination in order to heal. In taking responsibility myself for what was right for me as a doctor and healer, I felt a great deal more strength and satisfaction even though initially I was really out on a limb and ostracized by many of my colleagues.

Fortunately, things are changing and the idea of "integrative medicine" is beginning to take hold. In the early 1990s, when I first started a program at the University of Maryland School of Medicine dedicated to scientifically evaluating complementary and alternative therapies and investigating their integration into a mainstream medical setting, we were pretty much lone wolves. Now, however, many medical institutions are taking up the challenge (including the National Institutes of Health) and have centers or programs looking at integrative medicine. The academic institutions with integrative medicine centers have also formed a consortium to promote the advancement and understanding of integrative medicine with committees focused on research, education and clinical care. This is an important first step and opens the way for a cooperative effort to look at the best of both worlds, conventional and alternative, in order to transform medicine.

The Chinese have a character, *Wei Ji*, which translates as "crisis." This character can be broken down into two parts, the top part meaning "chaos," and the bottom part "opportunity." Health care in the United States and many other Western countries is at a point of crisis. Increasingly it has become depersonalized, expensive and overly focused on drugs and technology. In facing its own adversity and chaos, however, the medical establishment has its own unique opportunity to look beyond its boundaries to seek positive change. By exploring that which is unfamiliar or foreign, medicine may have the opportunity to rediscover meaning in its own practice; a practice that not only incorporates new tools that may be gentler and less invasive, but one that also puts the patient, the individual, squarely back into the center of focus. By and large, it is people such as those who have shared their stories in this book who are driving the greatest changes in medicine. They are demanding to be seen as whole, complex and multifaceted individuals who wish to be in control of their lives, know about their choices, and be involved and valued as partners in a healing relationship.

Brian Berman, M.D.

INTRODUCTION:
"How I recovered."

If you met me today, you would probably think that I was a typical mother of two teenagers: I drive, cook, swim, work as a freelance writer, walk the dog, even play golf (badly) with my very tolerant husband and kids.

You would probably never guess that just after Christmas in 1995, during routine surgery to replace a failing heart valve, I had a stroke that completely paralyzed my left arm and weakened my left leg to such an extent that my doctors thought I would not walk again. In fact, in the hospital hallway, a well-meaning doctor told my already devastated husband, "Your wife will *probably* walk, but of course we don't know." Thank goodness no one told me.

I recovered. During my journey back to health, I learned about the power of combining conventional medicine with alternative (also called "complementary") health treatments. I also discovered that despite being surrounded by a loving family and skilled doctors, there was no single wise person who could tell me how to get better. Conventional surgery had saved my life. Conventional physical and occupational therapy helped me regain some use of my limbs—up to a point. But I soon realized that I was alone in this body, that how much I recovered was up to me: The stroke had robbed me of the left side of my body. I wanted it back, but I knew that this was not going to happen by itself. I needed to take some responsibility for my own recovery: to *own my health*.

This is the book I wish someone had given me the day I woke up with half my body paralyzed. If you or someone you love has ever had a frightening diagnosis, a devastating injury, a debilitating illness or an unrelenting pain, this book is for you. Even if you have had none of these health problems, but just feel that you'd like to rejuvenate your body, improve your diet, learn about health options for midlife and beyond, lose that weight, stop smoking, reduce your stress and get more joy out of life, this book is for you, too. This book is different from other health books. Not only does it give you valuable health information, advice and research evidence, it also introduces you to real people—patients, doctors and alternative practitioners—who share with you their unique, often riveting, personal experiences as well as some fascinating life journeys.

In each chapter you will find stories of men and women who transformed their lives and overcame seemingly insurmountable health problems by finding and combining many forms of health care, from advanced pharmaceuticals and surgical techniques to the ancient healing traditions of China and India. In these stories as well as in the "Closer Look" sections between each chapter, you will also meet passionate healers, including physicians, surgeons, bodywork therapists, energy workers, yoga and meditation teachers, acupuncturists and herbal medicine experts. Woven throughout the book are easy-to-understand summaries of research data, as well as advice from medical and scientific experts, to give you the facts you need to choose the most effective treatments and lifestyle changes. In the last chapter, which answers the question "What do I do now?" you learn how to find holistic physicians who combine "the best of both worlds," competent, accredited alternative practitioners and insurance companies that provide coverage for complementary medicine. Appendices define all of the major forms of complementary and alternative medicine and include additional information, resources, books and Web sites.

I was lucky: I found that combining alternative treatments with my conventional medical care (and by always keeping both my doctor and my practitioners fully informed) I could actually make a difference in my recovery. While not everyone's condition will respond in the same way, I hope that this book will help you discover your own power to heal.

My Body Betrays Me

When I woke up from open-heart surgery to replace a failing mitral valve and realized that I couldn't move my left arm, my first reaction was detached puzzlement and a mild curiosity. What was this about? It was not as if my arm was feeling weak; I simply had no connection to it. I could see it lying on the bed. I could feel it if someone touched or moved it, but I had no idea of how to move it myself. Trying to lift my arm or even wiggle a finger seemed as futile as trying to levitate the chair that was at the foot of my bed in the cardiac intensive care unit.

Doctors came and went, posing various theories of what might be causing the problem. The most popular view was that my arm position during the surgery had caused a temporary paralysis. My husband, Michael, looked dubious. Soon, the neurologists arrived. They would pick up my flaccid left hand and say, "*Try to move it,*" almost as if I were stubbornly refusing to cooperate. After several such visits, I finally became frustrated and said to some poor resident who was only trying to help: "Why don't you try to use *your* brain to move this arm? That's how hard it is!" I felt trapped and helpless in my own body. And angry, too. This was becoming ridiculous. Why was this happening to me? Everyone had told me this valve replacement was a "routine" surgery, and those ominous consent forms about the chances of death or disability (including stroke) were "just formalities."

By this time, a few hours had passed in the intensive care unit. The doctors decided to do a magnetic resonance image (MRI) scan of my brain, to see what might be going on. By that time, the neurologists had determined that my left leg was weak, although I could move it. And, when they asked me to smile (something I was decidedly not inclined to do), the left half of my mouth drooped slightly.

The next day, a trio of neurologists appeared, arranged themselves in a row of chairs next to my hospital bed, and regarded me solemnly through the bars of the raised bed railing. "We think you have had a stroke," said the most senior one. The others nodded. "We don't know how permanent the damage is," he continued. "People often regain some function over time." But after that first dizzying sentence, I wasn't really paying attention. I knew what a stroke meant. I had often written on the subject for the publications of my hospital clients.

"But you don't understand," I said. "I have two children. I play the piano. I'm learning the cello. I write at a keyboard. I carpool. I cook. I *need* my left hand, and I need to be able to walk." They nodded and said a few more things about the possibility of recovery, but, of course, no one could be sure. And then they left. As I watched them walk away, I began to feel a growing fury at the uselessness of these doctors. What good did it do for them to tell me that I had had a stroke if they weren't going to do anything about it?

Often called a "cerebral-vascular accident" or CVA, a stroke means that some obstruction, usually a blood clot, prevents oxygen-rich blood from flowing to part of the brain. Without oxygen, the deprived brain cells—neurons—die, and the bodily functions they control either stop completely or become impaired. Over time, other neurons might take over the functions of the dead cells, and the brain develops new "pathways" to communicate nerve impulses to the rest of the body. But there is no way to predict how or when this will happen.

A stroke is indeed an accident—in my case, a disastrous side effect of surgery—and is perhaps more appropriately referred to as an "insult" to the brain. My stroke was probably caused by a tiny piece of heart tissue that broke off during the surgery, traveled through blood vessels and lodged in my brain, causing a blockage to the neurons that controlled the left side of my body.

I felt like my body had betrayed me. During my life I had faced many health challenges and had always somehow bounced back, but this felt like a catastrophe. "My life is ruined," I remember saying to Michael, my loyal husband of more than twenty years. He had been spending day and night with me, sleeping in a chair in the intensive care unit and despairing that all he could do for me was feed me ice chips. A vigorous and athletic trial lawyer with a passion for long-distance bicycling, he is accustomed to attacking problems and finding solutions.

But there was nothing to attack here. No impassioned argument or clever negotiating could make these invisible threats go away. The only answer was "wait and see." So we waited. On New Year's Eve, Michael arrived bearing a bottle of sparkling cider that he cheerfully offered to the nurses on duty at midnight, insisting that I take a sip, too. I was in pain and feeling sorry for myself, but I sipped as we watched the ball drop in Times Square on the television hanging from the ceiling. "Next year it will be champagne," he promised me. (And he was right.)

Something Wakes Up

The day after New Year's, the real work began. Two energetic, bubbly young women—an occupational therapist and a physical therapist—seemed to burst into my hospital room, sweeping aside all possibility of self-pity with a firm "let's get down to business" attitude. The contrast between their optimism and the team of glum neurologists was stunning. One of them attached my useless left arm to a plastic form in a sling, arranging the fingers over a curved hand rest. "So that the muscles won't atrophy and tighten up, which happens when they stop receiving signals from the brain," she explained cheerfully. "And so it will be easier for you to move them again." Sounded good to me. That was the first hopeful thing I had heard so far.

They visited me often, moving and massaging the arm and giving me exercises to do with my weakened leg. After a couple of days, they decided it was time to get out of bed "just to see about walking." It was a good thing they were on either side of me, because my left leg collapsed under me as soon as I tried to put weight on it. "Just weak," they said. "At least you can move it. We'll practice." And so we did. After another couple of days, I could walk around the halls with a four-pronged cane, and even tackle stairs. Despite the fact that there was still no signal from my left arm, it was decided that I was medically stable enough to go home with continued daily physical and occupational therapy visits.

Spiritual Energy

About two weeks after I got home, the occupational therapist said during one of my daily sessions, "I feel something in your shoulder." She had been moving and massaging my useless, flaccid arm every day, seemingly trying to "teach" it what movement felt like again. I was feeling hopeless. Nothing was happening, despite her best efforts. She was a young woman from Australia, who always wore mystical looking beads and many silver bracelets and who talked about "spiritual energy." I thought she was exotic and interesting, but never really took her "spiritual" side too seriously. But this time, she seemed riveted on my left shoulder. "Some energy is trying to wake up in there," she said. I felt absolutely nothing and thought she was just trying to make me feel better.

Later that night, as I was sitting on the couch watching a movie with Michael and my mother-in-law, Lora, I suddenly "felt" a muscle in my left shoulder. With great effort, I could make a shrugging motion and drag the whole arm across my lap. Michael and his mother watched, then they both burst into tears. I was too excited to do anything but try it again . . . and again and again. When the occupational therapist came the next day, she said (almost smugly), "Of course. I told you. Now we have to get more control over the movement."

Slowly . . . slowly . . . over several weeks, other muscles began to "wake up," progressing down the arm, into the hand and fingers. I was clumsy, slow and awkward in my movements, but at least I could connect with my arm again. It seemed like a miracle and inspired me to redouble my efforts. I would lie in bed awake at night, lifting the arm up and down, trying to touch the thumb to each finger (sounds easy, but it wasn't!), over and over again.

❖ ❖ ❖ ❖

Now, several years later, I have almost fully recovered from the stroke. I believe that my recovery was due to what is now being called "integrative medicine," as well as the love and support of my family. The term integrative medicine originated in the late twentieth century to describe the combination of conventional (also called "allopathic" or Western) medicine and alternative, or complementary health practices. That sounds impersonal, but it is not. This is what integrative medicine means to me:

The high-tech world of modern surgery and a titanium heart valve saved my life. But when I had a stroke, the world of conventional medicine was not enough. Alternative methods such as yoga and acupuncture gave that life back to me by helping me regain the use of my body and strengthening my spirit. But it was only the combination, the *integration,* of these two worlds that has enabled me to fully live.

I did not have a book like this to help guide me in my recovery process. At the time, I had never heard of the term "integrative medicine." I just knew that I needed to find ways to get better. I learned by trial and error, making some mistakes, before finding methods that worked for me. This book is to share what I have learned—from my own experiences, those of other patients and from experts—about combining conventional medicine with alternative methods; to explain what some of the most useful alternative practices are; and to tell you the stories of remarkable people who creatively combined conventional and alternative medicine to regain their health. It took me a long time to be able to write this story. I was used to writing about *other* people's illnesses and the sophisticated medical research that helps them. My own story seemed far too personal. But thanks to many people I now understand that others may be helped by what I have learned. Happily, my communication skills (located in a different part of the brain from the area that controls muscle movement) remained intact!

Why I Believe in Combining Complementary and Conventional Medicine

My mitral valve failed because of a genetic disorder called Marfan syndrome. First described by a French doctor in the nineteenth century (named, of course, Dr. Marfan), this syndrome is a rare inherited disorder of the connective tissue throughout the body, seen with a frequency of one in every ten to twenty thousand people. Different from muscle tissue, connective tissue—which includes tendons and ligaments—is what holds our bodies together, the "scaffolding" that gives structure and shape to organs, muscles, blood vessels and in turn the entire body. (For example, scoliosis—curvature of the spine—is often caused by Marfan syndrome.)

Recently, it was discovered that the disorder is caused by a defect in one or more genes that are responsible for producing the protein "fibrillin" which gives connective tissue its elasticity and strength. This defect results in less fibrillin, and therefore less elasticity in the connective tissue, but to varying degrees, so the complications can be more or less serious, even within the same family.

The most serious potential problem of this condition involves the heart. Stretching of the tissue in blood vessels, heart valves, or the aorta (the main blood vessel leading away from the heart) can cause the thinning tissue to rupture or tear. In the aorta, such ruptures can cause sudden death. An aortic rupture killed my father (from whom I inherited the gene) at the age of thirty-six.

In addition to having scoliosis, my particular condition involved not the aorta but the mitral valve, which leaked slightly and caused me to have less energy than other people. I always knew that, over time, as the tissues stretched, the leak might become large enough so that the entire valve would have to be replaced. This finally happened in 1995, when I was forty-three years old, and it was during that surgery that the stroke occurred.

Growing up with chronic health problems spurred me to venture outside of the world of conventional medicine in search of ways to overcome them. My search led to alternative practices and eventually set me on the path toward integrative medicine. During both college and graduate school, I had already begun to dip a toe into the world of alternative medicine, beginning with a yoga class, which I found helped with strength, balance and posture, while putting no undue stress on my floppy joints. I also found the deep, meditative breathing to be relaxing and calming, and it just helped me feel better about my body.

The Fork in the Road: Making the Choice to Own Your Health

My experience of surgeries, physical limitations and, finally, a devastating stroke is not so unusual. Most of us will face a health challenge during our lives—either to ourselves or someone we love. Challenges may come in the form of an accident or trauma, cardiovascular problems such as heart attack or stroke, diseases such as cancer or multiple sclerosis, or just simply getting older.

We may be dealing with pain, reduced bodily function, the changes of menopause, sexual problems or anxiety and depression.

At some point, each person dealing with a health problem has to make a choice. For me, that moment came after a few months of conventional occupational and physical therapy for the stroke. My therapists told me that I had "plateaued." I could walk, but slowly and without good balance. I could use my left arm to pick up larger objects, but it was still very hard to pick up a vitamin pill or a penny, button a shirt, turn a doorknob or a faucet, or manipulate a fork. They suggested that I probably wouldn't improve much more and should now turn my attention to "adapting" to my limitations. This would mean buying buttonhole fasteners, shoes without laces, kitchen tools that would hold down a tomato while I sliced it, perhaps even walking with a cane for long distances. There were even adaptive devices for the car. (Disability management seems to be quite an industry!)

Western, conventional medicine was done with me. In that world, I was to accept my limitations and learn to adapt. The therapy was basically over. The only problem was that "adapting" was not what I wanted to do. *I wanted my old life back.* I thought back to the days right after my surgery, when my world-renowned heart surgeon paid me a brief visit. He breezed into my room, seeming, as usual, to be on his way somewhere else and said, "Oh, sorry you stroked, but heart-wise you're fine." (As my longtime physician pointed out, "So, okay, you don't need to have dinner with the guy. You didn't hire him for his bedside manner. You hired him for his technical skill." True.)

Well, heart-wise I was fine. That sturdy titanium mitral valve was clicking steadily and reassuringly with every heartbeat. But months later, here I was, sitting at my kitchen table laboriously working on my occupational therapy "homework": moving some small balls of putty from one piece of paper to another, one by one. (Using only my left hand, of course. No cheating!) I was frowning with intense concentration: This simple task was excruciatingly difficult. My fingers just wouldn't pick up the tiny objects, and when I did happen to get one between my thumb and forefinger, it was equally hard to release my grip and let it drop.

Elizabeth, my then-nine-year-old daughter, was cheering me on. "A daughter always needs her mother," she said to me. "But sometimes, a mother needs her daughter, too." Her way of coping with the scary prospect of a mother who couldn't move her arm was to take on the role of helper. She felt very important when she could guide my arm into a sweater or tuck me into bed. But her favorite job was to supervise my arm and hand exercises, probably because, as she saw me improve, she could begin to believe that she'd get her mommy back again. But as vigilant a personal trainer as she was, we both knew that she couldn't help me move those balls. I was the only one who could do that, and at that moment I really felt like giving up. This is where the choice comes in.

I felt that I needed to decide—right at that moment—how I was going to handle this insult to my body. As I sat there, I actually began to visualize a road that forked off in two directions. If I chose one branch, it would mean giving in to despair, disability and perhaps becoming an invalid. The other path would mean that I would continue to fight back. Because the paths diverged after the fork and grew further and further apart, I could see that choosing one would make it more difficult to change my mind as time went on.

Staring at those silly putty balls, I decided not to give in. **At that moment, I made the decision to "own my health."** Every patient I interviewed for this book described a similar experience and decision. Although it might be expressed differently, the meaning is the same: At some point, we all made the choice to take charge of our health and our recovery. I knew where the path to despair and disability would end up, and I didn't want that. This meant, of course, that I had to choose the path of fighting back. I didn't know (and still don't know) where that path will eventually lead, but the journey is certainly more satisfying.

I know I would not have had the courage to choose the path of struggling back to health without the loving support of my family and friends, all of whom never doubted for a moment that I would recover, and who never tired of telling me so. It's a hard road to go alone, and I now understand that the love and *belief* of others in my recovery was as important as almost any other medical intervention (well, maybe except high-tech surgery). It gave me the nourishing "juice" I needed to keep up that lonely battle.

I remember a time at home when I was still having trouble making my left arm do what I wanted it to. I was tired of being dependent on others to help me get dressed or hang up my clothes. I had decided that I was going to fold a blanket by myself, without asking Michael to help me. But, hard as a tried, I could not do it. My left hand was still not strong enough to grip and hold onto even the slight weight of the corner. After long minutes of frustration, I collapsed on a couch in our bedroom in tears. Michael heard me from the next room, came in and sat down next to me. He put his arms around me and we cried together. "We'll get through this," he said. That was all I needed to hear. We folded the blanket together.

The Integrative Medicine Pathway

Once I had made the decision to fight back to recovery, it was almost as if the pathway opened up for me. I had read that the practice of acupuncture was used in traditional Chinese medicine for the treatment of many illnesses and conditions, including stroke. Acupuncture is a treatment that dates back more than 3,000 years. It involves the (usually painless) insertion of thin needles into special points of the body to restore the flow of what is believed to be our life force, called "qi" (pronounced "chi"). This life force flows through invisible channels in our bodies, called "meridians." It is believed that blockages in the meridians that obstruct the flow of qi lead to disease, and that the insertion of acupuncture needles into strategic points along the meridians removes the blockages and restores the flow.

I was impressed with the fact that traditional Chinese medicine—which also includes herbal treatments and systems of slow movements and exercises—takes a completely different view of disease and the role of the doctor or healer than does conventional, Western medicine. At this point in my recovery, conventional medicine did not have options other than physical or occupational therapy to offer me, and my insurance company was telling me that I had now used up my allotted "covered" sessions. The message, at least from the insurance company medical administrator, was that I should now accept my physical limitations and learn to "adapt" to them—that the problem was dead neurons in my brain. I did not believe it—or maybe I just could not accept the possibility. In any case, I needed to find another way. As one Chinese doctor (trained in both Eastern and Western medicine) told me, "We believe that imbalance within the entire body creates the disease and, with the proper help, the body can cure itself." Thus began my journey into the world of alternative medicine. Now, of course, I realize that the most powerful approach is one that combines the best of both worlds.

By this time I had "graduated" from my home-based occupational and physical therapy visits to becoming an outpatient at a rehabilitation clinic. On a typical day I would use the exercise bicycle, lift weights and bounce balls while balancing on one foot. But my progress seemed to be slowing down. One day, I mentioned to the physical therapist that I was interested in acupuncture. "Funny you should say that," she answered. "There used to be a physiatrist here but she left to become an acupuncturist." I was very interested. A physiatrist is an M.D. with a specialty in rehabilitative medicine. Here was a Western-trained, conventional doctor who knew about stroke rehabilitation and also about acupuncture.

Before doing anything else, I consulted with my brilliant and very open-minded Harvard Medical School-trained cardiologist, Eugene Lindsey, M.D., who is as conventional a doctor as they come, but with some important qualities: He really listens, he sees me as a complete person, not just a collection of symptoms, he respects my opinion about what I need (within reason, of course), and he is not afraid to admit that he does not have all the answers. (To read more about Gene and his practice of treating the whole person, see "A Day with a Cardiologist," in chapter 4.)

For me, having a doctor like Gene made it very easy to explore alternative methods and to combine them with conventional treatment. "I really thought that after your stroke you might be permanently impaired," he told me recently. "But now I think you somehow *willed* neurons to grow in your brain." His openness to other healing modalities, combined with his (and my family's) belief in my recovery, helped give me the strength and the will that I needed.

ALTERNATIVE TREATMENTS THAT I FOUND MOST USEFUL

When I embarked on my journey into alternative medicine, I seemed to find each of my teachers and healers when I most needed to receive what they could offer. At first I thought this was just coincidence, but now I believe that if we are open to possibilities, we seem to get what we need. Here is a list of what I found most useful. (Appendix I contains brief definitions of the most common complementary methods. Subsequent chapters, as well as the "Closer Look" sections between chapters, provide more detailed explanations of each of these methods. *Please note that it is very important to inform both your doctor and any alternative practitioner of all of your health care treatments.)*

Acupuncture. Acupuncture sessions are very relaxing, almost meditative. You lie on a table and the practitioner inserts the thin needles into very specific body points. Then you lie quietly for twenty to thirty minutes. Often, I actually feel a flow of something—almost like energy—going through my body. I become very peaceful and might even go into a half-sleep state. After the session, I feel rested, refreshed, almost as if I've been on vacation.

Yoga, qigong, tai chi. These are forms of exercise that involve slow, meditative body movements and deep breathing to improve posture, coordination, balance, strength, and general well-being, as well as treat specific conditions. Yoga comes from "Ayurveda," the ancient Indian system of health, and uses special postures and breathing to treat conditions that range from stress to asthma, arthritis and heart problems. Qigong and tai chi are ancient practices of traditional Chinese medicine.

Here's a little related "integrative medicine" anecdote: During the time that the physical therapist was visiting my home every day just after my stroke, I broached the subject of yoga to her. She had never done it, but was interested, so I showed her some of the postures I remembered. Soon, she was showing up at my house in exercise clothes and getting down on the floor to do yoga and deep breathing with me! She said, "I usually just stand there and count while people do leg lifts. This feels so much more involved." After our sessions ended, she actually signed up for a yoga class and began trying to incorporate the postures into her conventional physical therapy treatment with other patients.

(continued)

Therapeutic massage. There are many different forms of therapeutic massage that help release muscle tension and reduce pain. I found deep tissue muscular therapy, Shiatsu massage and Ayurvedic massage particularly helpful for increasing range of motion and reducing pain. (Please see "Four Ways to Feel Better.")

The Alexander Technique. This is an extremely powerful method of using your body effortlessly, created at the turn of the twentieth century by a Shakespearean actor, F. M. Alexander, who had lost his voice. By watching himself closely in the mirror as he prepared to speak, he developed a technique of "non-doing": of freeing tension throughout the body, especially in the head and neck, to promote effortless movement in all activities. I began studying the Alexander Technique after my stroke to help me reconnect with my left arm, but I learned so much more. My first lessons involved simply sitting down and standing up. In the very first lesson, the feeling of rising easily, almost weightlessly, from a chair convinced me that this was worth pursuing. My teacher, Debi Adams, would gently place her hands on my shoulders, neck or torso as I did these activities, calling my attention to unconscious patterns of movement. I was tightening muscles that I did not need for the movement, hunching up my shoulders, for example, in preparation for standing up. These kinds of habits can become ingrained over time, causing pain and making it more difficult to move. Alexander lessons helped me become more conscious and aware of how I moved my body, yet the learning seems to take place almost on an unconscious level, as Debi gently taught my body directly how it feels to move in a different way. I am still surprised by little improvements that keep happening—seemingly automatically—almost every day. (Please see "A Closer Look at the Alexander Technique.")

The Pilates exercise method. Created at the beginning of the twentieth century by Joseph Pilates, this is the exercise method of choice for dancers and actors who need to be strong and look good, too. It is also the choice of anyone dealing with reduced physical function or who wants to build strength while avoiding stress on the joints. Pilates is based on a system of weight-bearing and resistance exercise—using springs attached to pulleys and moving platforms—to stretch and strengthen muscles throughout the body without stress. It is almost like doing yoga on machines. You don't necessarily "bulk up," you get longer and stronger. (Please see "A Closer Look at Pilates.")

(continued)

Meditation and relaxation techniques. I believe in meditation. I think taking twenty minutes during the day to focus on your breathing and slow down is a good thing to do. There are many different forms of meditation and I have found a few that work for me. There is nothing mysterious about meditation. I just think of it as a small "vacation" from the hubbub of daily life, television, computers, phones and conversation. Studies have shown that the "relaxation response" induced by regular meditation actually lowers blood pressure, slows down brain waves, and has many beneficial health effects. I believe this is true because I have felt it. (Please see "A Closer Look at Meditation.")

Of course everything I do is combined with regular exercise—swimming or walking, and regular monitoring by my conventional physicians. Although herbal supplements and nutritional guidelines have been helpful to many people, I need to be careful with herbs or vitamin supplements to make sure there are no adverse reactions with the conventional medication I take for my heart.

Please do not try any of the practices mentioned in this book without first checking with your doctor. And make sure to keep both your conventional doctor and your alternative practitioners fully informed.

How to Use This Book

A cornerstone of the integrative philosophy is that optimal healing occurs when *everything* affecting you as the patient is addressed. To quote the late Sir William Osler, renowned physician and teacher, "It is more important to know what sort of patient has a disease than what sort of disease a patient has."[1] Fundamental to the integrative model is the relationship between you and your doctor or other caregiver. Integrative practitioners recognize that they are not the sole sources of healing. By combining complementary/alternative and conventional medicine in a relationship that treats you as a whole person, they

---

[1] Sir William Osler was a Canadian, the personal physician to Queen Victoria, the most noted physician of the early-twentieth century, and the author of the most influential textbook of medicine of the times. According to Eugene Lindsey, M.D., "Osler was the heart and soul of what made Johns Hopkins Medical School famous. He was the Babe Ruth, Michelangelo, Shakespeare and Lincoln of medicine and supposedly the greatest bedside physician and teacher who ever lived."

can help you discover, or actually rediscover, your own innate capacity for health. And while the tools of conventional medicine—including surgery, diagnostic techniques and advanced medicines—are powerful, integrative physicians believe that these interventions are most effective when they are delivered in the context of a humane, caring doctor-patient relationship as well. So you can and should expect such a relationship from your health-care providers, and you should also be an active partner in choosing complementary therapies consistent with your own values or philosophical beliefs.

Throughout this book are references to many practices that may be unfamiliar to you. As you think about "owning your health" by combining complementary practices with conventional medicine, it might be helpful to have a more detailed idea of the range of choices in the complementary or alternative "world." Appendix I is an expanded glossary of most of the major complementary modalities, and can be used as a reference as you read the rest of the book.

The design of this book allows you to pick and choose the information that interests you.

- To learn more about particular alternative modalities, look for this symbol ⚯ marking the "Closer Look" sections between chapters.
- For health tips from the experts, look for this symbol ✓ marking the "Take Action" sections.
- For research on what works and what does not, look for this symbol ⚕ marking the "What's the Evidence?" sections.
- In various places in the book, you will also see "sidebars" in shaded boxes that give you extra information about what is in the main text.

Andrew Weil, M.D., who has written many books about natural healing, stresses the importance of careful exploration of complementary and alternative practices: "When you venture out of the world of standard medicine to look for alternative treatments, it is even more important to be an informed consumer. Alternative medical practices range from those that are grounded in long traditions of careful work to those that are nonsensical."[2] I hope that the information in this book will help you and your doctor create your own integrative, personal prescription for health.

---

[2] A. Weil, *Spontaneous Healing*. (New York: Knopf, 1995), 238.

A NOTE TO DOCTORS

Almost every patient whom I interviewed for this book made similar comments when they talked about the conventional doctors who were *not* helpful to them. The comments were usually made about specialists or surgeons whom they had just met, not their primary care doctors (with whom they already had long-standing relationships).

The comments were these: "The doctor never looked me in the eye." And "The doctor never asked how my spouse or family was coping with my illness." As one patient said, "[The doctor] kept looking at her watch while she was talking to me. I felt like I wanted to hold onto the hem of her white robe to keep her in the room with me." I have had these kinds of experiences myself.

Before my heart operation, when we first met the surgeon—a world-renowned expert in replacing and repairing defective heart valves—he assured me (in between taking phone calls about his upcoming lecture tour in South America and his dinner plans for that evening), "It's just like getting your hair done. You come in early in the morning and we take care of everything." He bustled my husband and me out of his office (the phone was ringing again) before we had time to ask any more questions—certainly before I could voice the terror I was feeling at having my chest cut open and a piece of metal installed in my heart.

The patients also commented on their appreciation when a doctor *did* look them in the eye and *did* show an interest in their husbands or wives. "I felt heard/ understood/seen" were some of the comments here. And the husband of one patient burst into tears when a doctor finally asked him how he had been holding up. "During the months of my illness, when my husband was taking over the house and family responsibilities and worrying about me, no one had ever seemed to care about him before," said the patient.

Every patient interviewed for this book also talked about the importance of their loved ones in their recoveries. I know that I felt better just knowing that Michael was in the hospital with me. Later, his steady presence in my life helped me to recover. And this valuable medicine is free! But few doctors seem to recognize the toll that such caregiving and nurturing takes on family members. If these people are as important to the patient's recovery as I believe they are, the medical profession should care for their emotional needs as well, or at the very least, acknowledge them.

(continued)

When Michael was still reeling from the news that I had had a stroke, one of the staff doctors said to him, "You have to be strong for her," during a rare moment outside my room when he allowed tears to well up in his eyes for the first time. Says Michael now, "I didn't mind her saying that. What bothered me was that was *all* she said. It would have been helpful if she had acknowledged how hard this was for me, as well."

1

ONE WOMAN ON OWNING HER HEALTH

"I decided I was going to live."

J anet Madden McCourt of Pembroke, Massachusetts, hit what she describes as "rock bottom" in 1997, when she was fifty-five. Both kidneys had failed— one of the effects of a deadly bone marrow cancer called multiple myeloma. She suffered from near constant pain in her bones and from an eruption of shingles on her legs (a searing rash caused by the same virus that causes chicken pox in children). She needed kidney dialysis (a several-hour procedure that uses a machine to perform the blood-cleansing work of normal kidneys) three times a week, which left her weak and nauseated for the entire day following the procedure. "I couldn't even walk up the stairs," she says. To make matters worse, her construction company was on the verge of failure because she was too ill to manage it.

She could not tolerate chemotherapy for the cancer because of her failed kid-neys, so her doctor prescribed steroids. "The steroids tore a hole in my stomach, ruined my esophagus and blew me up to a size twenty-six," she says. "I gained so much weight that I could barely fit into extra large sweatpants. I hated to go out because of the stares and whispered comments about women who 'let themselves go.' I couldn't believe that as a former model I had once thought that appearance defined who I was." As a final indignity, she had to cut off her long blonde hair because it kept getting in the way of the vomiting.

She knew she did not have long to live: After a bone marrow scan, her doc-tor had asked her if she wanted to know the truth. "I guess you've just told me," was her answer. She later learned from another doctor that her life expectancy was less than one year. As the weeks went by, her weakness, pain and despair grew. "You get to the point where you either want your life back or you just want it to be over," she says. Then, in October 1997, Janet's oldest daughter called with news: She was pregnant. "Right then, I decided that I was going to live long enough to see my first grandchild born," says Janet. "I had been a success-ful businesswoman all my life, able to do anything I set my mind to. I decided that I could conquer this illness, too."

It is now four years later. Janet has not only one, but *three* small grandchil-dren. Her cancer has been in remission most of that time, and she has a healthy new kidney, transplanted from her sister. At age fifty-nine, she once again has the long, silky hair and striking features that earned her modeling jobs in New York at nineteen. But today, that hair is coppery red instead of naturally blonde. "When I realized a few years ago that I wasn't going to die after all," says Janet, "I decided it was time for a new color."

❖ ❖ ❖ ❖

Janet Madden McCourt is one of a growing number of people who are seek-ing creative solutions to serious, even life-threatening health problems by com-bining the best treatments available from the worlds of conventional medicine and complementary or alternative therapies. This book tells the stories of sev-eral women and men who recovered from injury, disease and trauma, managed chronic pain and other health problems through each stage of life, and took care of their families and children in the same way. Their methods may be varied, but they share one important quality: At some point during the course of the illness, they made a decision to take charge of their health care by broadening their search for the physicians, practitioners and particular treatments that would help them. They made the decision to own their health.

Later in this chapter, you will learn how Janet, for example, battled "incurable" cancer by adding meditation, other mind/body techniques and nutritional supple-ments to her conventional cancer treatment. She then became the first person in the world with multiple myeloma and kidney failure to undergo a life-saving experimental kidney/bone marrow transplant at one of the finest conventional hospitals in the world. (The procedure has since been used successfully in other patients.) She knew that neither conventional medicine nor alternative health systems alone would save her life: She wanted both. By taking charge of her health care the way she had always taken charge of her life—and "owning" her health— Janet embodies the concept of the "patient as healer" who works in equal partnership with caregivers in the search for health. I hope that the stories of patients, physicians and alternative practitioners in this book will resonate with you, and that in reading them you will gain insight, ideas and, perhaps, hope.

Health Explorers

An increasing number of people feel, like Janet, that their greatest chance for good health lies in combining the best that conventional medicine has to offer with alternative or complementary therapies. In most cases, these people are like "health explorers"—entering largely uncharted territory: Outside the world of conventional medicine, the health care choices are overwhelming and often confusing. Which to choose? Meditation? Yoga? Acupuncture? Which herbal supplements? What *kind* of massage? How to combine the various possibilities? And what to tell my doctor?

Why are these people "explorers"? Because, despite the fact that more than 40 percent of all Americans now use some kind of complementary or alternative medicine (CAM) treatment, they are, for the most part, making these health-care choices on their own.[1] More than 70 percent of them do not inform their conventional doctors. In 1993, David Eisenberg, M.D., of the Harvard Medical School, reported that there were more annual visits to providers of alternative medicine (425 million) than to all U.S. primary care physicians (388 million), at a cost of $13.7 billion.[2] In 1998, Eisenberg and his colleagues found that between 1990 and

---

[1] D. M. Eisenberg, et al., "Trends in Alternative Medicine Use in the United States, 1990–1997: Results of a follow-up National Survey," *Journal of the American Medical Association*, 280 no. 18 (1998): 1569–1575.
[2] D. M. Eisenberg, et al., "Unconventional Medicine in the United States: Prevalence, Costs, and Patterns of Use, *New England Journal of Medicine* 328 (1993): 246–252; and D.M. Eisenberg, "Advising Patients Who Seek Alternative Medical Therapies," *Annals of Internal Medicine* 127, no. 1 (1997): 61–69.

1997 annual visits to CAM practitioners went from 400 million to more than 600 million, and the amount spent on these practices rose from nearly $14 billion to $27 billion, most of it not reimbursed.[3] People seem to be patching together (and paying for) medical care from two separate worlds.

A visit to any major bookstore in search of health-care information can be an overwhelming experience. One group of shelves—with titles such as *Your Guide to Illness and Surgery* or *The Complete Family Medical Encyclopedia*—gives you information about conventional medicine. The group of shelves next to it is filled with such titles as *Meditation Is Good Medicine*, *Herbal Remedies* or *The Complete Book of Chinese Healing*. On these shelves you will find information about alternative forms of treatment.

But few if any books help you combine *both* types of medicine: conventional and alternative. That is the purpose of this book. First, let's look at the difference between these two "worlds" of medical treatment.

Conventional Medicine*

The world of conventional or allopathic medicine includes powerful and well-funded academic medical centers—perhaps epitomized by the vast and imposing Greek architecture of the Harvard Medical School and its teaching hospitals. Conventional medical education, research and clinical care are supported by billions of dollars from the National Institutes of Health, as well as private infusions of funds from the biomedical and pharmaceutical industries in search of ever more effective medicines.

Some doctors trained in this world deliver their services in sleek medical institutions, filled with the high-tech tools of the trade: magnetic resonance imaging (MRI) machines capable of "seeing" blood flow and brain activity inside the human body; chemotherapy infusion centers delivering the latest chemical weapons against cancer; new laboratories capable of high-speed identification of disease-causing genetic defects in human DNA; gleaming operating

---

[3] Eisenberg et al., "Trends in Alternative Medical Use."
* With special thanks to William Benda, M.D., Brian Berman, M.D., and Andrew Weil, M.D., for interviews and material that contributed to the explanations of CAM and integrative medicine in this chapter.

rooms equipped for minimally invasive microsurgery. Other conventional doctors practice family medicine in community health centers and small private practices, even providing services from vans on the street to the homeless.

Public health relies on conventional medicine to prevent and treat disease. Conventional physicians/researchers are identifying the origins of disease at the cellular level, scrutinizing even the genetic information contained in the DNA within our own cells. They then use this information to design ever more specific treatments, targeting disease-causing cells while sparing healthy cells. In the treatment of cancer, for example, such methods hold the promise of less destructive, more effective chemotherapy treatments. Conventional medicine is the method of choice for the treatment of trauma infectious disease and surgical care (If you have a heart attack or are injured in an automobile accident, a conventional hospital emergency room is where you want to be!).

Those who practice conventional medicine are justifiably proud of the achievements of their profession—especially the diagnostic, pharmacological and surgical advances of the twentieth century. Conventional medicine has limitations: It cannot treat most viral infections or cure most chronic, degenerative diseases, allergies or autoimmune diseases. Treatments can be toxic. It is ineffective in treating diseases that are psychosomatic, and it still cannot cure many forms of cancer. Perhaps the most visible limitation of conventional medicine is in its delivery through an unwieldy and expensive managed care system. Despite efforts to control costs and improve services, the managed care system often puts tremendous economic stress on doctors and hospitals, resulting in hurried relationships between patient and caregiver that do not promote healing.

Complementary and Alternative Medicine (CAM)

Practitioners in the world of alternative medicine are trained in much smaller schools in this country or around the world. (For the purpose of this book, I use the terms "alternative" and "complementary" interchangeably, although there is a growing preference for the latter term, since most of these practices are considered as "complements" to conventional medicine, rather than "alternatives.") Often, the medical traditions date back several thousand years—for example, Chinese medicine and Ayurvedic practice. In addition to the more widely known Oriental techniques such as acupuncture, alternative disciplines include homeopathy; energy medicine; such mind/body techniques as meditation, guided imagery and the Alexander Technique; herbal and botanical therapies; neuromuscular therapies such as craniosacral work, Trager and Shiatsu, and therapeutic massage techniques; and specialized exercise methods such as Pilates. (Please see Appendix I for a more complete listing and description of CAM services.)

CAM remedies are usually less toxic than conventional medicines, and the techniques used by CAM practitioners are almost always less expensive than conventional treatments. CAM methods can help people cope with the effects of chronic illness and often focus on healing rather than curing; on the health of spirit and mind as well as body. There is also a strong emphasis on disease prevention. CAM therapies are generally less effective in treating serious infectious illness and often are no substitute for surgery.

Growing numbers of patients are turning to alternative remedies, often because of dissatisfaction with aspects of conventional medical care. And the world of conventional medicine is beginning to pay attention. In 2001, the National Center for Complementary and Alternative Medicine (NCCAM), part of the National Institutes of Health, had a budget of $92 million (up from $2 million in 1992) to fund studies on the effectiveness of alternative remedies, including gingko biloba to prevent Alzheimer's disease, yoga for insomnia and massage for lower back pain.

FINDING OUT WHAT WORKS

As of this writing, NCCAM provides funding to twelve medical research centers around the country that are evaluating alternative treatments for many specialty areas or chronic health conditions including: addictions, aging, arthritis, cancer, cardiovascular disease, chiropractic, craniofascial disorders, neurological disorders, neurodegenerative diseases and pediatrics. The centers are designed to efficiently evaluate promising alternative medical practices by establishing mechanisms for investigators to have their research ideas reviewed, developed and executed in a scientifically rigorous manner. NCCAM then makes information available to the public. (A list of resources, including Web sites, with much of this information, can be found in Appendix II.)

In 1996, NCCAM funded the establishment of a complementary medicine field in the Cochrane Collaboration to answer the questions of patients, doctors, health insurance companies and health policymakers about alternative practices and their effectiveness. Cochrane is an international network of more than six thousand individuals in sixty countries who work collectively to compile up-to-date systematic reviews of evidence regarding the benefits and risks of all health-care practices. The Cochrane Library, which contains all of these reviews, is one of the most highly regarded sources of quality information on medical practices. It is updated quarterly and is available on CD-ROM and on the Internet at *www.cochrane.org/*. (This book cites several research studies from the Cochrane Collaboration.)

Integrative Medicine: The Best of Both Worlds

Increasing numbers of health-care consumers want the best of both worlds: They want the technological arsenal of conventional medicine to take care of traumatic injuries, provide lifesaving intervention for heart attacks and strokes, and treat serious illness both medically and surgically. They want the latest techniques emerging from clinical research studies, the most highly trained, skilled doctors and the best, most advanced equipment.

But they also want caring, compassionate and prevention-oriented relationships with caregivers. They are growing increasingly intolerant of the frequent tendency of conventional doctors to consider CAM treatments as archaic or ineffective, and of the resulting divisiveness between those who favor alternative therapies and those who oppose them.

Physicians who practice "integrative medicine" (a term coined at the end of the twentieth century) address these concerns. While they may incorporate aspects of both conventional and alternative therapies, they do not uncritically accept either. The integrative physician explores a wider range of options to select the most effective, least invasive, least toxic and least costly medical interventions that are appropriate to the patient's situation, regardless of whether these methods are conventional or alternative. And most importantly, integrative physicians create relationships with their patients that are compassionate partnerships, in which the physician recognizes and respects the patient's goals, health-care preferences and autonomy. Studies have shown, in fact, that the more patients feel that they "own" their own health care, the better the outcomes. (See box, opposite page, "Patient as Healer.") There are, of course, many conventional physicians (my own among them) who practice this kind of "partnership medicine" as well.

PATIENT AS HEALER

"Your health is in your hands," says Ester R. Shapiro, Ph.D. "Although you may not have control of the course of an illness, how you respond to that illness—drawing on the support of family, community, your own beliefs and spiritual values—can help you heal." A psychologist, researcher, writer and teacher, Shapiro notes that only approximately 10 percent of health outcomes are produced by any contact with the health system. As many as 90 percent are due to your lifestyle, economic resources, social support, and a sense of power in determining the course and condition of your life and the lives of your family and community. "Patients who feel a sense of control—of ownership—of their health actually do better clinically than those who feel that they are helpless victims of their illness," she says.[4] Even the Institute of Medicine's recent publications are addressing the high cost and poor results of an illness-oriented system of care by proposing collaborative models that highlight behavioral determinants of health, patient-centered care, improved communication and greater emphasis on community-based services.[5]

Shapiro's publications focus on the way in which people and their families deal with extraordinary life challenges, including illness and death. She edited the Spanish-language translation and adaptation of *Our Bodies, Ourselves,* which many consider the ultimate book on patient empowerment (at least for women)[6] and teaches patient empowerment in community groups and workshops. "I am interested in how people incorporate the challenge of illness into their lives and the lives of those around them," says Shapiro. "How do people succeed in

(continued)

---

[4] For research on "self-efficacy" (the effects of patient empowerment), see *Self-Efficacy*, by Albert Bandura or the 2002 edition of *Health Psychology* by Shelly Taylor (see Appendix II for full citations). Both are evidence-based health promotion researchers.

[5] Institute of Medicine, *Health and Behavior: The Interplay of Biological, Behavioral, and Societal Influences* and *Crossing the Quality Chasm: A New Health System for the 21st Century,* National Academy Press (2001), http://www.nap.edu/books/0309070309/html.

[6] E. Shapiro, coord. ed. with Boston Women's Health Book Collective, *Nuestros Cuerpos, Nuetras Vidas/Our Bodies, Ourselves* (New York: Seven Stories Press, 2000).

overcoming adversity? What resources in their environment—family, religion, culture and community—combine with their own personal resources to build *resilience?* Resilient people know how to look for things that might help them recover from illness, while others might feel overwhelmed and defeated. How can we teach that?"[7]

Shapiro is associate professor of psychology at the University of Massachusetts at Boston (UMB) and research associate at the Mauricio Gaston Institute for Latino Public Policy and Community Development. As Practicum Coordinator for the Clinical Psychology Doctoral Program at UMB, she helped found a clinical training program dedicated to delivering urban services from cultural, developmental, interdisciplinary and health promotion perspectives. She is the author of *Grief as a Family Process: A Cultural and Developmental Approach to Integrative Practice,* 2nd edition (Guilford, in press).

In addition to providing the best conventional care, integrative medicine focuses on the preventive maintenance of health by attention to diet, exercise, stress management and emotional well-being, according to Ralph Snyderman, M.D., Chancellor for Health Affairs, and Andrew T. Weil, M.D., Director, Program for Integrative Medicine at the University of Arizona College of Medicine. In an article in the *Archives of Internal Medicine* (March 2002), Snyderman and Weil identify several characteristics of integrative medicine, including an insistence that patients become active participants in their own health, and that "doctors view their patients as whole persons—minds, community members and spiritual beings as well as physical bodies." They also note that, "Most Americans who consult alternative providers would jump at the chance to consult a physician who is well trained in scientifically based medicine and is also open-minded and knowledgeable about the body's innate mechanisms of healing, the role of lifestyle factors in influencing health, and the appropriate uses of dietary supplements, herbs, and other forms of treatment, from osteopathic manipulation to Chinese and Ayurvedic medicine."

---

[7] E. Shapiro, "Chronic Illness as a Family Process," *Journal of Clinical Psychology* (2002), in session.

David Spiegel, M.D., of the Stanford University School of Medicine, points to a weakness in conventional, Western medical practice as one reason for the increased interest in complementary medicine:

"By and large, doctors no longer conceive of talking, comforting, guiding, and educating patients as 'real' interventions. Rather, it is something to do until the injection is ready. An illness can be a lonely journey and patients crave people who understand what the journey is like and can stay the course with them. Thus, the apparent appetite for complementary and alternative medicine is stimulated by the vacuum of modern medical care. This vacuum, by the way, is being intensified by the business managers of modern North American medicine who pump even more time and energy out of the doctor/patient interaction by saddling doctors with more patients per hour, reducing their autonomy, and treating them like assembly line workers instead of professionals."[8]

---

[8] D. Spiegel, "Complementary Medicine in North America," in *Encyclopedia of Stress* (London: Academic Press, 2000), 512.

TRAINING NEW PHYSICIANS

The momentum of integrative medicine is spreading across the country. For the past four years, the University of Arizona's Program in Integrative Medicine, founded by Andrew Weil, M.D., has been offering two-year fellowships to physicians who have completed residencies in primary care specialties. The program also provides clinical services to patients and conducts basic research on CAM modalities, but its main focus is the restructuring of medical education.

During the past two years, colleagues at a number of health centers around the country have been meeting and sharing ideas intended to foster the rational introduction of integrative medicine into medical education and practice. They have formed the Consortium of Academic Health Centers for Integrative Medicine (chaired by Brian Berman, M.D.) to address the gap between what patients expect and want and the realities of the medical profession. This group includes representatives from the following medical schools: Albert-Einstein Yeshiva, Columbia, Duke, Georgetown, Harvard, Jefferson, and the Universities of Arizona, California (San Francisco), Maryland, Massachusetts, Michigan and Minnesota. The intention of the Consortium is to include as members enough schools until it can speak for one-fifth of the country's 125 medical schools. The goal is to become a significant voice in the call for fundamental changes in the way future physicians are trained.

As we think about the value of compassion and autonomy in health care, we should also think about the importance of being kind to ourselves. People who still struggle with illness despite their best efforts to draw on both conventional and alternative healing treatments and methods sometimes feel a sense of guilt and failure: "Perhaps I didn't visualize health strongly enough"; "I'm making bad decisions"; or "I must still be harboring negative emotions." It is important to understand that hard as we try, there are still physical events that are beyond our control. Just as we ask health providers to offer us compassion and kindness as we struggle, we must do the same for ourselves. Guilt has no place in the search for good health.

Finding a Reason to Live

Guilt and a sense of failure were certainly not part of the many emotions that washed over Janet Madden McCourt when she was finally diagnosed with bone marrow cancer. "I was at first in complete denial," she said. "But eventually I accepted it. In my life, I had accomplished more than I had ever imagined. I had raised my children as a single parent, and they were almost grown. I guess I felt that I could go now. But all that changed the day I learned my daughter was pregnant. I decided I was going to live."

In fact, it was the very way in which Janet had lived her life that prepared her to fight a terminal illness. As soon as she had a reason to live, she became galvanized into the kind of problem-solving that characterized her entire life. "I have always pushed myself to be an overachiever," she said. "I was abused as a child and wanted to prove that I could overcome—and maybe even block out—that part of my life." As a young woman, she had boundless energy, holding down a full-time job during high school and then a successful modeling career in New York. Her health was always good. "I watched what I ate and worked out in a gym almost every day for most of my life—at least whenever I had time and could afford it," she said. (She eventually left modeling because of the way photographers and advertising directors sexually exploited young women. "There had been enough of *that* in my life," she said.)

Back home to Massachusetts, she worked for a time as an X-ray assistant, but soon launched what would be the first of many agencies that supplied temporary help to client companies in health-care, corporate and technical services. By the time she was in her thirties, she had been married and divorced and was raising two children alone while running several businesses. In addition to the temporary personnel agencies, she had also started a detective agency and a security firm. "I just kept wanting to do more and then more," she said. "Every time I heard about a new kind of business, I would say, 'I could do that!' and then I usually did."

In the meantime, she was being recognized in the business community. She became one of the first female Rotarians, was on the board of the Small Business Association of New England and other organizations, and helped to build the New England Women Business Owner's Association. In 1985, she was nominated as the Small Business Owner of the Year. ("I think the award actually went to Ben & Jerry's that year," she said ruefully. "You can't compete with ice cream!")

By the mid-1980s, she had about two thousand people on her various payrolls. But then the recession hit, her client companies started declaring bankruptcy, and in 1990 she was forced to follow suit. "It was devastating to lose all that I had built," she said. But her style was not to give up. She took bookkeeping jobs, sold jewelry and other expensive items that she had bought, and invested with a partner in a small piece of residential property with the idea of building a house. She also went to work for a real estate company, studied for and passed the exam to become a construction supervisor, and launched her own construction company. "I had never touched a tool in my life," she said. "But I knew how to hire good contractors. If I ran low on cash flow to pay them, I would 'temp' myself out to other companies as a secretary, administrator or bookkeeper. Nights I worked as a bartender in an exclusive restaurant." She was fifty years old.

In 1996, just when the construction company was beginning to make a profit, Janet started noticing that she no longer had the arm strength to open wine bottles or carry trays in the restaurant. "I had also begun breaking bones for no obvious reason—I would lean over the arm of a chair and break ribs, or lean on my wrist and it would break. I even broke three vertebrae in a minor skiing tumble. But I just thought it was age," she said. She soon lost her job at the restaurant and then came down with what she thought was a stomach virus. "I couldn't stop vomiting and went to the emergency room of the local hospital," she said. "They gave me fluids and told me it was the flu." Two weeks later, still vomiting every day and feeling worse, she was back to the emergency room. "My eyes were turning yellow and looked sunken in and my skin was gray," she said. "But they just gave me more fluids and sent me home again."

Finally, at her mother's insistence, she saw a specialist, who ordered tests, determined that she was in kidney failure and had her admitted to another hospital for emergency dialysis. Further tests to find out why a relatively young woman with no history of diabetes should have massive kidney failure revealed the diagnosis of multiple myeloma—an incurable cancer of the bone marrow. "My doctor told me that I would have to remain on dialysis three times a week for the rest of my life," said Janet. "The bone marrow cancer made me ineligible for a kidney transplant that would make dialysis unnecessary. But I also learned that 'the rest of my life' was not expected to be more than one year."

Venturing into the World of Complementary and Alternative Medicine

After she had made up her mind to fight for her life, the first thing Janet did was to go to the library. "That's where I do my best work," she explained. "I read everything I could find on alternative therapies for cancer, although of course I intended to continue taking the steroids my doctor had prescribed." She learned about cancer-fighting diets and supplements, about therapies such as acupuncture and Reiki, about yoga, meditation and tapes that played messages of healing over and over again. "I tried everything, but eventually settled on a few techniques that seemed to work best," she said. "I was not afraid to ask my friends and family for referrals to practitioners." (Please see Appendix I for definitions of these and other complementary and alternative therapies.)

Eventually, she settled on a program of meditation, Reiki (a form of healing during which the therapist channels energy into the body of the patient), acupuncture and, most importantly for her, the constant use of "auto-suggestion" and "mind power" tapes repeating healing messages over and over again. "Some of my tapes had subliminal messages hidden in music or waterfall sounds. Some I made myself. I would wear headphones almost all day and all night to listen to these positive thoughts, even while I slept. I had a mission: Nothing was going to get into my head unless it was a positive or healing thought." (Please see "A Closer Look at Energy Healing, Spirituality and Therapeutic Touch" for more information about Reiki; as well as chapter 7 for information on biofeedback, visualization and auto-suggestion.)

The tape she made herself said, "Water is rushing in from the top of your head and flowing through your body with great force, washing and cleansing away all of the bad cancer cells—sending them out through your toes." Another tape repeated: "You are getting better. Each day that goes by you get stronger and stronger." Janet also believes in the power of prayer. "I prayed every day, and asked everyone I knew to do the same," she said. "I had family, friends, friends-of-friends and their clergy all praying for me—including people I didn't even know.

"I picked modalities that I could do with my mind, or that practitioners could do, since I couldn't do very much with my body, even yoga was too difficult and painful," she said. "I decided to strengthen my mind so that it could strengthen my immune system." As for pain, she found both Reiki and acupuncture helpful. "The pain in my legs from the shingles was excruciating, but after one Reiki session it was gone, although some bone pain remained," she said. "But I felt so good that I cancelled the appointment I had made at the pain clinic for that same afternoon." Acupuncture offered temporary relief from the pain in her bones, but she still needed conventional pain medication.

Janet continued combining alternative practices with conventional cancer and pain treatment for four months. At the end of that time, her doctor told her that the multiple myeloma had been in remission for more than a month. "Who can say which therapy or combination of therapies worked?" she said. "I was more interested in results."

The Next Step: Getting a New Kidney

"So now I'm thinking: The cancer is in remission. I can have a kidney transplant," said Janet. "I was really beginning to think that I could do this. I can beat it." But her nephrologist disagreed. "He told me that even though my cancer was in remission, you never get rid of multiple myeloma. It will always be in your body. He told me no one would agree to perform a kidney transplant."

Taking matters once again into her own hands, Janet scoured the Internet to find out "everything there was to know" about kidney transplants and myeloma treatment and research. "I was desperate to find the best hospital around," she said. Her search led her to Nina Tolkoff-Rubin, M.D., medical director of renal transplantation at the Massachusetts General Hospital (MGH) in Boston. "I had heard from other patients at the dialysis center that the MGH was an excellent place for kidney transplants, but I still needed to find a way to get my foot in the door of that hospital," said Janet. "I knew I just couldn't walk in without a referral." So she told a fib.

Waiting until her doctor was on vacation, she went to see the head nurse at her dialysis center and said, "Guess what? My cancer is in remission, and my doctor wants me to have a referral to the transplant coordinator at Massachusetts General!" The nurse was delighted for her and arranged the appointment. Janet had indeed found a way to "get her foot in the door" at Massachusetts General, but when tests revealed her history of multiple myeloma, she was turned down once again as a transplant candidate. Characteristically, she refused to give up.

"Dr. Tolkoff-Rubin initially said that I was not eligible for a kidney transplant because of the bone marrow cancer," said Janet. "But I said to her, 'Look, you've got to find a way to do this transplant because I'm taking myself off dialysis. I won't live like this anymore.'"

Janet's determination impressed Tolkoff-Rubin. "Janet hated the constraints of dialysis and would do anything to get off it," she said. "I knew we had to find some innovative, creative way to treat her if her life was to be saved, so I decided to investigate the work being done at our Transplantation Biology Research Center." After meeting with the team of surgeons and researchers at the Center, which is directed by David H. Sachs, M.D., Tolkoff-Rubin explained to Janet a new transplant procedure developed at the MGH. This involved simultaneously transplanting a kidney and bone marrow from a genetically matched, living donor.

One of the most difficult obstacles to successful organ transplantation is rejection: The recipient's immune system "sees" the transplanted organ as an "invader" and sends a patrolling army of T-cells (which are normally created in the bone marrow to target foreign attackers, such as viruses) to destroy it. In order to preserve the new organ, transplant recipients must take powerful anti-rejection (immunosuppressive) drugs for the rest of their lives.

Unfortunately, these drugs also make them more susceptible to opportunistic infections, cancer, diabetes and heart problems.

The MGH procedure involved mixing the donor's bone marrow into the recipient's immune system within a few hours of the organ transplant. It was hoped that the donor's bone marrow would "trick" the recipient's immune system into "recognizing" the donated kidney. This technique is called "mixed chimerism." (The chimera is a mythical animal with the head of a lion, the tail of a serpent, and the body of a goat.) The blended immune system is balanced to prevent both rejection of the transplanted organ and the development of graft-versus-host disease, in which donor marrow attacks the recipient's body.

"They told me the odds were unknown, since this had never been tried in a human," says Janet. "But when we found that my sister was an excellent genetic match and that she was willing to be the donor, I decided to go ahead and risk it. If I couldn't have the kind of active life I wanted, if I couldn't play with my grandchildren, I simply didn't want to live."

In September 1998, Janet Madden McCourt became the first human in the world with her type of cancer and kidney failure to receive the double transplant procedure developed by the MGH Transplant Team. (Similar techniques had been used in animal models.) Transplant surgeons A. Benedict Cosimi, M.D., and Francis Delmonico, M.D., performed the surgery, transplanting a kidney from Janet's sister. Following the kidney transplant, Thomas Spitzer, M.D., performed an infusion of the sister's bone marrow. Janet received anti-rejection drugs initially, but they were slowly tapered off. Eventually, her body accepted her sister's kidney as its own, and she has not taken any anti-rejection drugs since. As an added benefit, the infusion of her sister's bone marrow seems to have kept the multiple myeloma at bay. More than three years after the surgery, Janet's bone marrow cancer is undetectable and the kidney donated by her sister is functioning perfectly.

The anticancer effect of the blended bone marrow is still not fully understood, according to Dr. Spitzer: "This appears to be a graft-versus-tumor effect," he says, "which we need to explore through further research." Since then, the

MGH transplant team has successfully used the double transplant protocol on other patients, according to Sachs.

Janet Madden McCourt was determined to live, and chose the best treatments she could find from both worlds of medicine. "I believe that I would not be alive today without the help of my alternative practitioners and the skills of all of the doctors who did the research and surgery at Massachusetts General," she said. Janet is now a full-time student at the University of Massachusetts. She is studying art, photography, printmaking and architecture, and is planning to take courses in many other subjects, all while continuing to work part-time. "I decided to do two things that I never had time for," she said. "Get a college degree and develop some hobbies." She also does part-time accounting work for a local deep-sea fishing company.

I caught up with Janet recently during the midwinter break from college classes. She had just returned from Colorado, where her son lives, and an impromptu family reunion. "We were all together over the holidays," she says. "My children and their spouses and, of course, the grandchildren. It was wonderful." Back home, she tries to keep up with her exercising, walking regularly. This year, she bought a bicycle. She has no time to continue some of the alternative therapies that she used years ago, but still pays close attention to monitoring her food intake as well as her level of stress.

"I had taken some nutrition courses, and I remember one of my professors saying, 'Try to eat foods that grow out of the ground and avoid food that is processed or white,'" says Janet. "So I stay away from white flour, sugar and rice, as well as red meat. I eat grains, vegetables, fruits, chicken and lots of fish." As for stress, Janet is vehement on the subject. "From early childhood, I was never without stress," she says. "First, it was the abuse and the money struggles. Later it was my divorce, raising kids alone, building businesses, watching them fail and building more. I completely believe that the constant stress broke down my immune system. So now, if I feel stress overcoming me, I stop, sit back, evaluate my situation and do some yoga deep-breathing exercises. I believe that my weakened immune system led to the cancer that destroyed my kidneys and nearly killed me. I am *never* going to let that happen again."

A Closer Look at "Peeke" Performance:
Advice from an Outspoken Doctor

Pamela Peeke, M.D., M.P.H., first took on the medical establishment when she was in school: "I was a beginning medical student," she remembers. "One of my classmates said, 'Let's go check the gallbladder in 308.' I was appalled, and blurted, 'Is there a person attached to it? Or is it a green thing on a pillow?'" For Pam, this was only the beginning. "In my third year, during rounds, I asked a patient how her tummy was feeling," she says. "Later, the chief of obstetrics/gynecology said to me, 'I cannot believe you said tummy instead of abdomen. That was disrespectful to the patient.' He marched me back into the patient's room and said to her, 'Madam, this young doctor referred to your abdomen as a tummy. I apologize for the inappropriate use of the term.' The patient said, 'What's an abdomen? Of course that's my tummy.'"

On the first day of Pam's surgical rotation, she went into the women's locker room to change for an operation. (She was one of the only female doctors in the program at that time.) "The nurses told me to put on one of their uniforms," she remembers. "But there was no way I was going to freeze my behind during seven hours of open-heart surgery in a wraparound dress. So I went out in the hall and asked one of my friends to get me a medium bottom and a small top from the men's scrubs." Soon, the nurses were asking the laundry staff to put piles of men's scrubs in the women's locker room as well. "Scrubs are warmer and more comfortable than dresses," says Pam. "And that's how dresses disappeared from that hospital."

Since medical school, Pam Peeke's career has spanned internal medicine; critical care and trauma; laboratory work in psychoneuroimmunology (mind/body medicine) and molecular biology; and research into the influences of nutrition and metabolism on human health. She has also become a media spokesperson on nutrition, appearing frequently on CNN and the *Today* show, and she writes a monthly column, called "The Peeke Prescription," for *Prevention* magazine. She is the author of *Fight Fat After Forty* (Viking 2000), the first book to explain the stress-fat connection, based on her research. To date, the book has been translated into eight languages, including Chinese. She is currently at work on a second book on women's health. (More information can be found on her Web site: *www.drpeeke.com.*)

Before medical school, Pam had earned a master's degree in public health and public policy from the University of California at Berkeley. "My graduate work gave me a holistic framework in which to study medicine," she says. "So by the time I got to medical school, I was already open to thinking about medicine and health care in nontraditional ways."

After she graduated, Pam specialized in critical care and trauma. "I wanted to be challenged and to me that meant handling life and death situations all day long," she says. Very quickly, she began making some interesting observations. "By just looking at the personalities, lifestyles and attitudes of people who came into the emergency room, we could almost predict who was going to make it," she says. "My colleagues and I would ask ourselves, 'Who has the most mellow, realistic attitude about their illness or injury? Who has a lovely way of living, including exercise, a healthy diet and moderate stress? Who has the type of personality that can adapt to a catastrophic health problem? In a nutshell, *who can regroup?* It would break my own heart to see anger in a heart attack patient, for example. I would say, 'Hey, in the midst of this difficulty might lie opportunity. Maybe this is a good time to think about making some changes in your life.'"

A Serendipitous Meeting

Pam tried to talk to her mentors about these observations. "I would ask them why we weren't educating our patients more about nutrition, physical fitness and stress resilience. They told me that we are not taught this in medical school. This didn't make sense to me and the lack of emphasis on illness prevention through lifestyle and diet began to bother me more and more."

After about ten years in critical care and trauma, Pam was attending a conference and happened to be sitting next to a nutrition expert from the University of California. "We talked at length about my interests, and he offered me a research fellowship in nutrition and metabolism at a center for clinical research funded by the National Institutes of Health (NIH)," says Pam. "This felt right to me, so I gave up a lucrative career in critical care and moved to the University of California at Davis, moonlighting every weekend at the critical care unit and researching nutrition during the week."

Pam's interest in nutrition comes not only from her patient care experiences, but also from her own life. She has always been a serious athlete—a marathon runner, mountain climber, power weightlifter and hiker—as well as a member of the American College of Sports Medicine. "I wanted to learn how to fuel the human body, not only for sports, but also to help people better respond to illness and trauma," she says. "My interests naturally expanded to include the study of stress and its impact on health." Pam's research led her to George Chrousos, M.D., whom she describes as "one of the major experts on stress at the NIH." After reading his work, Pam called to ask for a meeting with him. "Three hours later I had signed up to move to Washington and become a senior research fellow in his lab," says Pam. "My assignment was to set up the first laboratory at the NIH to study human fat cells. I also began my most serious molecular biological research into mind/body medicine, focusing specifically on stress, nutrition and *psychoneuroimmunology.*"

This term describes a relatively new field in medicine that explores the connections between our minds, emotions and health. One example is the relationship between stress and disease. Professor Candace B. Pert, of the Georgetown University School of Medicine, writes: "Recent technological innovations have allowed us to examine the molecular basis of emotions, and to begin to understand how the molecules of our emotions share intimate connections with, and are indeed inseparable from, our physiology."[9]

After about two years as a basic and clinical research scientist, Pam was asked to speak about nutrition at a conference. "The word somehow got out that there was a doctor at the NIH who was also an expert on nutrition," says Pam. "That's when the media got interested. I learned very quickly to translate complex science into TV sound bytes, as in, 'You have thirty seconds to talk about calcium, Dr. Peeke.'"

One day, Pam was invited to speak on an NIH panel and met Joseph Jacobs, M.D., the first director of the newly formed NIH Office of Alternative Medicine. "This was the beginning of a brand-new era at the NIH," says Pam. "And right away my 'Berkeley detectors' perked up. I said to myself, how can I be a part of this? I talked to Dr. Jacobs, and he invited me to come over and help out. So the next thing I knew I had two jobs. I would wear my white coat to study molecular biology and nutrition in the laboratories of NICHD (National Institute of Child Health and Human Development) then take it off, run across the street to the Office of Alternative Medicine to help develop research protocols to determine whether macrobiotic or vegan diets had effects on cancer, or whether chelation therapy helped heart attack patients." Pam also visited research centers around the country to evaluate proposals for research projects to investigate complementary and alternative treatments. (That office has since become NCCAM—the National Center for Complementary and Alternative Medicine within NIH.)

In addition to conducting her own research in nutrition and mind/body medicine, Pam is now assistant clinical professor at the University of Maryland School of Medicine, teaching complementary medicine and nutrition science. "Can you believe that nutrition is still not a required course in most medical schools?" she asks incredulously. "My goal is to teach these future doctors to incorporate what we now know about nutrition, metabolism and the mind's connection to the body into the practice of integrative medicine."

---

[9] C. B. Pert, *Molecules of Emotion: Why You Feel the Way You Do* (New York: Scribner, 1997), quoted in M. Gearin-Tosh, *Living Proof: A Medical Mutiny* (New York: Scribner, 2002), 18.

On a typical day, Professor Peeke might present the class with a case history like this one and ask her students to discuss what they would do: "A forty-five-year-old woman weighs about two hundred pounds and hasn't seen the inside of a gym since she was a kid. All of her physical and emotional energy goes to taking care of her family; there is little left to take care of herself. She comes to see us because she is burnt-out, stressed-out, exhausted and, to top it off, she's having all kinds of menopausal symptoms that are making her miserable. We examine her and find out she also has high blood pressure, high cholesterol and she is pre-diabetic. She says that she's heard about herbs and vitamins for menopause and weight loss, and by the way, what's this cabbage soup diet all about? But she doesn't know what to do or whom to believe about what is best. How do you advise her?"

More often than not, says Pam, the medical students are at a loss. "These kids can crack a chest and repair an aorta but they can't get this woman out of her mess," she says. "So we talk about how they can help this patient understand the effects of stress on her body, how yoga and meditation and simply getting some exercise will help her feel better, how proper nutrition and herbs can help with weight loss, cholesterol and menopause symptoms, how she can expose her kids to yoga and proper eating. I tell these students, 'You'd better understand that fruits, vegetables and grains are like a medicine cabinet, and that mind/body medicine is a powerful tool.'" (Please see chapter 10 for more about the treatment of menopause.)

In another case history, Pam presents a young man who has been in a serious car accident. "He's in post-op intensive care, and his situation is precarious. What are they going to do?" Pam uses this scenario to talk about the importance of belief systems, spirituality and even prayer. "The stronger the belief system the patient has, the greater the chance for recovery," she says. "These kids know I'm a doctor, that I have worked in trauma and have also taken care of patients as an internist. So they seem to listen and pay attention."

(For information and research data on nutrition and the use of mind/body medicine for specific conditions, please see the chapters on cancer, heart disease, children's health, pain, trauma and women at midlife, as well as "A Closer Look at Energy Healing and Spirituality" and "A Closer Look at Healing Herbs.")

✓ Take Action: Best Ways to Have a Stress-Resilient Life ✓

Toxic stress is defined as any stress you perceive as being associated with feelings of hopelessness, helplessness and defeat. Build up your stress resilience by managing stress better. Dr. Pamela Peeke suggests ways to reduce and manage stress:

1. Get a massage on a regular basis. Massage therapy reduces stress-hormone levels and calms the mind as well as the body.

2. Create a support system of people who care about you as you encounter life's challenges.

3. Tap into your spirituality. Explore your meaning in life and your belief systems.

4. Give to others each day. Volunteer on a regular basis, and complete the circle. What is given to you is given back to others.

5. Laugh a lot. See many of life's adventures as associated with wit and humor. Laughing reduces stress hormone levels.

6. Find your pockets of peace each day. Rest, rejuvenate and relax your mind and body throughout the day, to allow greater clarity of thought, reduced stress and greater energy levels.

7. Get up and move throughout the day. To complete the mind/body connection, it's imperative to do something as simple as walk frequently each day. This physical activity reduces stress-hormone levels, and keeps you mentally and physically fit.

8. Eat regularly and eat high-quality food. A well-nourished body is integral to a healthy mind and lifestyle.

9. Keep tabs on your waistline. The new science shows it's all about keeping your waist-to-hip ratio within normal limits. Too much fat deposited deep inside the abdomen is toxic weight and life-threatening. It's the only fat associated with heart disease, diabetes and cancer. Eat appropriately, stay physically active and minimize toxic stress to eliminate toxic weight.

Stress Resilience: What's the Evidence?

The following books and research studies support Dr. Peeke's advice:

Benson, H. with M. Stark. *Timeless Healing: The Power and Biology of Belief.* New York: Scribner, 1996.

Berg, R. L. and J. S. Cassells, eds. *The Second Fifty Years: Promoting Health and Preventing Disability.* Institute of Medicine, Division of Health Promotion and Disease Prevention. Washington, D.C.: National Academy Press, 1990.

Bjorntorp, P. "Visceral Obesity: A 'Civilization Syndrome.'" *Obesity Research 1,* no. 1 (1993): 206–222.

Chrousos, G. P. and P. W. Gold. "The Concepts of Stress and Stress System Disorders: Overview of Physical and Behavioral Homeostasis." *Journal of the American Medical Association,* 267, no. 9 (1992): 1244–1252.

Dugmore, L. D. et al. "Changes in Cardiorespiratory Fitness, Psychological Well Being, Quality of Life, and Vocational Status Following a 12-month Cardiac Exercise Rehabilitation Programme. *Heart* 81, no. 4 (1999): 359–366.

Healthy People 2000: *National Health Promotion and Disease Prevention Objectives.* DHHS Publication No. (PHS) 90–50213.

LaRoche, L. *Relax—You May Only Have a Few Minutes Left: Using the Power of Humor to Overcome Sress in Your Life and Work.* New York: VIllard, 1998.

Sapolsky, R. M. *Why Zebras Don't Get Ulcers: A Guide to Stress, Stress-Related Diseases, and Coping.* New York: W. H. Freeman, 1994.

2

THE "VITAL FORCE"

"Are we more than a collection of molecules?"

What makes us the people we are? Some would say that we are simply the sum total of our physical parts: the bones, muscles and internal organs, and the cells and molecules that make them up. Others might argue that there is something more, something invisible—which might be called the soul or spirit—that exists within us as well. This question is important in any discussion of complementary and alternative health practices. Most, if not all, of the methods described in this book are based on the second premise: the belief that there is, in fact, some non-material "life force" within us that is the essence of our personalities and that may also play an important role in the health of our bodies.

What is this hard-to-define and mysterious quality? It has many names in different cultures. Perhaps the easiest concept to grasp is that of "energy" or "life force." Although we can't see it on an X ray or touch it, many people believe that it affects the way we think, feel, interact with our world and react to disease. Practitioners of traditional Chinese medicine—a system that is thousands of years old—call this energy *qi* (pronounced "chee"). It is believed that qi— which is also thought to pervade everything in the universe—pulses through our bodies, much like the blood, through invisible but well-mapped pathways called meridians. Blockages in the flow of qi lead to disease or pain, and much of Chinese medicine is directed to removing these blockages, freeing the flow of energy so that the body can heal itself. (The Japanese word for life force is *ki*.)

"Western scientists do not acknowledge these energies, although some would acknowledge that there is a life force, a spirit, or a soul that breathes life into bodies," writes Herbert Benson, M.D., in his book *Timeless Healing*. Benson, who is associate professor of medicine at Harvard Medical School and founder and director of the Mind/Body Institute at Beth Israel Deaconess Medical Center in Boston, goes on to explain, "Many cultures have named and believe in a mysterious healing energy. The ancient Egyptians called it 'ka,' the Hawaiians 'mana,' and the Indians 'prana.' In these cultures, people believe that healers can direct and restore these healing forces."[1]

The belief in a universal life force has been present throughout recorded human history. More than five thousand years ago, Ayruvedic healers and yogis in India referred to prana as energy that, like the Chinese concept of qi, is not only within us, but also in the world around us. In his book, *How We Live*, Sherwin Nuland, M.D., professor of surgery at Yale Medical School, describes how, in the middle of the nineteenth century, "many authorities, and virtually all plain people too, believed that living things were possessed of an unknowable form of energy . . . commonly called 'the vital force.'" He notes that Aristotle, in the fourth century, B.C., identified a life force in humans with the psyche. Despite the eventual supremacy of scientific thought in medicine, Dr. Nuland notes that "the general notion of vitalism, attenuated though it may be, lives on in the minds of any and all who refuse to believe that there is not some form of still-unexplained energy that brings more to the phenomenon of life than can be accounted for by a series of chemical reactions."[2]

According to Ted J. Kaptchuk, O.M.D., assistant professor of medicine at Harvard Medical School and a renowned authority on Chinese medicine, practitioners of most alternative healing believe that this "vital energy" is the source of their intervention. "One can almost speak of a faucet that pours out healing juice," he writes.[3]

Rather than trying to explain qi (or whatever we choose to call it) as an invisible but powerful physical force—such as gravity, for example—Kaptchuk sees qi as a metaphor for explaining how the phenomena of life—whether our

---

[1] H. Benson with M. Stark, *Timeless Healing: The Power and Biology of Belief*. (New York: Scribner, 1996), 157.

[2] S. B. Nuland, *How We Live* (New York: Vintage Books, 1997), 66–67.

[3] T. J. Kaptchuk, in *Fundamentals of Complementary and Alternative Medicine*, ed. M. S. Micozzi (New York: Churchill Livingston, 1996; 2000).

bodies, emotions, minds or the world we live in—are all connected. "I look at vital energy as a way of understanding interrelationships and change," he says. "How the oxygen we breathe and the food we eat become transformed into our thoughts and our creative work; and in nature, how rocks become minerals; or how seeds become plants. And in Chinese medicine, how energy blockages or deficiencies can cause disease."

In an article written for conventionally trained physicians, Kaptchuk and his coauthor, David M. Eisenberg, M.D., explain the "attraction to and acceptance of alternative medical therapies" that prompt many patients to seek out this "healing juice": "Alternative medicine offers a person threatened by illness or disease a connection with fundamentally benign, lawful, coherent, potent, and even meaningful powers," they write. "When illness isolates, alternative health care allows a rescuing connection to life-supporting cosmic forces." In addition to the forces of qi and prana described above, Kaptchuk and Eisenberg point out other examples: "[H]omeopathy speaks of a 'spiritual vital essence,' chiropractic refers to the 'innate' . . . and new age healing practices work with 'psychic' or 'astral' energies."[4]

Kaptchuk, a trim, intense man with longish hair, which he wears tied back in a ponytail, is an engaging public speaker and the author of *The Web That Has No Weaver*, a comprehensive and readable explanation of Chinese medicine. A New York native who describes himself as "a product of the sixties who wanted to do something outside the system," Kaptchuk has a degree in Oriental medicine from a medical school in China and is a scholar of science, anthropology and the history of medicine. After many years of practicing Chinese medicine in both China and the United States, he now lives in Cambridge, Massachusetts, and teaches alternative medicine at Harvard Medical School. He spends the bulk of his time researching and writing about alternative medical practices and their integration with conventional medicine.

"I can see, smell, feel and even taste qi, in the same way that I can sense true and real things about my child or my wife that no one else can see and that would be undetectable by scientific instruments," said Kaptchuk in an

---

[4] T. J. Kaptchuk and D. M. Eisenberg, "The Persuasive Appeal of Alternative Medicine," *Annals of Internal Medicine* 129, no. 12 (1998): 1062.

interview. "Even though qi may not be reproducible, measurable or verifiable by any scientific methods that we have now, I believe that it exists on a different level of reality."

Qi: The Vital Force in Traditional Chinese Medicine

One of Cheng Xiao Ming's most vivid memories early in his medical career was the day he examined a woman who had been injured in a car accident. He was working in a hospital in Hongzhou, China, after having graduated from a Western-style medical school (also in China) with a degree in orthopedic surgery. "She had a blockage in the flow of blood in her leg that had created a large stasis (pool of blood), the size of a tennis ball, and hard as a rock," he remembers. "We could not help her with Western methods of surgery." In most Chinese hospitals, Western-trained physicians practice alongside doctors of traditional Chinese medicine (TCM) and this was the case in Cheng's hospital.

"I watched as a TCM doctor gave the patient herbs and used his hands to move the stagnant blood," says Cheng. "In time, the herbs and the deep 'acupressure' of his hands completely resolved the stasis. This made a very deep impression in my mind." The impression was reinforced as he later watched other TCM doctors repair complex bone fractures, not with surgery, but by using their hands to put the tiny bones back in place. "They trained to do this by covering broken chopsticks or pieces of wood with an ox skin or another thick piece of leather, and then trying to put the broken pieces back together from the outside of the covering," he says. "This type of practice increased the dexterity and sensitivity of their hands."

After these experiences, Cheng decided to return to medical school, this time to study TCM. "I wanted to learn how to treat people without the side effects and pain of Western surgery," he says. Four years later he graduated with a second medical degree and expertise in a system that was completely different from Western medicine. "Chinese medicine understands the body as a complete system—every organ and tissue has a relationship to every other, to the body as a whole, and also to the environment and even the universe," he says. "Western medicine understands the body only in relation to itself, which is of course useful in the diagnosis and treatment of trauma and acute problems, but limited in the treatment of chronic conditions."

Cheng now lives in Boston where he has a highly respected TCM practice, including acupuncture and Chinese herbal medicine. Thanks to many years of teaching experience, he is accustomed to explaining TCM philosophy and theory to the Western mind. "I ask my students, 'Who lives longer, the rabbit or the turtle?' They all answer, 'The turtle, of course,'" Cheng says. "Then I ask them, 'So does this mean we should all live like turtles?' 'Of course not!' they say. 'We'd never get anywhere.'"

At this point, his eyes twinkle. "Then I say to them, 'On the outside, we should be like a rabbit, strengthening our muscles, exercising our bodies and running when we need to. But on the inside, we should be like a turtle, breathing slowly and deeply, slowing the heart when it is at rest, creating a peaceful internal environment. Just like we have to train our bodies to be strong, we must also train our minds and internal organs to relax. When you are peaceful, you can logically and calmly resolve any problem, even if there is turmoil around you.'"

Cheng himself seems to radiate inner peace, organizing his busy treatment and teaching schedule with equanimity, always seeming to be able to fit in someone who needs to see him. Several mornings a week, he rises at 3:00 A.M. and spends two hours meditating and practicing qigong and tai chi exercises—slow, graceful movements that he calls "internal training" that help to slow down the mind and move qi inside the body. By changing the inner environment of the body, both of these forms of exercise are thought to improve the actual functions of organs and tissues. People usually learn qigong and tai chi under the guidance of a master teacher. But in most cities, classes in both techniques are also available in specialized centers, adult education programs and even in conventional health clubs. (Please see chapter 7 for more about the use of qigong for pain; chapter 11 for the benefits of tai chi in improving balance and preventing falls in older people; and chapter 6 for the use of both methods in the treatment of chronic illnesses.)

As noted above, it is the flow of qi along pathways called "meridians" inside the body that is the focus of all Chinese medical treatments. Even though meridians are invisible, thousands of years of practice and observation have resulted in clearly mapped diagrams of their routes within the body. Like most practitioners of Chinese medicine, Cheng has large drawings on the walls of his office showing the elaborate network of meridians throughout the body. If you have ever had acupuncture and felt the tingling sensation along a meridian when a tiny needle is inserted into just the right spot, you would think that the meridians must indeed be as visible and tangible as your blood vessels. "The needles don't cure disease," explains Cheng. "They adjust the qi, reinforcing it, reducing it where necessary, moving stagnant or 'stuck' energy. With the free flow of energy restored, the body can heal itself. After all, our bodies fight off viruses and bacteria every day. TCM methods increase that ability."

Other TCM methods include the use of Chinese herbs, taken internally or put directly on the skin, deep tissue massage (called *tui na*), and qigong massage (during which the practitioner uses the hands to transmit and move qi energy, with the patient fully clothed). (Please see "A Closer Look at Oriental Bodywork," for more about Chinese massage.) Because of his dual training, Cheng believes in the combination of TCM with conventional, Western medicine. He works regularly with patients who are also receiving conventional treatments for many conditions, including orthopedic problems, pain, cancer and stroke. (Please see research section for studies of TCM.)

In China, almost all hospitals have a system called "three legs walking," explains Cheng. "One leg is pure Western methods, one pure Chinese and one combined. Usually, the combined approach uses Western diagnostic methods and TCM treatment. But there are even differences in diagnosis: Western medicine diagnoses and treats a disease. TCM diagnoses by symptom, using more than twelve different wrist pulses, the condition of the tongue, and palpation (feeling) of muscles and other tissues along meridians.

Many problems diagnosed in Chinese medicine are said to relate to imbalance between "yin" and "yang" energy in the body. Yin energy is represented by the more "quiet" characteristics of organs and structures in the body. It nourishes the inside of the body. Yang energy is more active, causing change or activity. "You can't have one without the other," said Cheng. "A car, for example, can't run (yang activity) without the gas (yin nourishment). For good health, the yin and yang energies need to be in harmonious balance. (Detailed descriptions of yin and yang energy can be found in chapter 6.)

What happens when the yin and yang energies are out of balance? If one or the other is too strong or too weak? Cheng gives an example: One of his long-time patients, whom we will call "Harold," began seeing him at the age of forty. He was married, with a three-year-old son, and had a full-time office job. He had severe allergies, asthma and bronchitis. At the office and at home, he was forced to use an inhaler to restore his breathing almost once an hour, and he was hospitalized two or three times a year for pneumonia and severe bronchitis.

In Chinese medicine, the three meridians that relate to lung function pass through the spleen and kidney as well as the lungs, Cheng explains. "For Harold, the first step was to build up the yin (nourishing) energy inside the lungs," he said. "We do this with special herbs. When the lung energy is stronger, we use acupuncture in all three meridians to move it around. This improves the breathing function."

After three months of weekly visits, Harold's lungs inhaled and exhaled smoothly. His asthma and allergy symptoms slowly began to disappear. Now, at age forty-six, he comes to see Cheng only once a month and uses the inhaler only at the beginning of a cold (which he gets rarely). He has a second child, and has not been in the hospital for six years.

"In order for a person to get sick, the body must first have an energy deficiency, according to Chinese medicine," says Cheng. "If your body is strong everywhere, you won't get disease." Using osteoarthritis as an example, Cheng explains that internal yin deficiencies permit cold and damp to enter the body as pathogenic (disease-causing) infectors. "So we nourish the inside of the body with herbs so that it is strong enough to repel the cold and damp. Then we use acupuncture to restore the active (yang) function of the joints and limbs."

Traditional Chinese Medicine: What's the Evidence?

Nearly every chapter in this book discusses research studies evaluating the use of some aspect of TCM—whether acupuncture, energy work, herbal medicine or massage—for a variety of conditions. Here, we will look at the evidence for TCM in general.

Traditional Chinese medicine is a well-developed, coherent system of medicine that has been practiced in China for thousands of years. "As an extensive and established medical system, TCM is used by billions of people around the world for every condition known to humankind," writes Lixing Lao, Ph.D., L.Ac., associate professor in the Department of Complementary Medicine, University of Maryland School of Medicine.[5] Lao has surveyed the literature on TCM, noting, "Modern research on TCM is still in its infancy." Still, he identifies several studies that indicate TCM's usefulness as both primary and complementary therapy. These include research findings that TCM is useful in the treatment of addictions, back pain, muscle spasms and neck pain, eczema, osteoarthritis and to improve well-being.

As a therapy used in conjunction with conventional medicine, acupuncture has been found effective in such conditions as cancer pain and nausea and vomiting, fibromyalgia, ischemic heart disease, migraine and stroke rehabilitation. Lao also notes that the "World Health Organization has listed over forty conditions for which acupuncture is listed as a primary or adjunctive therapy." (Please see chapter 8 for additional research about acupuncture for stroke and spinal cord injury, and for evidence that spinal cord injury patients preferred massage to acupuncture for pain; chapter 7 on the use of TCM for other kinds of pain; for a consensus report from the National Institutes of Health listing conditions for which acupuncture is and is not effective; and for research on the potential adverse effects of acupuncture; and chapter 5 on the use of acupuncture to reduce the side effects of chemotherapy.)

Lao's most poetic citation, however, comes not from the modern research literature,

---

[5] L. Lao, "Traditional Chinese Medicine," in *Essentials of Complementary and Alternative Medicine*, eds. W. B. Jonas, and J. S. Levin (Baltimore, MD: Lippincott, Williams & Wilkins, 1999), 228.

but from *The Yellow Emperor's Inner Classic,* thought to be the first classic work on traditional Chinese medicine, dating back to 2697 B.C.:

> *In a peaceful calm,*
> *Void and emptiness,*
> *The authentic qi*
> *Flows easily.*
> *Essences and spirits*
> *Are kept within.*
> *How could illness arise?*

References

Berman, B. M. and J. P. Sawyers. "Complementary Medicine Treatments for Fibromyalgia Syndrome." *Baillieres Clinical Rheumatology* (London) 13, no. 3 (1999): 487–492.

Berman, B. M., et al. "Is Acupuncture Effective in the Treatment of Fibromyalgia?" *Journal of Family Practice* 48, no. 3 (1999): 213–218.

Cheng, X., ed. *Chinese Acupuncture and Moxibustion,* 1st ed. Beijing: Foreign Languages Press, 1987.

Christenson, B. V., et al. "Acupuncture Treatment of Severe Knee Osteoarthritis: A Long-Term Study." *Acta Anaesthesiologica Scandinavica* (Copenhagen) 36 (1992): 519–525.

Claude Larre, S. J. *The Way of Heaven: Neijing Suwen,* Chapters 1 and 2. Cambridge: Monkey Press, 1994.

Coan, R., et al. "The Acupuncture Treatment of Neck Pain: A Randomized Controlled Study." *American Journal of Chinese Medicine* 9, no. 4 (1981): 326–332.

Dundee J. W., et al. "The Role of Transcutaneous Electrical Stimulation of Neiguan Anti-Emetic Acupuncture Point in Controlling Sickness After Cancer Chemotherapy." *Physiotherapy* 77, no. 7 (1991): 499–502.

Hu, X. M., ed. *Chinese Medicine Secret Recipes.* Shanghai: Wenhui Publishers, 1989.

Johanson, K., et al. "Can Sensory Stimulation Improve the Functional Outcome in Stroke Patients?" *Neurology* 43 (1993): 2189–2192.

Loy, T. T. "Treatment of Cervical Spondylosis—Electro-Acupuncture Versus Physiotherapy." *Medical Journal of Australia* 2 (1983): 32–44.

MacDonald, A. J. R., et al. "Superficial Acupuncture in Relief of Chronic Low Back Pain." *Annals of the Royal College of Surgeons of England* (London) 65 (1983): 44–46.

Melchart, D., et al. "Acupuncture for Idiopathic Headache." *Cochrane Database Systematic Review* 1 (2001): CD001218.

Naeser, M. A., et al. "Real Versus Sham Acupuncture in the Treatment of Paralysis in Acute Stroke Patients: A CT Scan Lesion Site Study." *Journal of Neurologic Rehabilitation* 6 (1992): 163–173.

Richter, A., et al. "Effect of Acupuncture in Patients with Angina Pectoris." *European Heart Journal* (London) 12 (1991): 175–178.

Shoukang L., "Treating Arthralgia with Acupuncture." *International Journal of Clinical Acupuncture* 2, no. 1 (1999): 71–76.

Sheehan, M. P., et al. "Efficacy of Traditional Chinese Herbal Therapy in Adult Atopic Dermatitis." *Lancet* 340 (1992): 13–17.

Smith, M. O., et al. "Acupuncture Treatment of Drug Addiction and Alcohol Abuse." *American Journal of Acupuncture* 10, no. 2 (1982): 161–163.

Thomas M., et al. "Importance of Modes of Acupuncture in the Treatment of Chronic Nociceptive Low Back Pain." *Acta Anaesthesiologica Scandinavica* (Copenhagen) 38 (1994): 63–69.

Vickers, A. J. "Can Acupuncture Have Specific Effects on Health? A Systematic Review of Acupuncture Antiemesis Trials." *Journal of the Royal Society of Medicine* (London) 89, no. 6 (1996): 303–311.

Vincent, C. A. "A Controlled Trial of the Treatment of Migraine by Acupuncture." *Clinical Journal of Pain* 5 (1989): 305–312.

Zhu, C. "Use of Point Yinmen (UB 37) for Treatment of Acute Lumbar Sprain." *Shanghai Journal of Acupuncture and Moxibustion* (China) 2 (1984): 17.

Prana: The Vital Force in Ayurvedic Medicine

Every time you breathe, according to the teachings of Ayurvedic medicine, you are bringing the life force called *prana* into your body. (Prana corresponds to the qi that is referred to in Chinese medicine.) Ayurvedic practitioners believe that everything in the universe—whether organic or inorganic—is made up of five elements: space (also called ether), air, fire, water and earth. Prana is the essence of the air element, says Dr. Vasant D. Lad, author, teacher and an authority on Ayurvedic medicine: "The flow of consciousness, from one cell to another cell in the form of intelligence, is called *Prana,* the principle of the air element," he writes. "Prana is a vital life force that is essential for communication on all levels of body, mind, and spirit. . . . [S]ensory stimuli and motor responses are the subtle movements of the air principle. Even the movements of the heart, respiration, peristalsis [in digestion], and other involuntary movements are governed by *Prana.*"[6]

Ayurveda is an ancient system of healing that has its roots in the Vedic knowledge of ancient India, explains Lad in an interview. "The goal of Ayurveda is to foster a deep connection with the true essence of our being." A Sanskrit word that means the science of life, Ayurveda is thought to be the oldest tradition of knowledge having to do with health. "Many believe that Ayurvedic practices were actually in use eight to ten thousand years ago, in India, and passed down in oral traditions," he says. "About five thousand years ago, they were written in ancient texts called the Vedas." Ayurvedic practices, including meditation, massage, breathing exercises (*pranayama*), yoga and the use of special foods, gemstones and herbs are all designed to strengthen the prana within us, he explains: "The prana is what drives life. It is everywhere in the universe. We consume it. As long as the prana, the life force, is within you, you are alive."

The ancient seers who developed Ayurveda were searching for a way to understand the creation of all things and the purpose of life, according to Lad. (In addition to teaching and writing, Lad is the founder and director of the Ayurvedic

---

[6] V. D. Lad, "Ayurvedic Medicine," in *Essentials of Complementary and Alternative Medicine*, eds. W. B. Jonas and J. S. Levin (Baltimore, MD: Lippincott, Williams & Wilkins, 1999), 202.

Institute of Albuquerque, New Mexico.) "The human body is a miniature version of nature," he says. "In nature, the five elements—space, air, fire, water and earth—correspond to elements that make up our bodies. Ayurveda helps us understand the unique body, mind and consciousness of each person, including which diseases we are prone to, and which changes in nutrition and lifestyle will help us avoid them. According to Ayurveda, this basic knowledge of body, mind and consciousness is the foundation of health and happiness."

Ayurvedic doctors diagnose ailments by closely observing each patient's physical, emotional and spiritual constitution, called a *dosha* (see box for a description of the three main types of *doshas*) as well as by a system of Vedic medical astrology and palmistry. "The word for Vedic medical astrology means 'light,'" says Dr. Lad. "We use Vedic astrology, as well as palmistry, as 'the light of life,' to guide us toward an understanding of our physical and emotional strengths and weaknesses. (Please see "Fibromyalgia: Answers from Ayurveda" in chapter 6 for more about Ayurvedic medicine, including Vedic palmistry and astrology.)

"Suppose your dosha indicates, for example, that you are prone to heart disease," continues Lad. "We can advise you to eat certain foods, avoid others, take special herbs, and make lifestyle changes that may prevent the disease before it occurs. Ayurveda gives us guidance toward perfect health."

"I found that there is art in medicine, as well as science"

When Vasant Lad was a young boy, growing up in India, his grandmother became very sick with kidney disease. "Her body was swollen all over. She was dying," remembers Lad. "But then a friend of my father's who was an Ayurvedic doctor, came to the house. He examined her and gave us Ayurvedic medicine. Even though I was only about nine years old, I was the one who nursed her and gave her the medicine regularly. She recovered. To me, the Ayurvedic doctor had performed a miracle, so when my father told me that I must become a doctor, I was happy to agree, even though I wanted to be an artist. But I have found that there is art in medicine, as well as science. Art never dies within us. It comes in teaching others and caring for patients."

Lad graduated from Pune University in India with a degree in Ayurvedic medicine. His curriculum was unique in that it combined allopathic (Western) and Ayurvedic medicine. He taught and practiced an integration of both kinds of medicine in India for almost fifteen years, becoming medical director at University Hospital in Pune, India, an integrative hospital that combines allopathic and Ayurvedic medicine. He moved to the United States in 1979, taught at several schools of natural medicine, and then founded the Ayurvedic Institute in New Mexico. He now teaches the principles of Ayurvedic clinical medicine, including herbology, pharmaceuticals, pharmacology and psychology. The institute also has a clinic, which offers patients Ayurvedic treatments, including detoxification (*panchakarma*) and rejuvenation (*rasayana*) therapies.

WHICH *DOSHA* ARE YOU?

In his comprehensive book, *The Best of Alternative Medicine: What Works? What Does Not?*, Kenneth R. Pelletier, Ph.D., M.D. (hc), former director of the Stanford University School of Medicine Program in Complementary and Alternative Medicine, cites Dr. Shri K. Mishra—researcher of Ayurveda, professor of neurology and dean of the School of Medicine at the University of Southern California—as a source of information for his chapter on Ayurvedic medicine.

As noted earlier, each living organism is a microcosm that reflects the macrocosm of the entire cosmos, and all of creation is made up of five elements: space, air, fire, water and earth. "From the five elements come three essential, overriding qualities that are present in all things," writes Pelletier. "The relative balance of these three qualities in each person determines that person's unique physiological constitution and functional body type."[7] According to Ayurvedic theory, while each person has some of the qualities of all three *dosha* types, usually one or two predominate. When *dosha* energy is out of balance, disease occurs.

The three *doshas* (a summary of characteristics identified by Pelletier, Mishra and Lad):

Vata represents the elements of air and space. *Vata* people tend to be active, changeable and energetic. They are usually tall and slender. They can be anxious, unpredictable, alert and restless. When their prana is out of balance, *Vata* people are prone to conditions that include nervous system problems, insomnia, arthritis, sciatica, lower back pain, constipation or intestinal gas. (In conventional medicine, this body type is called "ectomorphic").

Comments Lad: "*Vata* people can be hyperactive. They like to walk and talk quickly. They like jogging and running around. If there is nothing to do, a *Vata* person might start trying to fix furniture. We can use special food choices as well as herbs, meditation and breathing exercises to help them stay calm."

(continued)

---

[7] K. R. Pelletier, *The Best of Alternative Medicine: What Works? What Does Not?* (New York: Simon & Schuster, 2000), 232.

Pitta represents the elements of fire and water. *Pitta* people represent transformational energy. They are aggressive, explosive and efficient. When their prana is out of balance, *Pitta* people are likely to have liver and gallbladder problems, gastritis, hyperacidity, peptic ulcer, inflammatory disease, and skin problems, including hives and acne. ("Mesomorphic" in conventional medicine.)

Comments Lad: "The fire element in *Pitta* people often gives them reddish hair, bright eyes and fair skin that is sensitive to the sun. They have brilliant minds, but can be rather judgmental and critical. *Pitta* people should avoid hot, spicy foods, citrus fruit and excess sun exposure."

Kapha represents the union of earth and water. *Kapha* is the densest of the three qualities. *Kapha* people tend to be slow-moving, conservative, stable and sometimes overweight. They can also be tranquil, stubborn and procrastinating. They tend to have slow digestion, a strong appetite and enjoy easy, deep sleep. (They often think they need coffee in the morning to help them get going—but of course there are alternatives!) When their prana is out of balance, *Kapha* people tend to suffer from bronchitis, sinusitis, tonsillitis and lung congestion. ("Endomorphic" in conventional medicine.)

Comments Lad: "Although *Kapha* people are blessed with strong, sturdy bodies, their tendency to sit and eat might lead to weight problems. They should avoid cheese, milk, yogurt, ice cream and cold drinks. In addition to respiratory problems, *Kapha* people are also prone to allergies and gallstones."

Ayurveda for Hypertension and Type II Diabetes

How might a patient make use of Ayurvedic medicine? Dr. Virender Sodhi teaches Ayurveda at the Bastyr University School of Medicine in Seattle, has degrees in both Ayurvedic and Western medicine and practices both modes of treatment with his patients. Sodhi describes a fifty-five-year-old attorney diagnosed with Type II diabetes and hypertension. "This patient was also overweight, under stress from work and family and had high cholesterol, in addition to a blood-sugar level that was three times the normal," says Sodhi. "His main reason for coming to see me was to avoid having to take insulin, since the conventional diabetes medications (Glipizide and Glucophage) his endocrinologists had prescribed were not working. He was very motivated: He would do anything to avoid insulin.

"This man had a *Pitta/Kapha* constitution, primarily *Pitta* imbalance but with *Kapha* imbalance as well," says Sodhi. "We began by recommending a *Kapha*-pacifying diet for his obesity, as well as a *Pitta*-pacifying diet for his anger and stress. (Please see box for descriptions of the *Vata, Pitta* and *Kapha doshas.*) We also used specific Ayurvedic herbs that are known to control blood sugars and activate the pancreas to make more insulin. We encouraged him to walk three miles a day and change his diet to lower his cholesterol levels. He cut out red meat, reduced his carbohydrates and balanced his diet with vegetables, beans, fish and chicken. He also began a daily yoga practice and Ayurvedic deep-breathing exercises." (Please see "A Closer Look at Yoga" for more about the practice, as well as research studies on its health effects.)

Within three months, reports Sodhi, the patient's blood-sugar levels had dropped from 300 to between 120 and 140. His glycosylated hemoglobin level dropped from 13.4 to 6.7 (normal level), and his total cholesterol dropped to 170 (from a high of 270). He has kept up this lifestyle for one and a half years and so far has avoided the need to take insulin.

Another patient was a twenty-nine-year-old computer programmer with a very stressful job writing software for a stock-trading company. "He developed a malignant hypertension," says Sodhi, "which is the most serious kind of hyper-tension. It can kill you." The patient's blood pressure soared to 200/120, and stayed high despite a month in the hospital taking beta blockers, ACE inhibitors and diuretics. After he was discharged, he came to see Dr. Sodhi, who diagnosed his constitution as *Pitta/Vata* and prescribed an Ayurvedic regimen (after consulting with his conventional doctor), to pacify both his *Pitta* and *Vata* imbalances.

"We did a blood chemistry analysis and found that his kidney function was abnormal," says Dr. Sodhi. "The high blood pressure and the rupturing of small blood vessels in his eye were both symptoms of this underlying problem. Further analysis revealed that the true cause was acute stress from his job. I suggested that he take several months off from work, which he was able to do using disability leave. We then did Ayurvedic cleansing and detoxification procedures (*Panchakarma*) and started him on Ayurvedic herbs, meditation and a yoga practice. Within the first month, his blood pressure started to come down and was soon back to normal—120/80. His kidney function improved, and the eye symptoms started to disappear. He has since left his job and started a much less stressful home-computing and consulting business."

 ## Ayurvedic Medicine: What's the Evidence?

Is it possible to test the efficacy of medical systems—such as Ayurvedic medicine and traditional Chinese medicine—that are thousands of years old, are based on philosophies very different from those of Western medicine, and that use medicines and treatments that are developed in other cultures? Yes, but there are complications, say the experts.

When trying to evaluate Ayurvedic treatments for particular diseases, one of the difficulties that arises is the different diagnostic methods, points out Srinivasa N. Raja, M.D., professor of anesthesiology and director of the Pain Division in the Department of Anesthesiology and Critical Care Medicine at the Johns Hopkins School of Medicine. "Are we evaluating the same disease entity or not?" he asks. (For similar reasons, diagnostic differences also complicate research into traditional Chinese medicine.)

Another problem comes from the Ayurvedic medicines that are used. "Some of these medicines and herbal treatments are not available in this country," says Raja. "It is easier to do this research in India, where the medicines are prepared." Another problem with Ayurvedic research is the difficulty of designing randomized controlled trials of specific substances, according to Pelletier. "As with all clinical practices, Ayurvedic treatment is individualized for each patient, and consists of extremely complex combinations of interventions."[8]

Raja does not practice Ayurvedic medicine, although he is originally from India and familiar with the system. (Please see chapter 7 for an interview with Raja on his pain

---

[8] Ibid., 239.

research at Johns Hopkins.) In Raja's opinion, the way to evaluate this ancient school of medicine is more rigorous collaborative studies with medical schools in India. This has already begun to happen. In this country, Raja is interested in obtaining funding to research Ayurvedic treatments for pain. "The first study we would like to do is on osteoarthritis," he says. "My other interest is in neuropathic pain, such as diabetic neuropathy. (Neuropathic pain originates in the nervous system. Please see the explanation in chapter 7.) Patients with long-standing diabetes have pain because the diabetes affects nerves in their limbs and hands, giving them a tingling and burning sensation. The pain after shingles is another example of neuropathic pain."

Despite these research complications, Ayurvedic medicine has been studied in this country. With respect to research on Ayurvedic herbal products, however, Kenneth Pelletier points out that in the opinion of Dr. Shri K. Mishra of USC, "much of this research is controversial, since it may be biased by a business agenda."[9]

All of that being said, here are the results of some Ayurvedic research, as reported by Kenneth Pelletier:[10] (Please see "A Closer Look at Meditation," and "A Closer Look at Yoga," for specific research on these practices.)

Ayurveda is beneficial for some chronic diseases

A 1989 pilot study suggested benefits from Ayurvedic treatments for several chronic diseases, including rheumatoid arthritis, sinusitis, bronchitis, asthma, eczema, psoriasis, diabetes, hypertension, constipation and headache.

Lower risk factor for heart disease after *panchakarma*

Three months after panchakarma (an Ayurvedic internal cleansing treatment), 80 percent of thirty-one adults were found to have improved function of their circulatory system, reduced total cholesterol, a reduced measure of free radical damage and significantly reduced anxiety, all of which indicated reduced risk factors for heart disease.

Better quality of life and lowered health-care costs

An NCCAM-funded demonstration project compared three groups of healthy people (a total of eighty-three people) in a randomized controlled one-year trial. One group received no treatment; one group received Ayurvedic treatment in the form of

---

[9] Ibid., 239.
[10] Ibid., 240.

meditation, Ayurvedic diet and yoga; and one group received a Western program of relaxation training, a low-fat, low-salt diet and aerobic exercise. At the end of the year, both of the treatment groups reported improved quality of life, with greater improvement in the Ayurvedic group in health perceptions. In the Ayurvedic program, people who closely followed the program showed a decrease in depression. "Estimated health care costs over the year of the study were more than double for the untreated group, compared with the two treatment groups. Researchers concluded that the health promotion programs, especially the Ayurvedic intervention, were effective." This study was carried out by Dr. David Simon at the Sharp Institute for Human Potential and Mind/Body Medicine in San Diego.[11]

More evidence about chronic disease, blood pressure and hypertension

Dr. Vasant Lad of The Ayurvedic Institute of New Mexico has reviewed research on Ayurvedic interventions for chronic disease. "Ayurveda believes it can effectively treat these conditions with diet and lifestyle recommendations, cleansing programs, Ayurvedic massage, and rejuvenation," he writes. He stresses, however, that for these treatments to be effective, the patient must make a commitment to take responsibility to follow through with lifestyle changes and to have a genuine desire to heal.[12]

Lad cites laboratory and human experimental studies that have indicated benefits of Ayurvedic products in conditions such as Alzheimer's disease, Parkinson's disease and rheumatoid arthritis. "These studies have also helped to identify potential toxic substances and drug-herb interactions requiring knowledge and careful use of Ayurvedic products."[13] There are also several studies of transcendental meditation (TM), a specialized meditation technique derived from the Ayurvedic tradition, showing benefits such as lowered blood pressure and hypertension.

---

[11] Ibid., 241.
[12] Lad, "Ayurvedic Medicine," in *Essentials of Complementary and Alternative Medicine*, 211.
[13] Ibid.

References

Janssen, G. W. H. M. "The Application of Maharishi Ayur-Veda in the Treatment of Ten Chronic Diseases: A Pilot Study." *Nederlands Tijdscrift Voor Geneeskunde* (Amsterdam) 5 (1989): 586–594.

Schneider, R. H., et al. "A Randomized Controlled Trial of Stress Reduction for Hypertension in Older African Americans." *Hypertension* 26, no. 5 (1995): 820–827.

Sharma, H. M., et al. "Improvement in Cardiovascular Risk Factors Through Panchakarma Purification Procedures." *Journal of Research, Education and Indian Medicine* 12, no. 4 (1993): 2–13.

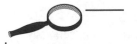

A Closer Look at Yoga:
Discovering the Music of the Body

To walk into the large, airy studio at the beginning of Carol Nelson's yoga class is to feel instantly calm. The students—women and men of varying ages—remove their shoes in the hallway, greet each other cheerfully, collect rolled-up blankets or pillows from a pile in the corner and settle themselves comfortably on the special yoga mats neatly arranged in two rows. They are wearing loose pants or leggings, T-shirts or sweatshirts, and some have already begun to gently stretch out their backs and legs.

Carol, a regally tall, attractive woman with wavy dark hair to her shoulders greets students at the door wearing a black T-shirt, black leggings and bare feet. When everyone is settled, she begins the class by saying, "This is our time to relax. One of the gifts of yoga is that we take the time to be with our bodies: the 'vehicles' that take us through our day. Often, we don't pay much attention to our bodies until they start giving us problems." She asks the students to assume what she calls "the constructive rest position," lying on the back, legs bent, eyes closed, arms relaxed, breathing quietly and noticing the breath as it enters and leaves the body. The class is not organized by levels of experience. Each student works at his or her own pace, with Carol's guidance, doing only what feels right.

Later, in an interview, Carol explains that she uses the constructive rest position to guide students back into their bodies. "Closing the eyes, turning inward and connecting with the natural rhythm of the breath helps to let go of that busy chattering mind that is obsessing about a phone call or errand you need to take care of later." To her students, she says, "The next hour and a half is your time. You can't take care of any of the things you are thinking about anyway, so let's just focus on the breath and the body."

She then uses the constructive rest pose as preparation for a series of yoga positions. These may include sitting, standing, lying or twisting poses—always with the reminder to *breathe!* The work is slow and extremely gentle. Carol demonstrates the postures and then walks among the students helping them with a suggestion or a gentle touch on an arm or leg. "After twenty-five years of study and practice, I believe that a very gentle approach to the body is best, along with being aware, alert and attentive to how each pose feels," says Carol. "I don't believe in pushing or pulling. Forcing postures can cause injury." Although she has studied with many teachers (the well-known B. K. S. Iyengar, for example, whose methods can be more strenuous, almost athletic workouts), her favorite teacher was Noelle Perez

Christian, in Paris, with whom she worked for many years.

"Noelle had been one of Iyengar's first Western students and had seriously injured her body by forcing yoga poses," says Carol. "She has since written many books about her experience and her own philosophy of yoga that evolved from it. When I studied with her, I heard, over and over again, *'doucement, doucement,* softer, quieter, gentler. Why are you so tense, Carol?'" Carol has modeled her teaching style on Noelle's philosophy. "I don't think of yoga as a 'fitness fad' or even a technique," she says. "If you have a body, you can practice yoga, regardless of your fitness or flexibility. I have even taught people in wheelchairs."

The practice of yoga is believed to be about three thousand years old. It originated in India as part of the ancient Ayurvedic system of health. (Please see chapters 2 and 6 for details about Ayurvedic medicine.) The word yoga comes from the Sanskrit word *yuj,* which means to yoke animals (such as oxen) together. Some interpret this to mean the joining of mind and body in a harmonious whole. Carol thinks the word also means to "harness" the universal energies of the sun and moon. "There is solar and lunar energy that flows through all of creation, of which we are a part," she says. "When we practice yoga, we are tapping into that energy by joining it with our individual energy. We become aware of the music of our own bodies and how we fit into the music of the world around us. Iyengar called it 'the union of consciousness and nature.'"

While different types of yoga are practiced throughout the world, the three most common methods in the West are the poses (*asanas*), breath control (*pranayama*) and meditation. Together, these are often referred to as "hatha yoga." The different yoga postures increase the body's store of prana, or vital energy. The concept of prana is similar to the concept of qi on which traditional Chinese medicine and health practices are based.

The teachings of the ancient yogis in India (who were held in reverence) refer to energy centers of the body, called chakras, which are located in ascending order from the lowest part of the pelvis, through the lower belly, upper belly, waist, heart area, throat, brain and the "third eye," located in the center of the forehead. Each energy center has a color, a sound, an animal and a lotus flower with a certain number of petals assigned to it. Beautiful ancient drawings often show the chakras and their locations in the body. "In modern medicine, the chakras correspond to particular glands of the endocrine system," Carol points out, "including the adrenal, pineal, pituitary and thyroid. And studies are beginning to show that certain postures actually stimulate the related glands, increasing circulation in those areas. Of course, the yogis knew all of this thousands of years ago."

Carol has dedicated her life to teaching yoga because she believes that every person can benefit from it. "The Dalai Lama once said, 'if you have a body, you have a condition,'" says Carol. "Life is not free of pain, on the physical, emotional or spiritual level. The teachings of yoga give us some ways to ease our discomfort, whatever it may be. It may not eliminate your arthritis or your depression, but it may make you feel more comfortable, even if it is just for that hour and a half. It gives you the message that you can step away from the pain or emotional distress, and perhaps you can bring that message with you when you leave the class and step into your everyday life: Comfort is possible."

One of Carol's students, when asked to describe a class, says: "Carol tells us to release the arms into their sockets. Release the thighs into the hip sockets. Extend the neck. The mouth, jaw and cheeks are relaxed. She gives specific, detailed, down-to-earth directions in a melodious, hypnotic voice. And as you follow each little direction, you're suddenly in a position you never thought you could be in. In the end, it happens, but not by force. Today, my body just somehow opened from the spine. I was astounded at how easily it came."

A Story of Yoga and Life

"Music and yoga have been intertwined in my life since I was a teenager," says Deborah Dunham, who has played her double bass on numerous occasions with the Boston Symphony Orchestra and held positions of principal bass in other ensembles around the country and in Europe. She says that yoga was one of the best ways— aside from high doses of prescription drugs—to alleviate the pain of a pinched nerve in her neck (originally misdiagnosed as carpal tunnel syndrome), which for two years had prevented her from practicing the bass for more than twenty minutes at a time. It also helped her overcome "nightmare" stage fright during solo performances and auditions. And finally, it was the clarity of mind that she gained in the practice of yoga that gave her the courage to face personal challenges and move with more purpose in her life.

Raised in the Pacific Northwest, Deborah studied music at the Leopold Mozart Konservatorium in Augsburg, Germany, and the California Institute of the Arts near Los Angeles. Deborah has smiling eyes and an infectious laugh that comes easily. "I chose to play the bass partly because of my height," she says, "and I also liked the deep, resonant sound." Although she had taken yoga classes since high school, in Germany Deborah began to integrate meditation with the breathing and postures.

At that time in Germany, she was twenty-three years old, in an unhappy marriage and the mother of a three-year-old daughter. "The combination of the yoga, breathing and meditation helped me to become calm and clearheaded," she says. "I was able to look at my life and face the fact that my marriage wasn't working. I'd married in a state of enchantment at the tender age of eighteen and truly didn't know the man who made me his wife. At the time of my realization he refused to seek counseling with me, and instead of sitting around complaining, I took action. But I was also afraid of leaving. I needed to confront my fears about the probability of raising my daughter alone, and about whether that would hurt her in any way later on. Somehow, the yoga and the quiet time in meditation gave me the strength to make this huge life change."

She left the marriage and Germany at the same time, returned to the United States with her daughter, started working a nine-to-five job and once on her feet went back to school. "It was stressful trying to balance this new life," she says. "I literally watched myself make mistakes, and there were a lot of them, but in those days there were no role models to turn to. I know, however, that without the help of yoga and many wonderful and compassionate friends, things would have been much worse." Soon, she began playing the bass professionally as a freelance musician, balancing life at home with life on the stage. Five years after leaving her first marriage she met her current husband, James Dunham, a divorced single parent with a young daughter who attended the same school as Deborah's daughter. "You could say that we met through our children," she says. "We've been devoted to each other ever since."

Now happily living in Houston with James—a violist, former member of the Grammy-winning Cleveland Quartet, and currently tenured professor at the Shepherd School of Music at Rice University—Deborah is freelancing with orchestras in Houston, Boston and elsewhere around the country. She has also begun to work toward a Doctor of Musical Arts degree in Performance.

The Power of Yoga: Clearing Pain

When Deborah and James moved to Rochester, New York, for his new position as violist with the Cleveland Quartet, yoga became even more important in her life. In the process of pushing furniture around her new home Deborah pinched a nerve in her neck. The pain from the injury radiated down her arms to her wrists. Her doctor misdiagnosed the cause, attributing it to carpal tunnel syndrome. "I didn't even consider a second opinion at the time, since the diagnosis made sense," says Deborah. "I'd been practicing hard for an audition, and the doctor, having dealt with other musicians, thought my symptoms looked like carpal tunnel. Not only that, but some of my musician friends in previous years had suffered from this malady. Their complaints sounded like mine."

The only good news for Deborah was that she was forced to focus her practicing, since she could only practice for twenty minutes at a time. "I clearly saw the parallel between practicing music and practicing meditation," she says. But the pain in her arms and wrists was unsettling, and she was unhappy with the side effects of pain pills. A colleague in the orchestra invited her to a yoga class in Rochester and also introduced her to a place in the Berkshires called Kripalu Center for Yoga and Health in Lenox, Massachusetts, near Tanglewood, the summer home of the Boston Symphony.

"I fell in love with the Kripalu style of hatha yoga," says Deborah. "I felt some relief right away from their interpretation of the postures, and I loved the care and slow pace of their classes." Kripalu was only a five-hour drive from Rochester, and Deborah began spending as much time as she could spare at the Center. Her daughter even fell for the place after taking a "coming of age" program for young teens. "My body got stronger, and my posture was more aligned," says Deborah. "I seldom needed painkillers any more. Then the pain moved to my neck and shoulder area and *away* from my arms and wrists. That's when I finally realized that the problem had been a pinched nerve all along. Through chiropractic treatment and more yoga, however, the remaining pain cleared completely. And my playing had changed as well." By this time, Deborah had a tenured position with the Philharmonic and was gaining respect as a private teacher in the area.

"Knowing what yoga had done for me I decided to obtain a basic-level yoga teaching certification from Kripalu," says Deborah. "I wanted to pass on the postures and breathing techniques properly to my students, some of whom suffered greatly from tension, overly harsh self-criticism and crippling stage fright. I originally had no intention of teaching classes to the general public."

The Power of Yoga for the Older Adult

However, a month after receiving the certification, Deborah got a call from "The Yoga Room" in Rochester. A Monday morning teacher was needed. Since Monday is typically a musician's day off, she gladly accepted the position knowing she would be getting a yoga session at the same time. "But I didn't stop to think who would be taking a Monday morning class," says Deborah. "Imagine my surprise on the first day when I looked out into the faces of my first public class and saw that nearly all of them were senior citizens. A good-natured bunch, but many couldn't raise their arms over their heads. There was stiffness in knees, and some had difficulty with the hip area." Deborah had to get creative in a hurry, and also invited any of her students who had difficulty with the postures to sit them out until they had spoken with their doctors about doing yoga.

"We had a long session of warm-up movements first," says Deborah. "Then we did as many of the easy postures I could remember. I offered the option of using chairs and pillars in the room for stability. At the end of the class I realized I'd have to seek out advice and do more research in order to accommodate the needs of the class. I spent a lot of time at the beginning of subsequent classes breathing and warming up with these young-at-heart charges; we began to repeat the postures over and over for short periods, which seemed to work well. Most of the class could not hold postures for very long at first and the repetition helped strengthen them and build confidence. I kept modifying the postures, and by the end of six weeks I started seeing hints of transformation. Those who practiced yoga regularly were looking more fit. Wrinkles seemed to soften."

Deborah says that watching her students improve steadily over the weeks and months made her a true believer in the power of yoga. "The regular attendees who couldn't get their arms up over their heads in the beginning could now raise them high in the air. They were less stiff, more flexible; they had more color in their faces—they just looked so beautiful at the end of each session! Their energy levels were up. They would come into the yoga studio before class and the room was full of a sound like gentle chatting of happy children. That touched me, too, seeing how a yoga class promotes trust and a sense of community."

After ten years in Rochester, their daughters left for college, the Cleveland Quartet disbanded, James was invited to teach at the New England Conservatory of Music in Boston and Deborah became a substitute bassist for the Boston Symphony Orchestra, also playing as a freelancer for the Boston Pops and other local ensembles. The pace of life and performance picked up dramatically, and Deborah began neglecting her regular yoga practice.

"About three months after we moved, I started feeling tired, achy, a little depressed and I'd put on some weight," says Deborah. "I couldn't figure it out. I went to our new doctor who asked me first what I had been doing in my life and after a battery of tests, which all came back negative, he had the presence of mind to ask me what I had not been doing. When I mentioned yoga his face brightened and without any hesitation he said, 'You know, we don't know how yoga works, but we do know it works for many of our patients.' Touchdown! Within weeks of a renewed yoga routine I was back in business. What a great personal revelation to experience falling out of a practice! If I was to do any more teaching as a yoga instructor, this would be most useful."

The Power of Yoga for the *Younger* Adult:
Stretch, Breathe and Drink Lots of Water

As if on cue, the New England Conservatory of Music called Deborah shortly after this revelation to ask if she would be interested in picking up a yoga class for their young students. "Pleased and charmed by the timing of this, I accepted," says Deborah. "But again I was not prepared for whom I was about to meet. I walked in and found a group of young, beautiful college students. After introductions, we delved into why they were in the class. Many complained of stage fright and concentration difficulties. One had rotator cuff problems. Many had tight hamstrings and back pain. Some had carpal tunnel syndrome and tendonitis. Warming up on the carpet in the room I was struck by the resemblance of this class to the first class in Rochester with the 'older' crowd. *Déjà vu.* These kids were so tight they could hardly relax! Imagine seeing someone in his twenties not being able to get his arms and hands overhead."

Deborah worked slowly with her young students, focusing on breathing, relaxation and stretching those tight muscles through modified postures. She asked those with ailments to refrain from certain postures and movement until they had checked with their doctors, and just breathe. "It was apparent that students, especially string and piano majors, develop the habit of not breathing—holding their breath in or out—during performances," says Deborah. "This is the kind of habit that carries over into one's everyday life until the quality begins to deteriorate. I looked at my own habits and realized I had firsthand experience."

After that first class Deborah went into the restroom and wept. "I tried to understand what was going on with these young people," she says. "I knew the pace in Boston and other American cities, and I had felt and seen the competitiveness that comes with such a pace from my new colleagues. This same environment was already causing these young adults the kind of stress that created the physical problems I'd just witnessed. What could teachers do to guide them?"

Once again, the students who came faithfully to class began to show improvement. They had less pain and tightness, and many were calmer and had less stage fright during performances and auditions. "We went on in the classes to talk about the importance of good nutrition and watching one's water intake," says Deborah. "The Kripalu training made me aware of how critical it is to keep the body hydrated. Here's a formula that's easy to remember. Take your body weight in pounds and divide that number in half. Use this number to determine the amount of water in ounces you'll need to drink daily. This does not include tea or juice or soda, just water. So if a person is 128 pounds, for instance, she should drink 64 ounces of water a day—eight glasses. Depending upon your weight you would drink more or less than this."

Instant Ease, Relaxation, Clarity and Focus

While in Boston, Deborah expanded her knowledge of yoga. She became interested in some of the Sanskrit texts, starting with the *Bhagava Gita* (Song of God), finding unexpected inspiration from them. She was introduced to Marshall Govindan and Babaji's Kriya yoga. "I learned invaluable techniques, especially the new breathing techniques, and was made aware of the texts and beautiful chants in Tamil," says Deborah. By the time James was offered a tenured, full professorship at Rice University in Houston, which he accepted, they had both also been introduced to Siddha yoga and heard a series of lectures given by the scholar Paul Eduardo Muller Ortega just after moving to Texas. "In his third lecture on the *Guru Gita* (Song of the Guru) he spoke of the Sanskrit word *agama*," says Deborah. "I had known this word to mean scripture, but Paul relayed to us that it also meant 'the source from which all scriptures flow.'

"Suddenly, I had a profound shift and understanding from within. I knew this *agama*. I'd felt it before. It had helped me change my life and enriched my performance of music: We all have this source, this *agama* in our lives, whether we call it prana, qi, Holy Spirit, Grace, the Universe, the Force or even just God. When we have tension, we can't get to this core of who we are and what we must do. But if we can relax, let go and trust in this *agama*—this source of inner wisdom—it will always be there. It is like a shower that's always on. For me, when I can release the tension, the things I don't need seem to drop away and I understand at once what is important. It is instant ease, relaxation, clarity and focus."

 Yoga: What's the Evidence?

The ancient system of yoga, which originated in India as part of Ayurvedic medicine, is becoming increasingly popular in the West. A recent Roper poll reported that more than six million Americans practice yoga. Yoga is used to treat stress, insomnia, headaches, anxiety, premenstrual syndrome, arthritis, back pain, and gastrointestinal, respiratory and cardiovascular problems. The practice is also used during pregnancy in preparation for childbirth. How does it help with such a wide variety of problems? "The regular practice of yoga induces a deep sense of relaxation, which is beneficial in itself, at least temporarily," writes Edzard Ernst. He describes the benefits of yoga that have been found, including suppleness, muscular strength and feelings of well-being. In addition, Ernst says, "Yoga breathing exercises counter the rapid breathing that accompanies the stress response and may in addition reduce muscular spasm and expand the available lung capacity." So when you are feeling stressed, deep yoga breathing may be a good way to calm down your body and your mind.

The research on yoga consists primarily of uncontrolled, observational studies, according to Ernst. In summarizing the results of these studies, Ernst reports that yoga practice by healthy people induces a deep sense of relaxation and has beneficial effects on mood, emotional well-being and perceptions of the quality of life. Physical effects include increased suppleness of body and muscular strength.

Yoga and heart disease

As we will see in chapter 4, "Healing More Than Hearts," yoga is an important part of many treatment programs for cardiovascular disease. "Yoga programs have shown the potential for helping to reduce heart disease by influencing such risk factors as blood pressure, anxiety, and unhealthy reaction to stress," writes Kenneth Pelletier. In the program to manage and reverse heart disease developed by Dean Ornish, M.D., and his colleagues, researchers found that those who benefited most were those who did yoga for at least two hours a day, reports Pelletier. (Author's note: Not many of us have that kind of time! I have found that even twenty minutes a day can help a great deal with stiffness and pain.)

Yoga helps with hypertension, asthma and osteoarthritis

The few controlled studies selected by Ernst suggest that yoga may have useful long-term effects in the treatment of hypertension, asthma and in reducing joint stiffness in osteoarthritis. In one study, eight weeks of yoga training improved pain, tenderness and range of motion.

The Vidanthan study, which is widely cited, demonstrates that yoga can help young adults with asthma. The study reports fewer symptoms and medication use.

Yoga helps healthy people get healthier

In addition, Pelletier points to an Indian study of forty male physical education teachers, already very fit, who practiced yoga daily for three months. They "showed a significant reduction in blood pressure, heart rate, respiratory rate, and body weight, with decreased autonomic or involuntary arousal," writes Pelletier.

In a controlled study of healthy female volunteers, Pelletier also reports, "One group of women practiced yoga, and a control group sat and read. There was significant improvement in the yoga group in psychological parameters." In addition, the heart rates of the readers slowed down, but rose again at follow-up, while the heart rates of the yoga group remained low.

There do not seem to be studies reporting any reason not to do yoga, but you should always check with your doctor before beginning any exercise program.

References

Collins, C. "Yoga: Intuition, Preventive Medicine, and Treatment." *Journal of Obstetric, Gynecologic, and Neonatal Nursing* (September/October 1998): 563–568.

Ernst, E., ed. *The Desktop Guide to Complementary and Alternative Medicine: An Evidence-Based Approach.* London: Harcourt Publishers Limited, 2001.

Garfinkel, M. S., et al. "Evaluation of a Yoga-Based Regimen for Treatment of Osteoarthritis of the Hands." *Journal of Rheumatology* (Toronto) 21 (1994): 2341–2343.

Nespor, K. "Psychosomatics of Back Pain and the Use of Yoga." *International Journal of Psychosomatics* 36 (1989): 72–78.

Patel, C. "Twelve Month Follow-Up of Yoga and Bio-feedback in the Management of Hypertension." *Lancet* 1 (1975): 62–64.

Pelletier, K. R. *The Best of Alternative Medicine: What Works? What Does Not?* New York: Simon & Schuster, 2000.

Schell, F. J., et al. "Physiological and Psychological Effects of Hatha-Yoga Exercise in Healthy Women." *International Journal of Psychosomatics* 41, nos. 1–4 (1994): 46–52.

Telles, S., et al. "Physiological Changes in Sports Teachers Following 3 Months of Training in Yoga." *Indian Journal of Medical Sciences* 47, no. 10 (1993): 235–38.

Vedanthan P. K., et al. "Clinical Study of Yoga Techniques in University Students with Asthma: A Controlled Study." *Allergy and Asthma Proceedings* 19 (1998): 3–9.

3

WHAT WOULD IT TAKE
TO CHANGE *YOUR* LIFESTYLE?

"I promised myself I would never
put my family through this again."

It was a beautiful fall day in 1997. Washington attorney Mark Soler was playing in his regular Sunday morning basketball game. He'd been getting
together with the same group of friends for years and was pleased that he could
keep up, since several of them were younger than he was. He thought he was in
pretty good shape, considering that this once-weekly game was his only form of
exercise. At fifty, Mark was youthful-looking, with a full head of curly salt and
pepper hair, a matching beard and penetrating pale green eyes. He was about
twenty-five pounds overweight, but his stocky build looked muscular and powerful. That morning, he had no concern about his health. In fact, the night
before, he and his wife, Andi, a psychologist, had gone to their favorite barbe-
cue place for dinner, and he had eaten his usual dish of pork spareribs.

Shortly after the game started, Mark was running toward the basket when
something happened. "I suddenly lost my breath," Mark remembers. "I stopped
running in the middle of the game and tried to catch my breath, but it didn't
work. Then I sat down and that didn't work either. There was no pain, but it felt
like an elephant was sitting on my chest. I figured I would just sit out the game
and see my doctor later in the day."

After a few minutes, he decided maybe that wasn't such a good idea. "When
it wasn't getting any better, my friends and I decided I had better get some
medical attention," said Mark. They made a plan: The friends would drive
Mark to his car, which was about twenty minutes away, and then he would

drive himself to the hospital. But that is not what happened.

"As soon as I got into the back seat of my friend's car, I realized that this was serious, because I really couldn't breathe, and I said, 'Get me to a hospital or I'm not going to make it.'" His friends called 911 on a cell phone, and this is what Mark remembers: "An ambulance was there in about sixty seconds. They knew it was an MI (myocardial infarction), gave me an aspirin to chew on, hooked me up to lines and took me to the *second* closest hospital, because that was the best one in Washington for cardiac care." Emergency staff at the hospital used a "clot-busting" drug to clear the blocked artery that had caused the heart attack and kept him in the emergency room, monitoring his condition closely.

When Mark's condition had stabilized, he was transferred to the intensive care unit. Cardiac surgeons performed an angioplasty (threading a flexible tube through the artery to clear out the blockage) and inserted a stent (a tiny expanding metal "scaffold" to keep the artery open and blood flowing freely).

Later, as he recovered in his hospital room, Mark used the time to confer with his office on the telephone and visit with friends. Sometimes he did both at the same time. One day a friend was visiting in the hospital while Mark was on the phone with his staff. "A nurse walked in and told Mark to get off the phone and rest," reported the friend. "When Mark said that he had to discuss a case with one of the lawyers, the nurse answered, 'If you had died would they be able to consult with you?'"

That comment had an impact on Mark: "I realized that if I didn't make a profound life change, I wasn't going to live very long," he says. Mark's father and paternal grandfather had died in their forties of heart attacks, and his other grandfather died of a heart attack at a later age. "I was still in law school when my father died," Mark says. "I was scared that the same thing could happen to me. Right then, I promised myself that I would never put my family through an experience like this again."

A Driven Lifestyle

Right up until the day of his heart attack, Mark had lived what he describes as a "driven" lifestyle. Twenty-three years before, he had helped to found the Youth Law Center, a public interest organization that represents children who are being abused in government-operated jails and juvenile facilities. He was working with staff lawyers in San Francisco and Washington, D.C., bringing lawsuits against institutions, traveling all over the country (and abroad) giving speeches and participating in panels about juvenile justice, teaching law school courses, testifying in Congress, consulting with Amnesty International and receiving national awards for his work. There was even a TV movie about one of his cases.

"I felt driven to do all of these things, to prove to myself that I could help kids wherever they were," says Mark. "I was the typical 'type-A' person: ambitious, hard-driving, preparing for whatever task I took on, whether it was lobbying, litigating, testifying or giving speeches. There was constant stress, and at least three trips a month around the country, eating hot dogs or hamburgers in airports and hotels, in between meetings or catching flights."

In short, Mark was a busy guy. Too busy to worry much about his health, even though he knew that the genetic odds were against him. "I have a great ability to compartmentalize," says Mark. "I did have a nagging feeling in the background that this wasn't the best way to live, that one basketball game a week wasn't enough exercise, that eating red meat and fried food almost every day was not a good diet, but I kept saying I'll change things in the future. I'll lose weight, eat better and start exercising—later. There just wasn't the emotional power and immediacy to change my life at that time. But after my heart attack, when I realized that if it had happened on an airplane to South Dakota instead of in the middle of Washington, D.C., I probably would have died . . . that scared me."

So the nurse's comment in the hospital got Mark's attention. "I realized that I had been given another chance: an opportunity to turn this experience around and live a long, healthy life," he says. "I didn't think there was any other choice if I wanted to stay alive." He then asked his cardiologists and nurses, "What do I have to do to make sure this doesn't happen again?" They were only too happy to tell him.

(For more information, please see "Take Action: Best Ways to Avoid Heart Disease," in the next chapter.)

After the Diagnosis, a Lifestyle Change

When Mark made the decision to change his lifestyle, he did so with his characteristic determination, and with the enthusiastic support of his wife, Andi. "Luckily, I was given a second chance to reclaim my health," Mark says. "We both realized that the unfolding process of our health would depend on the way we live." Together, they launched into a program of regular walking, then bought a treadmill to use at home. They completely changed their kitchen, using low- or nonfat substitutes for butter, cheese and snack foods. They cut out salt and red meat, and found recipes that used herbal seasonings, fish, turkey and vegetables. "What made it easier is that we were both committed to changing our way of living," says Mark. "We did it together."

Despite the seemingly unlimited number of health practices available outside of conventional medicine (see, for example, Appendix I), there is no need to try them all. Many people have found that incorporating just a few into their lifestyles makes a huge difference in their health. Experts recommend exploring those that interest you, perhaps starting with one or two that "feel right."

Mark Soler changed both his health and his life dramatically by combining a few complementary methods with his conventional medical care, always working in partnership with his doctor. Mark now takes conventional prescription medicines for blood pressure and cholesterol every day, as well as aspirin and a multivitamin. His doctor also recommended twenty to thirty minutes of aerobic exercise five times a week. The day Mark got home from the hospital, he and Andi started a walking program together. "That first day we only made it to the store down the street and back," says Mark. "That was it for the day. I was tired." During the following month, as he recuperated at home, Mark walked more every day. "First it was twenty minutes, then a little longer and faster. During the second month, I started alternating walking and jogging. I tried to push myself, not to settle for anything too easy."

After they bought a treadmill, they both started using it regularly. Three months after the heart attack, Mark was back playing basketball. "I was confident I could run, but the other guys weren't. They let me score at will that first Sunday. After that, they figured I could take it."

In addition to exercise, changing his diet and the medications, Mark uses visualization and guided imagery techniques to help him stay disciplined. "I'm still scared," he says. "Whenever I think about fried food or red meat, I visualize little milligrams of cholesterol going through my arteries, clogging them, and slowing down my blood flow. It doesn't help to cheat either, because you can't fool your body." As he does his visualization, Mark thinks about what might have happened if he had not been able to get to a hospital within an hour of the heart attack. "There wouldn't have been time to administer the clot-busting drug, and I know I wouldn't have made it," he says. "That knowledge helps keep the visualization real." (Please see also chapters 7 and 9, which describe the uses of guided imagery and visualization to control both pain and asthma.)

For the first year after the heart attack, Mark ate no fried food or red meat. Now, he will eat a "forbidden" food only about once a month, with a special treat on New Year's Eve. He maintains close contact with his conventional physician, who checks his cholesterol and blood pressure regularly. About six months after the heart attack, he noticed some shortness of breath once again, this time while on the treadmill. A medical exam revealed a second, smaller artery was clogged, requiring a second angioplasty and stent operation. Now at fifty-five, nearly five years after the heart attack, Mark has kept up his health routines, and he has had no further problems. "I've lost about twenty-five pounds and kept it off," he said. "I'm in almost the same shape I was in when I got out of law school, and my cholesterol numbers are great."

In fact, Mark's last stress-echocardiogram test (which measures heart function during activity) was so good that his doctor told him he didn't need a test next year, just an office visit. "I looked at the part of my heart that had been 'attacked' on the sonogram," says Mark. "It actually looked stronger than it was a year ago. Now, when I play basketball, I can still guard and run with guys who are fifteen to twenty years younger. This has given me tremendous confidence.

The physical wellness has wonderful psychological benefits." Mark's friends took careful note of his experiences as well: "Apparently, my heart attack had an impact on some of the guys I play basketball with," he says. "When I came back in really good shape, several of them began to change their behavior and diets. They had never seen anyone have a heart attack before, and it scared the hell out of them."

Both Mark and Andi still work full time but with an important change: "We began to think carefully about what is really important in life," says Mark. "For me, the biggest change was the realization that I don't have to prove anything any more: I no longer have to show people that I can close down a jail that is abusing children, win a lawsuit or an award. I can say 'no' to speaking engagements. I can cut down on my travel. Andi works a more reasonable schedule as well. We both feel that our time is much more precious, and we want to be careful how we use it."

Health Management or Disease Management?

Cardiologist Martin "Marty" Sullivan, M.D., whom you will meet again in the next chapter, has this to say about coronary artery disease (the cause of Mark Soler's heart attack):

"Atherosclerosis—caused by 'plaque' buildup in the arteries leading away from the heart and also called coronary artery disease—accounts for 48 percent of all deaths in the United States." In about half of the cases of heart disease, in fact, the first symptom is sudden death, says Marty, formerly of the Duke Center for Integrative Medicine and now founding director of the Institute for Healing in Society and Medicine. The Institute offers educational services and consultation to physicians and organizations in the practice of integrative medicine. As part of its program, the Institute seeks to educate health-care practitioners on their own mind/body/spirit connections.

"We know from epidemiological and crosscultural studies that in most cases this disease is preventable—it is almost entirely related to *lifestyle and culture*. We also know from research that diets like the 'Mediterranean' diet, low in saturated fats, high in fruits and vegetables and monosaturated fats, are known to reduce cardiac 'events' by 70 percent in patients who have had heart attacks." (Please see the research section in the next chapter for more evidence about diet and heart disease.)

"Drugs, angioplasty and bypass surgery alone address only the symptoms of atherosclerosis. For many patients, there is no evidence that drugs or surgery actually prolong survival rates. Why? Because they do not address the root causes of the disease," says Marty. "You can correct lesions in an artery surgically, but what about all the other arteries that are also coated with atherosclerosis? When another one becomes fully blocked, it will cause another heart attack. The best way to reduce or prevent plaque buildup is through lipid-lowering medications, diet, exercise and stress management. We know that all four of these interventions alone can reduce cardiac events by 25 to 70 percent. Studies using the combined approach show much lower heart attack rates." A study in Hawaii, for example, showed that men over sixty-five who walk regularly three to four times a week live longer than men who don't. Regular, aerobic exercise for patients with heart failure has also been shown to reduce symptoms and hospitalizations. (This study, along with related research, is cited in the next chapter.)

So why is lifestyle counseling not standard practice in all treatment of cardiac patients? "Less than 15 percent of people with coronary artery disease have any formalized outpatient intervention, including exercise and nutrition counseling, smoking cessation, psychological or group counseling and stress reduction programs. And, to be effective, these need to be ongoing educational programs, with follow-up support," says Marty. "You won't learn to play the piccolo if I just hand you one and leave. And you won't know how to change your lifestyle unless the health-care system is committed to providing you with long-term educational and counseling support." Mark Soler bought books about coronary artery disease, asked for advice from his doctor and had the motivation (fear of death is always a good motivator) to keep up with his lifestyle change. But most cardiac patients in this country do not have either the opportunity or the motivation to do what Mark did.

"The conventional medical system is focused on medical and surgical intervention, despite the fact that science itself is showing us that these other interventions are more effective," says Marty. "Until we focus more on prevention, and until insurance will reimburse these lifestyle interventions, we will continue to have a system that manages disease rather than health."

The Five Pillars of Health

Alexa Fleckenstein, M.D., could not agree more. She has never met Mark Soler or Marty Sullivan, but what they had to say reminds her of the advice she has been giving to her patients in neighborhood health centers and walk-in clinics for more than ten years. Alexa is a mother and grandmother, but her silvery pale blond hair, clear green eyes and smooth skin give the impression of a much younger woman. When she is asked for her secret of youth, she laughs and says, "Cold water." (More about that later.)

Alexa's medical training and experience encompass not only conventional medicine—she is board-certified in internal medicine—but also a wide range of complementary therapies. Since completing internship, residency and fellowship in primary care and ambulatory medicine, she has been taking care of outpatients in Boston. In 1997, she returned for a sabbatical year to her native Germany to complete a certificate in European Natural Medicine, which in that country is considered part of "mainstream" conventional medical care—a subspecialty of internal medicine. European Natural Medicine is a health system that grew out of the work of a nineteenth-century Bavarian priest named Sebastian Kneipp, who developed a natural approach to health care in the nineteenth century that swept Europe and eventually became the foundation for the naturopathy system in this country. (Please see Appendix I for a description of naturopathy and other complementary modalities.) European Natural Medicine is based on the belief that the human body has an innate healing power that can be stimulated by following a certain lifestyle. (Please see box, "The Five Pillars of Health.")

A voracious reader, Alexa had already absorbed many of the principles of European Natural Medicine before her sabbatical year. In fact, a visit to her home in a suburb of Boston reveals both her interest in natural medicine and her passion for gardening and nature. The white cottage and its surroundings could have been airlifted from a small European village. Roses, iris, peonies, anemones, rudbeckia and all kinds of berries in various stages of unchecked growth surround the house with rainbows of pinks, blues and purples. A kitchen herb garden flourishes with chives, sage, burnet, sorrel, parsley, several kinds of mint, lemon balm, oregano and thyme. Another small garden is crowded with medicinal herbs—St. John's wort, comfrey, yarrow, lady's mantle and others. In the front yard, instead of the clipped hedges common in her neighborhood, she grows a large patch of European white asparagus.

"In the course of my research, I rediscovered the work of Sebastian Kneipp," says Alexa. Kneipp's work grew out of the need to save his own life. In 1849, when he was a twenty-eight-year-old theology student in Bavaria, he was near death from tuberculosis—considered an incurable disease at the time. In the seminary library he found a book about the supposedly therapeutic effects of cold-water exposure. Figuring he had nothing to lose, he began a program of "therapy" that seemed suicidal to everyone around him: Several times a week, in midwinter, he would hurl himself into the freezing waters of the Danube for a few seconds, then dress, rush home and jump into bed. The notion was that the sudden burst of cold water would stimulate the body, giving it enough strength to fight off infection and disease. ("Now we would call this 'strengthening the immune system,'" notes Alexa.)

The treatment cured his tuberculosis, and Kneipp went on to develop his own system of medical care based on a healthy lifestyle and the benefits of cold water. Soon people from all over Europe were flocking to him for his treatments. "Kneipp health spas" sprang up throughout Germany, Austria, Switzerland, Luxembourg, France and Southwest Africa. Today, Wörishofen, Kneipp's former hometown, is filled with spas offering hydrotherapy; the pharmacy carrying his name still continues to manufacture herbal products; and every town in Germany has at least one Kneipp Club that organizes winter swims (although Kneipp himself had stopped endorsing such harsh treatments.)[1]

---

[1] S. S. Haas, "Hydrotherapy and More: Adapting Kneipp's Natural Medicine to the U.S., *Complementary Medicine for the Physician* 5, no. 8 (2000): 57.

"I would never advise anyone to jump into the Atlantic Ocean—and certainly not Boston's Charles River—in the middle of winter," says Alexa. "But I do believe that Kneipp's ideas for a healthy lifestyle are worth considering." Using her knowledge of conventional medicine, European Natural Medicine and alternative practices, Alexa has adapted Kneipp's system into a practical method of creating a healthy lifestyle in the twenty-first century. Her patients have taken to the ideas with enthusiasm and excellent results.

✓ TAKE ACTION ✓

Building Your Lifestyle on Kneipp's Five Pillars of Health

1. **Cold Water.** A few seconds of cold-water exposure every day strengthens the immune system and benefits the cardiovascular system, glands, respiratory system and skin. Turning the shower to cold just before you get out is an easy way to accomplish this. If possible, use a "hand shower" to start at the feet and move up. (Studies on cold-water therapy can be found at the end of this chapter.)

2. **Movement.** "Even just two minutes of moving your body every day has physical and emotional benefits," says Alexa. "It's never too little, and it's never too late. Everyone can find the time to do a few minutes of some kind of movement. Then slowly work up to more." (See other chapters for the benefits of exercise for specific conditions, including heart disease and chronic illness.)

3. **Nutrition.** Alexa spends a great deal of time counseling her patients about healthy nutrition. ("I don't like starving my patients or putting them on fad diets," she says.) She helps her patients change the way they eat, emphasizing regional, seasonal organic foods, especially fruits, vegetables and grains; cutting down on fat and drinking plenty of water. (Information and research on nutrition for specific conditions can be found throughout the book, as well as in "A Closer Look at Peeke Performance.")

4. **Herbs.** Alexa believes in the healing and nutritional powers of herbs and plants. "Our bodies evolved along with the plant life around us in the same way that the shape of a flower evolved so that a bee could pollinate it," she says. "The

(continued)

plants and herbs in our environment fit like a key into the lock of our physiology and metabolism. When we look outside the window and say, 'What a beautiful landscape,' it is more than a pretty view. It is our nourishment and sustenance. It is how we exist. We are physically part of the nature around us. (Please see "A Closer Look at Healing Herbs" for more information as well as research.)

5. **A Balanced Life.** Creating balance in our lives is a necessary part of human health. In general, a balanced life might include some exposure to art, music and beauty; a spiritual connection of some kind ("Humans are 'hard-wired' for spirituality," says Alexa); living in harmony with the seasons ("It's okay to put on a few extra pounds and even 'hibernate' and become more inward-focused during the winter."); and trying to follow the natural cycle of day, evening and night to avoid the health-eroding effects of sleep deprivation. ("Grocery shopping at 3:00 A.M. plays havoc with our circadian rhythm and body chemistry.") And perhaps most difficult to achieve: a healthy balance among work, family and relationships.

Consider the story of Dorothy, an overweight woman in her forties who was also a smoker. She came to see Alexa complaining of a urinary tract infection. "Whenever I have patients with urinary tract infections, I always check for diabetes, since diabetics are prone to such infections," says Alexa. "And Dorothy did turn out to have an early diabetes that she was unaware of."

Alexa first prescribed antibiotics for the infection, then encouraged Dorothy to take a brief daily cold shower at the end of her warm shower to improve her immune system. "In my work with patients, I find that cold-water therapy is particularly valuable as a motivational tool. Because the positive effect on mood is immediate, patients become motivated to make other little changes as well—including nutrition and exercise—and also feel a good deal of confidence in their ability to participate actively in their own treatment. Besides, there is also no additional time commitment involved, since they are already in the shower."

There are certain people who should *not* use cold water showers, Alexa is quick to point out. These include anyone with high blood pressure that is not controlled by medication and people with Raynaud's disease. People with acute lower back pain or a high fever should also avoid the practice. "As with any alternative therapy, including herbs and vitamins, it is extremely important to consult with your primary care physician before doing anything," she stresses.

After Dorothy started her cold-water routine, Alexa brought up the subject of exercise. "I start with a minimal exercise program so that people cannot fail," says Alexa. "They can walk, and if they have an old piece of exercise equipment in the basement—an exercise bike, for example—they can use that, too." Dorothy happened to have one, so Alexa asked her, "Do you think you could do two minutes on the bike?" Dorothy answered briskly (perhaps emboldened by her new cold-shower routine), "Are you kidding, Dr. Fleckenstein? Of course I can do two minutes!"

"Fine," said Alexa. "I'd like you to do two minutes every day. If you get carried away and do twenty minutes, that's fine, but it doesn't count for the next day. You still have to do your two minutes." Dorothy agreed. After a few weeks, she reported proudly that her legs were feeling stronger, and that a feeling of well-being was creeping up through her whole body. Alexa then suggested that she take a ten-minute walk every day at lunchtime.

"I also teach my patients what I call 'micro-movements,'" says Alexa. These are small, almost snake-like 'wiggling' and stretching motions that originate from the spine, that allow them to also loosen up the shoulders, torso, arms, legs, head and neck. These can be done while sitting in a chair. Even frail or very old people can do them." The movements are designed to adjust the posture and prevent slumping. Alexa regularly says to her patients, "When I come into the room, I don't want to see you just sitting there, I want you to be *wiggling!*" Alexa herself took up what she calls "Zen running" at the age of fifty-six. "It's a kind of shuffling run that has low impact on knees, hips and ankles, but excellent aerobic benefits. It looks a bit odd, but who cares?" she says. "If people look at me and say, 'I could do that, too,' that would be marvelous!"

Dorothy continued to see Alexa once a month, even after the urinary tract infection was cured, to report on her exercise progress. Throughout this time, they

put olive oil
in frig,

flax seed
  grind + put
  in frig - put
  on salads -
  potatoes etc

Dr weil. com
  soy , flax
  salmon

3-16-04

mews fact

extra virgin olive oil

Dr Andrew Weil

8 weeks to optimum health

Spontaneous Healing

soy
ginger
tumeric

Breathing — spirit

virtual

talked about diet and nutrition. "I first encouraged her to cut out white sugar and white flour (which is just as bad, especially for diabetics)," says Alexa. Then she asked Dorothy, "What's your downfall?" "Pizza, sweets, soda," answered Dorothy. "I eat at midnight, Dr. Fleckenstein." Alexa pointed out that the laws of nature apply to all of us. "Actions have consequences. If you eat pizza, you will have a pizza body, but even small improvements in lifestyle can have a big impact."

So Alexa began by making one suggestion. "Let's cut out one thing. How about soft drinks? No soda or juice from now on. Drink water instead. This is something achievable. Something you can do. Then we'll try to cut out some other things." Dorothy agreed to give it a try. But there was another problem: She hated vegetables and never ate them. This, thought Alexa, had to be remedied. "I asked her if she thought she could try at least one new vegetable every month," says Alexa. "Every time she came to see me, I wanted to hear what vegetable she had discovered." Alexa also gave Dorothy specific herbs for the diabetes, along with coenzyme Q10 and magnesium. With Alexa's encouragement, Dorothy began to experiment with ways of cooking vegetables in appealing ways. "Olive oil and garlic can make almost any vegetable taste good," says Alexa. "And these ingredients are also good for the heart!"

Alexa feels strongly about eating plant foods (see also research recommendations about a plant-based diet to reduce cancer risk in chapter 5): "Sometimes I go into my garden and harvest leaves and petals from various herbs and plants to make a 'garden tea' from whatever I find in season. I sometimes even use a few pine needles," she says. "This is my 'power drink,' but you do have to know what you are doing! For example, several kinds of leaves are poisonous, including those from carrots, tomatoes and potatoes." And she is almost vehement about the benefits of fruits and vegetables, quoting freely from studies to bolster her position: Eating fruits and vegetables forces you to chew better, reduces the speed with which blood glucose rises (important for diabetics), lowers cholesterol, boosts digestive enzymes and immune strength, binds toxins and removes them faster from the gut, provides some natural antibiotics, decreases inflammation and helps protect against some cancers. If you're still not convinced, she has even more reasons.

And then there was Dorothy's smoking. "I usually ask my patients to buy an egg timer, and every time they want a cigarette, to meditate for five minutes, with the timer," says Alexa. "This can be just sitting quietly with focus on the breath. I have also used chewing gum, hypnosis, cigarette substitutes—whatever they believe in. But the meditation seems to work best. Often, people feel so good after the five minutes that they don't light up. But it is a struggle."

A difficult hurdle for Dorothy was achieving a more balanced life. "Staying up late and eating pizza at midnight disrupts normal sleep patterns, and the 'circadian rhythm' of our bodies," says Alexa, "not to mention the disruption of the digestive system." The circadian rhythm is an innate physiological twenty-four-hour cycle of waking and sleeping, based on hormones that include melatonin, and on external stimuli, especially light. "This natural twenty-four-hour cycle is not something our grandmothers made up," says Alexa. "It is something we can nail down biochemically: We know that sleep before midnight is more beneficial than sleep after. Our bodies are negatively affected by late-night TV and pizza at midnight. Studies have shown that even the smallest amount of light can affect the circadian rhythm and disrupt hormone production. The result is sleep deprivation and fatigue during waking hours."

"Our bodies are so closely tied to our environment that to ignore that connection can only invite harm," says Alexa. "Just as our minds and souls crave a connection to other people and to a community, our bodies fare so much better when we recognize our connection to the natural world." (Please see research in "A Closer Look at Energy Healing, Spirituality and Therapeutic Touch.") She points to the traditions of all human cultures that reflect the changing cycle of seasons. "Almost every religion has a festival of light during the dark time of winter, including Chanukah, Christmas, Divali and Kwanzaa. Physiologically, we tend to put on a little more weight in the fall, perhaps eat a bit more meat and fat, to get us through the winter. Nothing to get too upset about," she says. "We are biologically programmed that way, just as all of the world's cultures celebrate the renewal of life in the spring."

Over several months, Dorothy did manage to stop eating at midnight, cut down on the pizza and soft drinks, reduce her smoking (she has not yet quit completely), and expand her diet to include vegetables. She kept up with her walking and exercise bicycle. She was able to manage the diabetes without insulin, and very slowly began to lose weight. "I don't like my patients to lose more than one or two pounds per month," says Alexa. "Otherwise, the body goes into starvation mode and resents the weight loss. Even if they lose only one pound, we celebrate. At least they didn't gain anything that month!"

Dorothy saw Alexa for several years. She remained insulin free and developed no complications from the diabetes. Her diet has improved substantially and she has kept the weight off. She also keeps a close eye on her blood sugar and monitors it at home every day. "She's come a long way," says Alexa. "But it is not always easy to maintain a healthy lifestyle. We do our best, sometimes we lapse, but the important thing is that we try again. We are all works in progress!"

 ## Hydrotherapy: What's the Evidence?

The foundation of Kneipp's Five Pillars of Health is water, also called hydrotherapy. A large body of research in Germany now supports the effects of cold-water therapy,[2] and the German insurance system pays all or part of physician-prescribed treatments. The importance and therapeutic potential of water, and especially cold water, is now simply taken for granted by most people in Germany.[3]

The Benefits of Cold Water

"The daily practice of hydrotherapy supports a healthy immune system and strengthens a weak one, elevates mood and improves circulation," says Alexa Fleckenstein, M.D. It can lower cholesterol levels and blood pressure, reduce chronic pain, improve skin health and promote hair growth. Cold water also tonifies

[2] M. Bühring, *Naturheilkunde: Grundlagen, Anwendungen, Ziele [Natural Medicine: Basic Application and Goals]* (Munich: Verlag CH Beck, 1997).
[3] Haas, "Hydrotherapy and More," 61–64.

the muscles and tissues beneath the skin. The involuntary deep breath when the cold water hits your torso stimulates the lungs. Varicose veins and hemorrhoids benefit greatly, and recurrent colds can be prevented. Research supports these findings, although until recently, all of the research has been done and published in German. Some time ago, observational studies were done of children in orphanages in Germany. Cold incidence was compared between a group exposed to daily cold water during the fall and winter and a group without this exposure. Colds were substantially fewer in the cold-water group after one to two months of hydrotherapy, then returned to their former high levels within one to two months after daily cold water ended.

Boosting the immune system

One pilot study of immune effects from cold-water therapy with a small number of breast cancer patients found significantly increased disease-fighting cell counts in every category examined, including neutrophils, T-lymphocytes, B-cells and natural killer cells.[4]

Lowering cholesterol

A prospective study of sixty-eight patients with high cholesterol in London's Thrombosis Research Institute reported a highly significant reduction in both total and LDL cholesterol along with other benefits after three months of cold-water therapy.[5]

Reducing the perception of pain

In a study in Japan, cooling by ice water was one of the "competitive stimuli" that reduced the perception of the pain of a laser beam on the skin.[6]

---

[4] G. Kuehn, "Sequential Hydrotherapy Improves the Immune Response of Cancer Patients," in *Potentiating Health and the Crisis of the Immune System: Integrative Approaches in the Prevention and Treatment of Modern Diseases*, eds. A. Mizrahim et al. (New York: Plenum, 1997).

[5] F. DeLorenzo et al., "Central Cooling Effects in Patients with Hypercholesterolaemia," *Clinical Science* (Colchester Essex) 95 (1998): 213–217.

[6] R. Kakigi et al., "Pain Relief by Various Kinds of Interference Stimulation Applied to the Peripheral Skin in Humans: Pain-Related Brain Potentials Following CO_2 Laser Stimulation," *Journal of the Peripher Nervous System* 1 (1996): 189–198.

Improved circulation and function in the legs

A Swedish group administered three weeks of alternating cold and hot hydrotherapy to the legs of patients suffering from intermittent claudication (reduced blood flow) and found that improved systolic blood pressure in ankles and toes, reduced pain and markedly better walking ability went beyond the results of standard treatment and persisted for at least a year after treatment.[7]

Swimming in the winter?

Ten healthy subjects who regularly swim during the winter were evaluated at Berlin's Institute of Biochemistry at Humboldt University Medical School. Their blood and urine showed increased levels of antioxidants, which prevent cell damage, indicating their bodies' increased tolerance to stress.[8]

[7] S. Elmstahl, et al., "Hydrotherapy of Patients with Intermittent Claudication: A Novel Approach to Improve Systolic Ankle Pressure and Reduce Symptoms." *International Angiology* (Torino) 14 (1995): 389–394.

[8] W. G. Siems, et al., "Uric Acid and Glutathione Levels During Short-Term Whole Body Cold Exposure. *Free Radical Biology and Medicine* 16 (1994): 299–305.

A Closer Look at the Alexander Technique: Using the Mind to Free the Body

"Susan's" chronic back pain was so severe that she needed large doses of medication and almost daily epidural injections in order to numb her spine just to get through her day. She had endured this pain for ten years. Susan (not her real name), a psychiatrist in her early thirties, had seen many specialists, had numerous tests, but no one could identify the cause. Finally, one of her doctors suggested that she try the Alexander technique.

This method of using your body effortlessly was created out of necessity. At the turn of the twentieth century, a Shakespearean actor named Frederick M. Alexander had begun to lose his voice with increasing frequency whenever he stepped onstage. By watching himself closely in the mirror as he prepared to perform before an audience, he observed that he had developed a habit of tightening his head and neck muscles and contracting his head backwards into his shoulders before each speech. When he recognized this pattern, he used close observation to develop a way of "non-doing": of freeing tension throughout the body—especially in the head and neck—by releasing any muscles that were not necessary in the activity. The technique became a way to promote effortless movement in all activities.

All Alexander practitioners refer to themselves as "teachers" and the people who come to them for help as "students." The process is an educational one: "I don't 'cure' anyone," says Deborah Adams, who likes to be known as Debi. "I teach them, giving them the awareness and the tools to heal themselves.

"At the end of Susan's first lesson it became clear to me that she was making choices that were causing her difficulty," says Debi. "But these were choices that she was not even aware of." Debi had asked Susan to sit in a chair and simulate her movements during a psychotherapy session with her psychiatric patients. As Susan did this, Debi placed her hands on Susan's shoulders and back, in the area where she felt the greatest muscle tension, and simply waited. "As I wait, I have the intention of allowing her body to release any holding patterns and lengthen, and eventually, it did so," says Debi. Alexander teachers are trained to use their hands to "listen" for tension and to gently guide release in their students. The goal is to restore the natural relationship of the head, neck and back, as Alexander had discovered.

Moving with Effortless Ease

Watching Debi is itself a lesson in the Alexander Technique. Whether she is rising from a chair, walking across a room, or reaching up to get a book from a shelf, her body seems to move as one fluid whole. There are no wasted motions. The head is poised gracefully on the neck, and the whole impression is one of effortless ease—almost as if she were floating without the pull of gravity. And this is exactly what it feels like during an Alexander lesson with her. You want to package up that floating feeling, carry it off with you, and release it the next time you need to trudge up a flight of stairs. If you have the patience to stick with the lessons, you eventually learn to do just that.

As Debi worked with her, Susan began to notice that as she listened to her psychiatric patients, most of whom were in severe emotional distress, she had a habit of tightening her back (making it narrower and causing her head and neck to compress downward). For years, she had been unconsciously responding to her patients' distress by clenching her own back. Over the course of several lessons, she became aware of that habitual response, as well as the feeling of release when she let that response go. "The moment she learned to 'inhibit' her habitual tightening, I felt her back become wider and her spine actually lengthen," says Debi. "This freed her neck and head, as well. In time, she was able to remember that feeling of release during the course of the day, and she could make the choice to allow it to happen."

After several weekly lessons, Susan was gradually able to cut down on her pain medications. She no longer needs regular lessons and continues to be free of medication.

❖ ❖ ❖ ❖

Taming the "Mad Sweater-Wringer"

Debi Adams, a piano and Alexander teacher and the mother of two teenagers, learned about the power of the Alexander Technique when she was in her twenties because of her own experience with pain. She had begun to notice some discomfort and "clicking" in her wrist when she was an undergraduate majoring in piano performance. By the time she was working her way through graduate school, practicing piano several hours a day, waiting tables and working as an accompanist, the pain had become severe. "One day, I was hired for an accompanist job that required me to learn a great deal of music in a very short time," she says. "I shut myself up in a practice room and played for eight hours. When I came out, my left hand had swelled up and become so painful that I couldn't hold anything, not even a piece of paper."

The pain lasted, with varying degrees of severity, for several years. She went to a conventional doctor who prescribed anti-inflammatory drugs, painful testing and physical therapy, which Debi described as "incredibly degrading. They were doing what they needed to do on a physiological level—having me move beans from one bowl to another—but the rest of me was dying. They didn't take into account that I was a whole person and how traumatic it was for me only to be able to play the piano five minutes a day. They did not deal with what the loss of music meant to me."

Eventually, Debi met another musician who was studying to become an Alexander teacher and who encouraged her to start lessons. "This was the first time that anybody asked me to look at what I was doing, to see whether anything was contributing to the pain," says Debi. "I realized that my hand hurt the most during the winter, when I would wash sweaters in the kitchen sink and wring them out. This was important. It captured something about my personality: the 'mad sweater-wringer' who used excessive amounts of force when she was using her hands to do something." Debi realized that her determination to become a better pianist—like her determination to wring every drop of water from those sweaters—was causing her to exert more effort than she needed at the piano and in life. "When I became aware of what I was doing, I could sometimes choose to use only the effort that I actually needed to press the keys down, and the pain lessened." She says.

The pain lessened, but it did not disappear. There was more awareness to be had. "Another Alexander teacher finally asked me to think about my attitude as I approached the piano. He didn't give me an answer, just asked me to think about it," says Debi. "I went home, sat at the piano, and raised my arms to play. Just before my arms came down—in that millisecond—I realized that I was becoming in that moment someone else. Evidently, I had an image of what a pianist should be and in trying to attain that image, I was becoming someone that I was not. That artificial image of myself was so ingrained that I never even realized it was there—until that moment."

With that realization, Debi was able to let go of that image of herself, and felt her body immediately release its tension. "Habitual responses—like my image of myself as a concert pianist—often cause us to contract our bodies, pulling our heads and necks out of balance," she says. "When I realized what I was doing, I could let go of that response and could simply play the piano with freedom, letting my head and neck return to normal balance, and releasing the unconscious tension that had caused pain in my hand. From then on, as long as I let go of that image, I remained pain-free. That was ten years ago. What came to me in that moment was the power of this work. It was the right path for me."

The Alexander Technique: What's the Evidence?

The Alexander Technique is based on three main principles:

- Function is affected by use
- The organism functions as a whole
- The relationship of the head, neck and spine is vital to the organism's ability to function optimally;

What Is It Used For?

Conditions most frequently treated include chronic pain, osteoarthritis, stress and headaches. It is also common for musicians, dancers, singers and actors to use the technique to improve their performances onstage.

Does It Work? Yes, for Breathing, Chronic Pain, Daily Function, Parkinson's Disease and Anxiety

There are few randomized controlled trials of the Alexander Technique, but what evidence there is does seem to point to its effectiveness, at least temporarily, in reducing pain and anxiety and improving breathing function in normal people.

In his evidence-based survey of complementary treatments, Edzard Ernst cites several controlled trials (the "gold standard" of research) of normal, healthy subjects. These studies found that the Alexander Technique improved respiratory function, and the ability of elderly women to reach for things, reduced anxiety and performance in music students.

In uncontrolled trials (which do not use a control group for comparison), studies found that sixty-seven people with chronic lower back pain reported improvements that persisted for six months after treatment in a multidisciplinary program that included lessons in the Alexander Technique. In another "observational" study, seven patients with Parkinson's disease reported improvements in depression and the performance of daily activities. Ernst also reports "multiple" cases of successes with the Alexander Technique in people with learning disabilities and craniomandibular (head and jaw) disorders.

References

Alexander, F. M. *The Use of Self*. London: Gollancz, 1996. (An account of how Alexander developed the method.)

Austin, J. H. M., et al. "Enhanced Respiratory Muscular Function in Normal Adults After Lessons in Proprioceptive Musculoskeletal Education Without Exercises." *Chest* 102 (1992): 486–490.

Dennis, R. J. "Functional Reach Improvement in Normal Older Women After Alexander Technique Instruction." *The Journals of Gerontology. Series A, Biological Sciences and Medical Sciences* 54 (1999): 8–11.

Dennis, J. and C. Cates. "Alexander Technique for Chronic Asthma." (Cochrane Review) in *The Cochrane Library* 2. Oxford: Update Software, 2002.

Elkayam, O., et al. "Multidisciplinary Approach to Chronic Back Pain: Prognostic Elements of the Outcome." *Clinical and Experimental Rheumatology* (Pisa) 14 (1996): 281–288.

Ernst, E., ed. *The Desktop Guide to Complementary and Alternative Medicine: An Evidence-Based Approach*. London: Harcourt Publishers Limited, 2001.

Jones, F. P. *Freedom to Change* (formerly *Body Awareness in Action*). London: Mouritz, 1997.

Knebelman, S. "The Alexander Technique in Diagnosis and Treatment of Craniomandibular Disorders." *Basal Facts* 5 (1982): 19–22.

Maitland, S., et al. "An Exploration of the Applications of the Alexander Technique for People with Learning Disabilities." *British Journal of Learning Disabilities* (Oxford) 24 (1996): 70–76.

Stallinbrass, C. "An Evaluation of the Alexander Technique for the Management of Disability in Parkinson's Disease—A Preliminary Study." *Clinical Rehabilitation* (Oxford) 11 (1997): 8–12.

Valentine, E. R., et al. "The Effect of Lessons in the Alexander Technique on Music Performance in High and Low Stress Situations." *Psychology of Music* 23 (1995): 129–141.

4

HEALING MORE THAN HEARTS
"I don't think you need to go to church to feel peace."

Mike Siddall was in his mid-forties, working as a mechanic for Sarasota County Transit in Florida when his troubles started. "I was starting to lose my breath," he recalls. "Things just didn't feel right. I was working two physically tiring jobs at the time and was having trouble keeping up." A native of Canada whose favorite activity was playing hockey, Mike had what he describes as "a pretty bad drinking problem." He was also a heavy smoker and ate mostly fast-food burgers and fries. "I really didn't care what I ate—and it was party central with the drinking," he says.

At first, he tried to ignore his symptoms. "I just wanted to keep on going at top speed," he says. "But then I realized that where I was going so fast was downhill." Finally, his girlfriend, Carolyn, took him to the emergency room. "I spent awhile in the hospital," says Mike. "They said, you've got a major problem, buddy. You'd better stop drinking, smoking and living the way you're living or you're going to die." Mike was not really surprised. "But even though I knew I had been doing some things wrong, it was still a rude awakening," he says. "They said I was in congestive heart failure, and you could tell they were serious. I believed them. That was it. I quit smoking and drinking right then. I didn't want to die. I wanted to be with Carolyn. And she was behind me all the way with support, nagging, hitting me upside the head, you name it. In fact, we got married soon after."

After Mike got out of the hospital, he and Carolyn moved to Pittsboro, North Carolina, where he found a mechanic's job with the Chapel Hill Transit

Company. He also found a cardiologist, Dr. Beth Rosenberg, in Chapel Hill. "She put me on medications for the heart and to lower cholesterol, and she also told me about an eight-week program at Duke for heart failure patients, the SEARCH (Support, Education and Research in Chronic Heart Failure) study. I decided to sign up for the program and see what the deal was," says Mike. During September and October 2001, Mike and Carolyn went to the weekly SEARCH study group sessions with other heart failure patients and their family members. "At first it was a little strange, talking to other people, learning to meditate and doing these weird activities—like laughing," says Mike. "Have you ever sat with a group of people and someone tells you to just laugh as hard as you can? By the end, we were roaring. That made my day. It felt real good."

Then there was eating a cracker. "This was a 'mindfulness' exercise where they gave us a cracker and told us to focus on the smell and taste, to eat it slowly and savor the flavor on your tongue," says Mike. "At first I thought this was silly, but it's really true that by the time you were done, you really enjoyed it. Now I do it at home. I don't just shovel food in my face anymore, and I enjoy eating a lot more." Another mindfulness exercise involved focusing on the body. "I'm sitting there and thinking about my feet, my legs, how it feels to sit in the chair, and soon you get to thinking about how your body works together. I felt more aware, and all of these things helped me feel less stressed, but especially the meditation."

When Mike first found out that he was going to learn to meditate, he was not sure if this was for him. "I always thought that meditation was kind of weird," he says. "But we decided to learn it anyway. You sit there, focusing on your breath, and after a while I got to like it. Now I do it every day at work. I close the door of my office—I have one now that I'm a supervising mechanic—and take fifteen minutes to sit quietly and watch my breathing. After awhile I found that things were starting to go more smoothly at work. I don't holler so much anymore, unless people really mess up, but even then I get over it faster than I used to. And my wife is happy now because I used to come home from work nasty. Somehow, I just feel more peaceful."

Mike found the educational discussion groups took some getting used to as well.

"We learned things about heart disease, but we also talked about feelings," he says. "After awhile, you get to know some of the people, and you find yourself rooting for them because they're worse off. It's kind of nice to root for somebody else. You focus on your own problems less."

Mike has now been out of the program for several months, and, with Carolyn's help, is keeping up with much of what he learned. "I'm still taking heart medicines—I'll be taking them for eternity," he says. "And I'm meditating every day. I also try to walk the dog as much as I can, although I still get out of breath. My doctors told me to do what I can. I still find it really hard to exercise, and I miss playing hockey. Even though I'm a supervisor now, I sometimes also miss getting down and doing the real work. The diet comes and goes. Sometimes I eat what I shouldn't, but the wife keeps me in line. She hollers and cooks healthy food."

Mike says the SEARCH study program not only helped his health, it did something more: "It made me a better person, more mindful and aware of other people, especially my wife, more kind and thoughtful of them. Before, I didn't really care about other people. Now I do." he says. "Having less stress was worth it alone. Even though my life has changed and is more difficult now, and I can't do some of the things I enjoy, I accept life the way it is. I don't think you need to go to church to feel peace."

✓ TAKE ACTION ✓
Best Ways to Prevent Heart Disease

Suggestions from the Duke Center for Integrative Medicine on caring for your mind, body and spirit.

1. **Be smoke-free.** Tobacco smoke damages the interior lining of blood vessels and causes arterial blockages. Tobacco use is a leading risk factor for heart disease. STOP NOW. Ask your health-care provider for resource assistance.
2. **Maintain a healthy weight.** Being overweight or obese puts additional demands on heart muscle, and is a leading risk factor for heart disease. Body mass index (BMI), a measure of weight to height, should be less than 25 percent.
3. **Exercise regularly.** A sedentary lifestyle weakens heart muscle. Try to work up to thirty to forty-five minutes each day through walking, bike riding, swimming, dancing, or recreational sports like tennis, racquetball, soccer or volleyball. You'll look and feel better as your cardiovascular, pulmonary and musculoskeletal systems are strengthened, and stress and depression are relieved.
4. **Monitor your blood pressure and cholesterol.** Blood pressure greater than 130/80 mmHg indicates a heart under stress. If your total cholesterol is greater than 200 mg/dl or your LDL is greater than 100 mg/dl, you require modification in your diet and exercise, and you may need medication. Check with your health-care provider.
5. **Eat nutritiously.** Meals and snacks should be HIGH in fresh or frozen vegetables, fruits, whole grains and lean proteins, and LOW in meats, saturated fats, sodium and refined sugars. Limit alcohol consumption to less than two drinks daily. Dietary supplements such as coenzyme Q10, omega-3 fatty acids, antioxidants, calcium, vitamins and minerals have protective health benefits, but they may react with other medications so talk with your health-care provider before taking them. (See p. 106 in this chapter for data on coenzyme Q10.)
6. **Practice meditation daily.** Focus on the present. Don't spend unnecessary energy worrying about the past or the future. Learn to live fully in the present moment, seeing things as they really are. Choose to respond to each situation as it unfolds rather than reacting out of habit.
7. **Nurture your soul.** Pay attention to your spirit. Read spiritual literature. Seek out a spiritual director. Cultivate acceptance, compassion, forgiveness, love and peace.

(continued)

8. **Share your feelings.** Talk with someone you trust—a family member, friend, clergy or health professional—about what's going on in your life, and when things really bother you.
9. **Do something you enjoy.** Treat yourself to a massage, concert or evening out. Pick up an activity you used to enjoy but haven't had time for lately. Or take up a new sport or hobby you've always wanted to try.
10. **Laugh a lot.** It has great mental and physical health benefits: it produces endorphins which counteract stress hormones, relax muscles and improve self-esteem.

A Type-A Cardiologist in Recovery

Dr. Marty Sullivan, forty-seven, describes himself as "a Type-A cardiologist in recovery." He churned his way through college and medical school, earning his M.D. at twenty-two and then launching a successful research and clinical career. "I was a doctor who was having a love affair with the science of medicine and how we could use scientific knowledge to help people," he says. He became a research fellow in cardiology and over the next ten years published dozens of scientific papers on his special interests: heart failure, cardiac physiology and exercise physiology. All the while, he was taking care of heart patients.

"At that time, I was seeing all of my patients' problems through a biochemical lens," says Marty. "I still remember one incident, when a resident working with me said that one of our patients seemed to be depressed and might benefit from a referral to psychotherapy. I answered 'Why? It's just a biochemical abnormality in the brain that a drug can fix.' I didn't understand what I now do about the connection between mind and body, between emotion and health."

But after about ten years, things began to change. "I felt restless," Marty says. "I began to think that this was not a very satisfying way to practice medicine. Something was missing in my relationships with my patients." Something was also happening inside him. "I had begun to explore my own life—the connections I was making with others, with myself, my spirituality (or lack of it). The illness or death of a patient would prompt me to examine the meaning of life: what connects us to each other and to the rest of the world. Once you get bitten by that kind of thinking, you keep going back to it."

Marty describes the way he *used* to practice medicine, at the beginning of his career, as standard operating procedure for the profession. "About 40 percent of patients who go to a family practice doctor with a complaint—whether it is pain, gastrointestinal distress or just fatigue and a feeling of 'malaise'—have no objectively observable physical problem," he says. "Doctors do tests, find nothing, and may prescribe medication, or even do exploratory surgery, but this kind of medicine is not going to cure the underlying cause. Many people have physical problems because that is the only way their bodies can handle the stresses of life, anxiety or depression."

Marty points to a recent study of patients in Hawaii that demonstrated, for example, that people who were given the opportunity to talk about their problems and emotions in support groups led by mental health professionals used fewer medical services than those who did not. "Think of the savings in health-care costs if these kinds of interventions were covered by more health insurance companies," he says. "By addressing the emotional context of patients' physical complaints, you have a better chance of curing them. Pills or surgery just treat symptoms. They touch only the surface of people's lives."

After working for several years to build funding support from Duke and other sources, Marty helped create the Duke Center for Integrative Medicine in 2000. "I didn't want to be a medical 'technician,' one who fixes things," he says. "I wanted to accompany my patients on their healing journeys." Marty also began to question the strictly "scientific" view of medicine that had so enthralled him early in his career. "I now feel that biochemistry does not explain all of the phenomena of life," he says. "Limiting ourselves only to what we can discern through our five senses is a myopic way to look at the human condition. Two hundred years from now, I think we will have a science that will give us an explanation for the connection between mind, body and spirit."

For example, several studies published in major scientific research journals show significant clinical benefits as the result of "distant healing" or prayer. "These studies show that distant mental intentions do measurably affect living systems," says Marty. "But how does this work from the physics perspective? Or from the perspective of psychology? We have no language or scientific model yet to describe these kinds of events." (Please also see "A Closer Look at Energy Healing and Spirituality," to find out how both religious belief and community support have been found to reduce the risk of heart disease.)

At Duke, Marty worked with a group of physicians, nurses, psychologists and other health-care practitioners who are asking the same questions. In addition to offering medical care and lifestyle counseling to patients, they are conducting research studies to explore the relationship among stress, emotions such as anxiety or depression, spirituality and heart failure. One such study, funded by the Medtronic Foundation, is called SEARCH. This is the study that Mike Siddall (the patient described at the beginning of this chapter) participated in.

In 2002, Marty Sullivan founded the Institute for Healing in Society and Medicine, which he now directs. The Institute offers educational services and consultation to physicians and organizations in the practice of integrative medicine. As part of its program, the Institute seeks to educate health-care practitioners on their own mind/body/spirit connections.

Heart Failure: Treating Body, Mind and Spirit

Heart failure—a condition in which the heart muscle itself cannot pump enough blood to meet all of the oxygen and energy needs of the body—can be caused by high blood pressure, heart attack, heart valve abnormalities, congenital defects or other illness. Sometimes, the heart, struggling to meet the demands of the body, enlarges, making it an even weaker, less efficient pump, creating a condition called cardiomyopathy. "More than four and a half million people suffer from some form of heart failure every year in the United States," says Laura Wood, R.N., a former cardiac critical care nurse who now works as clinical research coordinator for the Duke Center for Integrative Medicine. "And this disease is associated with high rates of illness and death."

When it is not in an acute phase, sending people to the emergency room, heart failure is a chronic disease, says Laura. "The heart continues to pump, but not efficiently, so people have trouble keeping up with their daily lives: whether taking care of the house, their children or their jobs. They have very little energy, and often can't do many things that give them pleasure, whether playing golf, going shopping or even having sex. As a result, many become depressed or anxious and do not have a good quality of life."

The SEARCH study, which began in July 2000, invites chronic heart failure patients—and their spouses or caregivers—to spend two and a half hours in weekly small-group sessions with other patients, in an eight-week program. (Many patients are actually referred to the program by their cardiologists.) Laura stresses that these sessions do not replace regular medical care—whether medications or surgery—but are in addition to it. "For the first half of the SEARCH class, we teach people meditation skills for stress reduction and improved health," she says. This mindfulness-based meditation was adapted from the *vipassana* method, first described in Buddhist teachings centuries ago, and adapted for patient use by Jon Kabat-Zinn, Ph.D., when he was at the University of Massachusetts Medical Center. "The meditation method teaches people how to '*be*,' instead of how to '*do*,'" says Laura. "We encourage patients to give meditation a chance, to make a commitment to try meditating for thirty minutes every day, at least for the eight weeks of the program." (Please also see "A Closer Look at Meditation," for more about the seminal work of Jon Kabat-Zinn, as well as research evidence on the benefits of meditation.)

During the second half of the class, group leaders introduce educational topics for discussion, including "learned optimism," which, according to Laura, helps people talk about their own perceptions of their life and their health. "We encourage people to examine the ways in which they approach problems: Do you see the glass as half empty or half full?" she says. "People can learn to change their ways of seeing the world." Other topics include "healthy" grieving over loss of function; and the connections between spirituality and health. "For most people, a health crisis precipitates some very profound thinking about the meaning of life and death," says Laura. "It can be helpful to explore spirituality with other people in the same situation."

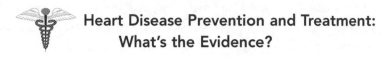

Heart Disease Prevention and Treatment: What's the Evidence?

Cardiovascular disease is the leading cause of death in the United States. Research has clearly identified ways to reduce your risk.

Good for your heart: stress reduction, meditation, spiritual belief and involvement with family and community.

In his book, *The Best Alternative Medicine, What Works? What Does Not?* Kenneth R. Pelletier, Ph.D., M.D. (hc) describes "a very significant finding reported by Dr. Joseph Blumenthal and his colleagues at the Duke University School of Medicine in 1997. Using a stress management program plus muscle tension biofeedback with heart disease patients, the results were more effective than the usual care exercise group," writes Pelletier. "Based on this stress management program, there were three fewer fatal heart attacks, three fewer bypass surgeries, and one less angioplasty. This savings of $70,000, or $2,100 per patient . . . were attained through improvement of health, not the denial of care."

(Please also see "A Closer Look at Energy Healing and Spirituality," for studies reporting that spiritual belief and close involvement with family and community are good for heart health; as well as "A Closer Look at Meditation," for the cardiac benefits of meditation, including the seminal work of Jon Kabat-Zinn, Ph.D.)

Can mind/body methods reduce hospitalizations and depression and improve the quality of your life? Stay tuned.

The SEARCH study at the Duke Center for Integrative Medicine—investigating whether mind/body methods reduce the risk of heart disease—will be completed in July 2003. "This is an empirically based research study in which we are collecting data from questionnaires we give to participants before they start the program, then again at three months, six months and one year," says Laura Wood. "We are trying to find out if the meditation, support group discussions and educational programs help reduce depression and anxiety, increase optimism and improve quality of life, as well as reduce the number of hospitalizations and the rate of mortality among participants. So far, our own observations and patient reports are telling us that people are feeling less depressed and anxious and developing increased personal awareness and an inner peace. They are learning to better enjoy their lives within the limitations of their illness. They are changing their focus from 'I can't' to 'I can.'"

Nutrition that's good for your heart: Eat more fruits and vegetables.

A new study in the journal *Lancet* has found that eating five or more portions of fruits and vegetables every day decreases systolic and diastolic blood pressure in a healthy population.[1] Lowered blood pressure means less risk of heart disease.

This study was a randomized, controlled trial to evaluate the effect of increased fruit and vegetable consumption among 690 healthy participants between twenty-five and sixty-four years of age. Participants in the intervention group were encouraged by a trained research nurse to consume five or more portions of fruits and vegetables per day. Follow-up phone calls and letters were used to reinforce this dietary message. Participants in the control group received the intervention after six months. All participants completed a food-frequency questionnaire at the beginning and at the end of the study.

At the six-month evaluation, participants in the intervention group demonstrated a significant increase in fruit and vegetable intake, elevated antioxidants (i.e., alpha-carotene, beta-carotene and ascorbic acid), and lower systolic and diastolic blood pressure compared to the control group.

"The falls in blood pressure in our study (4.0 mmHg systolic and 1.5 mmHg diastolic) would be expected to produce small clinical effects, but would substantially reduce cardiovascular disease at the population level," the researchers conclude. "A reduction of 2 mmHg in diastolic blood pressure results in a decrease of about 17 percent in the incidence of hypertension, 6 percent in the risk of coronary heart disease, and 15 percent in the risk of stroke and transient ischaemic attack."

Coenzyme Q10 (ubiquinone): Looks promising but more research needed.

In his review of the research on coenzyme Q10, Pelletier highlights studies that suggest that the supplement is effective as a protection against tissue damage in

---

[1] J. H. John et al., "Effects of Fruit and Vegetable Consumption on Plasma Antioxidant Concentrations and Blood Pressure: A Randomized Controlled Trial," *Lancet* 359 (2002): 1969–1974. The study reports previous evidence that high consumption of fruits and vegetables is associated with a reduced risk of cancer and cardiovascular disease. While some researchers speculate that this may be caused by an increased intake of antioxidant compounds, intervention trials of vitamin supplements have produced little evidence to support this hypothesis. Researchers are now beginning to consider whether the health benefits of eating fruits and vegetables may be caused by other mechanisms, such as lowering blood pressure. (For more information and this and other studies, see the Web site of The Integrative Medical Alliance *http://www.onemedicine.com/index.html.*)

heart disease[2] and beneficial to patients with congestive heart failure.[3] Coenzyme Q10, which is found in every cell in the body, is actually not an enzyme. It acts like a vitamin and works as a catalyst in chemical reactions. Its primary function is to help the body convert food into energy.

In the Chello study, forty coronary artery bypass surgery patients who received 150 mg of Q10 a day for even a few days before the operation showed less evidence of heart tissue damage and a lower incidence of ventricular arrhythmias (irregular heart-beat) during the recovery period. However, when used just twelve hours before surgeries, Q10 showed no positive effect.

In the Lampertico study, Q10 supplements produced improvements in a number of indicators of heart and lung function. However, cautions Pelletier, "the study had problems both in the design and the brevity of the treatment period." In another study, patients using Q10 "required less hospitalization for worsening heart failure, and episodes of pulmonary (lung) and/or cardiac asthma were significantly reduced."[4] Pelletier concludes that "research in this area is still in the early stages, and it remains uncertain."

Bad for your heart: high blood pressure, high blood cholesterol, smoking, obesity, diabetes and physical inactivity

A fifty-year study changed the way we look at cardiovascular disease (CVD). In 1948, the Framingham Heart Study—under the direction of the National Heart Institute (now known as the National Heart, Lung, and Blood Institute or NHLBI)—embarked on an ambitious project in health research. At the time, little was known about the general causes of heart disease and stroke, but the death rates for cardiovascular disease (CVD) had been increasing steadily since the beginning of the century and had become an American epidemic.

The objective of the Framingham Heart Study was to identify the common factors or characteristics that contribute to CVD by following its development over a long

---

[2] M. Chello et al., "Protection by Coenzyme Q10 of Tissue Perfusion Injury During Abdominal Aortic Cross-Clamping," *Journal of Cardiovascular Surgery* 37, no. 3 (1996): 229–235.
[3] M. Lampertico and S. Comis, "Italian Multicenter Study on the Efficacy and Safety of Coenzyme Q10 as Adjuvant Therapy in Heart Failure," *Clinical Investigator* 71, no. 8, Supplement (1993): S129–S133.
[4] C. Morisco et al., "Effect of Coenzyme Q10 Therapy in Patients with Congestive Heart Failure: A Long-Term Multicenter Randomized Study," *Clinical Investigator* 71, no. 8, Supplement (1993): S134–S136.

period of time in a large group of healthy people who had no symptoms and had not yet had a heart attack or stroke.

The researchers recruited 5,209 men and women between the ages of thirty and sixty-two from the town of Framingham, Massachusetts, and began the first round of extensive physical examinations and lifestyle interviews that they would later analyze for common patterns related to CVD development. Since 1948, the subjects have continued to return to the study every two years for a detailed medical history, physical examination, and laboratory tests, and in 1971, the study enrolled a second-generation group—5,124 of the original participants' adult children and their spouses—to participate in similar examinations. The Framingham Heart Study is now conducted in collaboration with Boston University.

Over the years, careful monitoring of the Framingham Study population has led to the identification of the major CVD risk factors—high blood pressure, high blood cholesterol, smoking, obesity, diabetes, and physical inactivity—as well as a great deal of valuable information on the effects of related factors such as blood triglyceride and HDL cholesterol levels, age, gender and psychosocial issues. Although the Framingham cohort is primarily white, the importance of the major CVD risk factors identified in this group have been shown in other studies to apply almost universally to all racial and ethnic groups, even though the patterns of distribution may vary from group to group. In the past fifty years, the study has produced approximately one thousand articles in leading medical journals. The concept of CVD risk factors has become an integral part of the modern medical curriculum and has led to the development of effective treatment and preventive strategies in clinical practice.

References

Astin, J. A., et al. "The Efficacy of Distant Healing: A Systematic Review of Randomized Trials." *Annals of Internal Medicine* 132, no. 11 (2000): 903–910.

Byrd, R. C. "Positive Therapeutic Effects of Intercessory Prayer in a Coronary Care Population." *Southern Medical Journal* 81, no. 7 (1988): 826–829.

Bruhn, J., et al. "Social Aspects of Coronary Heart Disease in Two Adjacent Ethnically Different Communities." *American Journal of Public Health* 56 (1966): 2493–2506.

Chello, M., et al. "Protection By Coenzyme Q10 of Tissue Perfusion Injury During Abdominal Aortic Cross-Clamping." *Journal of Cardiovascular Surgery* 37, no. 3 (1996): 229–35.

Cummings, N. A., et al. "Impact of Psychological Interventions on Health Care Cost and Utilization." HCFA Contract Report (1991):11-c-98334/9.

Framingham Heart Study: *www.rover2.nhlbi.nih.gov/about/framingham/index.html*.

John, J. H., et al. "Effects of Fruit and Vegetable Consumption on Plasma Antioxidant Concentrations and Blood Pressure: A Randomized Controlled Trial." *Lancet* 359 (2002): 1969–1974.

Lampertico, M., et al. "Italian Multicenter Study on the Efficacy and Safety of Coenzyme Q10 as Adjuvant Therapy in Heart Failure." *Clinical Investigator* 71, no. 8, Supplement (1993): S129–S133.

Morisco, C., et al. "Effect of Coenzyme Q10 Therapy in Patients with Congestive Heart Failure: A Long-Term Multicenter Randomized Study." *Clinical Investigator* 71, no. 8, Supplement (1993): S134–S136.

Pelletier, K. R. *The Best Alternative Medicine: What Works? What Does Not?* New York: Simon & Schuster, 2000.

A Day with a Cardiologist

Mrs. Pappas lies in a curtained cubicle in the emergency department. Her breathing is rapid and shallow, and she stares at the ceiling, oblivious to her surroundings. She is in her late seventies with rapidly advancing Alzheimer's disease and a history of heart problems. Her son, Charlie, a sturdy middle-aged man, is stroking her hair. Mrs. Pappas's elderly husband is in the cubicle as well, along with Charlie's wife, Francine, and his sister, Olympia—two women in their early forties. Mr. and Mrs. Pappas immigrated to Boston from Greece many years ago, but he still speaks very little English. The family called 911 late last night because Mrs. Pappas had become unresponsive, her respiration was rapid, about sixty breaths a minute, she had a fever of 103 and could move only stiffly and spasmodically. She is one of thirty patients that Eugene "Gene" Lindsey, M.D., will see today as the cardiologist on call for his group practice.

Recently, I spent a day accompanying Gene during one of his "on-call" days at a major Boston teaching hospital (with permission from his patients, whose names have been changed). Since graduating from the Harvard Medical School more than twenty-five years ago, Gene has been a staff cardiologist and internist at Harvard Vanguard Medical Associates, a multisite, multispecialty group practice. In 1997, he was elected chairman of the board of trustees of Harvard Vanguard. He freely admits that his knowledge of complementary and alternative medicine is limited. But that does not stop him from having a lively interest and respect for the possibilities of integrative medicine. He welcomes discussions with his patients about alternative care. "I see complementary practices as enhancing the health care I can give my patients," he says. "Over the years, I've learned as much from my patients about complementary health-care 'tools' as from books—maybe more." During the last few years, Harvard Vanguard instituted a new program that now offers services such as acupuncture, yoga, meditation and massage to its members. Gene enthusiastically supports the effort: "It is raising awareness of complementary therapies for all of us," he says.

Most importantly, in his own practice, Gene places great emphasis on the healing qualities of the relationship between patient and doctor, quite apart from any medical intervention. This sensitivity to the patient as a whole person—with a life, relationships and powerful emotions—rather than as a collection of symptoms, is one of the hallmarks of integrative medicine. He also believes in the value of patient autonomy, seeing himself as a consultant to his patients in their health care, working in partnership with them.

As soon as he arrives in the emergency department, Gene, who has known the family for many years, hugs Olympia and greets everyone else, looks quickly at Mrs. Pappas's chart and strides to the head of her bed. "Mrs. Pappas," he calls out to her. "It's Dr. Lindsey, can you hear me?" She groans and turns her head. "Ah, I think you know I'm here," he says. "We're going to take care of you. Let me listen to your heart." He leans over her, holding the stethoscope to her chest, connected to her not only through the rubber tubing, but by the hand he has placed on her shoulder as he listens intently. She lapses again into unresponsiveness. "Her heart sounds fine," he says, tucking the stethoscope back into his pocket. "Let's go out and talk."

The emergency department bustles with people and noise: Doctors are standing at computer terminals, filling out forms, or talking on the phone; patients are being wheeled about on stretchers; nurses are talking to worried family members; orderlies are cleaning out rooms between patients; frequent announcements from the hospital loudspeaker pierce any silences that might occur. There is nowhere to sit, let alone somewhere that gives even a semblance of privacy. Gene finds an unoccupied stretch of wall and gathers the family around him.

✦ ✦ ✦ ✦

Many patients look outside of the conventional medical system for the kinds of personal and humane relationships offered by most integrative physicians and alternative health practitioners. But it is important to recognize that even within the most conventional Western medical institutions—even in the world of managed care—there are doctors who take the time to connect with their patients—to learn what is important to them, what they are worried about, what they fear and what they hope. These doctors do this even as insurance pressures pack increasing numbers of patient visits into their days. Gene Lindsey is one of them. "Even if I am standing in the midst of a busy emergency room, I imagine a canopy coming down, enclosing my patients or family members with me and shutting out the rest of the world," he says. "I may see thirty patients in a day, but I may be the only doctor that each patient sees today. I want every patient to feel as if he or she is the only person I am thinking about. That is how I would want to be treated."

✦ ✦ ✦ ✦

Under the imaginary canopy, Gene begins to speak, "The symptoms and their sudden onset suggest an infection of some kind," he begins. "Another explanation is that the drugs she is receiving to help her brain combat the Alzheimer's symptoms may be poisoning her by causing some kind of negative neurological reaction. So we need to make some decisions about her treatment." He asks them to describe what had prompted them to bring her to the hospital last night. When Charlie finishes speaking, Gene looks searchingly at each family member. "We can support her medically with rehydration—getting some fluids into her—and broad-spectrum antibiotics for the suspected infection. We can also stop the neurological medication that may be affecting the connections in her brain. But if these measures do not work I will need guidance from all of you."

He pauses while the daughter translates for her father. As he continues to speak, the emergency room hubbub seems to recede, melting away. The small group standing together next to the wall seems to be alone in a world that has grown suddenly empty and silent. Now, Gene is turning to the daughter-in-law: "I know that you just lost your own mother to pancreatic cancer recently," he says. She nods without speaking. "That was easier to understand, wasn't it?" he continues. "We can see the physical effects of a disease like cancer, but it is harder to understand what course Alzheimer's disease will take. We do know that although we can't cure the disease, we can take the steps I mentioned before to make her comfortable." The two women have tears in their eyes. They hold onto each other. Until her illness, the elder Mrs. Pappas had been the family matriarch. Few decisions were made without her.

Gene pauses again for the translation before continuing: "More aggressive treatments might include a spinal tap to find the source of the infection or even putting a tube down her trachea to help her breathe. But we also must recognize that because of the Alzheimer's she is going to become progressively more incapacitated and dependent on others for her care, and there is nothing we can do to stop that. The question is, how aggressive should we be with treatments, which are invasive and uncomfortable? At some point we are going to have to decide what to do if, for example, her heart stops. Do we intervene or do we let nature take its course?" Translation pause again, then silence. Charlie abruptly turns so that he is facing Gene squarely. "Are we at that point now, Doctor?" he asks. "I think we might be," answers Gene quietly. "I don't think she is going to get better. We need to think about what she might want us to do."

The adult children confer with their father for several minutes. Finally, Olympia says. "We don't want her to suffer. Before this happened, she would talk about how she hated being helpless and dependent. My father doesn't want her to undergo a spinal tap, or anything like that. We think you should treat the infection, stop the medication, make her comfortable, but then let nature take its course."

❖ ❖ ❖ ❖

Gene has never worn the traditional doctor's uniform: the white coat. "It creates too much of a barrier," he explains. The only tools of his trade are the computer-generated list of patients he will see today and his stethoscope, tucked into the pockets of his sport jacket. "If I am to bond with my patients in a way that is truly therapeutic, I need to be not above or below them, but with them. I have some useful knowledge, and I'm pretty good at solving medical problems, but aren't we all just trying to figure out what life is all about anyway?" In the battered black appointment book he carries with him everywhere, he shows me a verse that he has copied from the Book of Psalms: *The days of our years are three-score years and ten; Or even by reason of strength four-score years; Yet is their pride but travail and vanity; For it is speedily gone, and we fly away.*" As he closes the book, he repeats softly, "We fly away . . ."

Later, Gene says, "In the case of the Pappas family, my job in those few minutes in the hallway was to help them arrive at a humane, moral and ethical decision about the care of their mother and wife. I try to present options and risks to them, as well as the likelihood of success, and I can tell them what other reasonable people have decided in that situation. My goal is to help them arrive at a decision that they will be able to live with after her death."

Once that decision has been made, the mood under the imaginary canopy changes. Gene's beeper is going off, but he ignores it. He is not yet finished. "I'll always remember that your mother once brought me handkerchiefs from Greece," he says. "No one ever gave me handkerchiefs before." They smile through their tears. "And she even brought me some Greek wine," he continues. The daughter translates, and her father says something in reply. "My father says we'll bring you wine!" she says. Nothing more can be done now except to order the hydration and antibiotics, stop the brain medication, watch her condition and wait. "I'll be in the hospital all day today," says Gene. "I'll be back to check in, and you can page me anytime. We'll work this through together."

The imaginary canopy disappears—for the moment. It is time to go upstairs to the hospital wards where more patients wait.

Mr. Doubletree is an eighty-three-year-old retired lawyer who has had two surgeries and a heart catheterization to repair damage caused by heart disease as well as chronic vascular and lung disease. Despite his surgeries, however, he has maintained his zest for life, walking every day near his home on Cape Cod, playing golf and generally staying active. But recently, several small strokes have begun to weaken him, slowing down his activity and causing difficulty in swallowing. Food particles found their way down his trachea to the lungs instead of the esophagus to the stomach, leading to infection and pneumonia. His deteriorating health contributed to the heart attack that brought him to the hospital a few weeks ago.

Today, as we stand in the hallway outside Mr. Doubletree's room, Gene says, "My goal is to rekindle his enthusiasm for life. Sometimes older people just need a reason to keep going on. He is someone who will be able to get back his life if he has the will to do so. To play to his strength, my message to him will be something like, 'Hey, the game is still going on! Do you want to be sitting on the bench?'"

As he walks into the room, Gene suddenly becomes jovial: He greets Mr. Doubletree's daughter, who is sitting by the bed, and then says in a hearty voice, "Mr. Doubletree! You're making a liar out of me. I thought you wouldn't be looking this good for another day or so. Look at you sitting up in bed like this!" The older man is clearly pleased and says rather gruffly that he knew he could do it. "So tell me about the swallowing problem," continues Gene. Mr. Doubletree says he is having some trouble with eating. Gene then begins to explain that since both the breathing and swallowing tubes are so close together, sometimes food can slip down into the lungs. "But we don't want this to happen, and the way to prevent it is for you to begin to move around, sit in the chair, try to walk and get stronger," he says. "This will help both your swallowing and your breathing." The patient and his daughter both listen intently. Before he leaves, Gene pulls out his stethoscope. When he has listened to Mr. Doubletree's heart, he smiles broadly. "You're in an ascendancy. You're going to take off like a rocket now," he says. The patient looks pleased again. "You're going to make it for me, aren't you?" asks Gene. "You bet," comes the answer.

Back outside in the hallway, Gene tells me that he was talking as much to the daughter as to the patient. "She'll repeat what I said to him for the rest of the day," he says. During the next eight hours, Gene will visit thirty more patients listed on a computer printout that he generated from the Harvard Vanguard Medical Associates database this morning. As the on-call cardiologist for the group practice, Gene will see not only his own hospitalized patients, but also those of the six other cardiologists he works with. In addition, he will handle all cardiac emergencies for the practice. His beeper emits its strident tone several times an hour as he progresses from patient to patient, interrupting the flow of his work with emergency calls or questions from residents. "I've become very good at multitasking," he comments.

The next patient is Mrs. Chase, a woman in her sixties who is ready to be discharged from the hospital today. Her recent angioplasty (a surgical procedure) to restore blood flow to a blocked vessel to her heart was successful, but she needs to maintain a healthy lifestyle at home. When we arrive, she is sitting on the side of her bed, fully dressed, holding her purse, and ready to go. She is overweight and has diabetes but is determined to stay healthy. She sighs when she sees Gene. "I thought I was doing everything right," she says. "I was on a diet, I was exercising. . . ." Gene is reassuring. "The relatively small coronary damage you had is a tribute to what you had been doing," he says. "But now we need to be even more diligent." She looks doubtful, "I don't understand," she says. He walks over to the small sink in her room and turns the faucet on full blast, then places his thumb over the opening. Some water still splashes into the sink.

"Your blood flow is like this water," he says. "Even with the blockage that you had, some blood continued to get through the vessel. Your coronary artery may have been only 50 or 60 percent obstructed for a time, and probably stayed that way longer because of your diet and exercise. At this level, you wouldn't necessarily notice any symptoms. Eventually, however, the plaque did increase, until it began to significantly reduce your blood flow: Once an artery gets to be 70 percent blocked, or more, you begin to experience angina (pain caused by reduced blood flow to the heart), and there is danger of a heart attack. This is why we did your angioplasty—to open up the vessel, restore the flow and improve your symptoms. Now we want to prevent any more blockages and keep that blood flowing freely." She nods. "So what should I do?"

Gene begins by explaining the importance of taking her daily medications, with the reason for each one. He then asks her about her exercise routine. She mentions having joined a gym. "Going to the gym sounds good," he says. "But I'd like you to exercise at least four times a week, not to the point of exhaustion, but until you feel pleasantly fatigued." She nods. And the low-fat, low-carbohydrate diet that we will give you is a good idea as well." She gathers up her discharge and medication information. They agree that she will call his office for a follow-up appointment next week. "I can't wait to get home and get started," she says.

Later, Gene says, "I always try to tell my patients that you can accomplish a lot through good health habits. The body wants to improve and will try to find ways to compensate for injury unless you continually abuse it." He describes several patients with coronary artery disease whose bodies developed "collateral" blood vessels as the result of regular exercise. These small vessels provide a way for blood to get "around" a blockage. "Imagine you are on expressway; there is an accident in front of you and traffic is at a standstill," says Gene. "You are near an off-ramp, so you get off, take a detour past the accident and get back on the highway on the other side. That is collateral blood flow. Of course, diet and exercise will also help reduce the plaque buildup that clogs arteries in the first place."

Despite the evidence that lifestyle change can reduce the risk of heart disease, many patients are still unwilling to modify their lives, according to Gene. "As an allopathic physician but one who is a maverick, I believe 100 percent in the ability of pills and procedures to help, but my own bias is that people rely on them too much," he says. "I made rounds in the hospital today on several people who had heart attacks and vascular disease but who refuse to stop smoking, or to begin exercising or change their diets. Bypass surgery and interventions such as angioplasty are seductive. They don't cure anything, but give you a 'patch job' and a stable period in which you can use diet and exercise, as well as medication, to change the conditions that caused your coronary disease in the first place. It can give you a second chance, even a third chance, but you have to take advantage of it by combining other methods of controlling the disease. If you depend on surgery and other interventions for salvation you'll be disappointed. In the same way, if you depend only on alternative methods, you'll be disappointed as well. We need both."

❖ ❖ ❖ ❖

After several emergency beeper interruptions and phone calls, we proceed to another floor and find ourselves at the bedside of an eighty-two-year-old woman wearing heavy makeup and with her hair dyed a glorious brown. She is a former endocrinologist from Russia who is scheduled for bypass surgery. She greets Gene cheerfully, and talks about her strange feelings of "euphoria" and tension. "Your body is preparing to have surgery," he explains, and is releasing hormones to prepare for the stress. But you probably know more about this than I do!" She nods in understanding, and says she hopes that the surgery will happen soon. She's ready now. Gene says he'll see what he can do.

Out in the hallway, he finds the surgeon, and urges that his patient be put on the operating room schedule for that afternoon. Today is Sunday, a day on which elective surgeries are not normally scheduled, but Gene persists. "She had chest pains again this morning and is emotionally ready to do this now," he says. "I don't think it would be wise to wait until Monday." After some negotiating back and forth, the surgeon agrees. Later, Gene tells me, "I call that bartering for my patient."

❖ ❖ ❖ ❖

As Gene goes from patient to patient, he displays facets of his personality that range from physician to motivational speaker, spiritual leader, personal trainer, family therapist and teacher. With the residents and nurses who are in charge of each patient, he can be team leader, mentor and consultant. His wavy silver hair and matching beard give him a scholarly air, made more pronounced by glasses framing lively hazel eyes that radiate interest, empathy and humor. This is a doctor who is not afraid to share something of himself. As he moves through the hospital, trailed by groups of respectful and attentive young residents, one can easily imagine the resemblance to his imposing and charismatic Baptist minister father. The six-foot-one frame that helped Gene win a college football scholarship has evolved over the years into the lean profile of a marathon runner. (Now in his mid-fifties, he runs almost every day and has completed more than forty marathons.)

❖ ❖ ❖ ❖

During the entire day at the hospital, Gene sits down only twice. Once is to eat a quick sandwich ("to avoid hypoglycemia," he explains). The second time is in the room of a man in his forties, who is recovering from a heart attack. "This is a patient who is medically stable but very anxious," Gene explains to me in the hallway. "I need to understand what his symptoms mean. And I don't want him to feel rushed." In the room, Gene pulls a chair up to the end of the bed, settles down and listens carefully as the patient describes his worries about asthma attacks, his occasional inability to speak audibly, his feelings of dizziness and disorientation, as well as his fear that the nurses will not respond quickly enough when he presses the call button. "You don't feel safe. You imagine being unconscious here and no one will know, is that it?" asks Gene. "Yes," says the patient, leaning back against his pillow. "You understand."

Gene examines his chart for several moments, then looks up. "I think some of these symptoms may be caused by too high a dose of the medications your doctors here prescribed," he says. "I'm going to discuss this with them and try to introduce some rationality in your medications. I'm also ordering a brain wave EEG for tomorrow to see if you have evidence of a seizure disorder." Seeing the anxious look on the patient's face, Gene then began a calm, slow explanation of what might cause seizure disorders, as well as how asthma might affect a person's voice. Only when he is satisfied that the patient fully understands and has no further questions does he push back his chair and stand up. "I'm going to tell your nurses and the doctor everything that we talked about and leave new medication orders," he says. "You can call me if you have any other concerns, and I'll be back to see you later." Out in the hall Gene immediately becomes a professor of medicine, explaining firmly and clearly to the resident and nurses in charge of the patient why the medication needs to be changed.

❖ ❖ ❖ ❖

Gene spends the rest of the day in the cardiac intensive care and post-surgical wards of the hospital, seeing patients who are recovering from recent heart surgeries. Most of these patients have large, full-color computer screens outside their rooms displaying detailed information about their heart rhythms and respiration rates. High-tech medicine. Gene scrutinizes these carefully but always pulls out his stethoscope anyway. "I like to hear what's going on for myself," he explains. "And it gives me a chance to have more contact with the patient. People feel more reassured when the doctor spends time examining them."

One elderly woman complains that her left arm feels weak. "Probably a little piece of tissue broke away during the surgery and temporarily blocked some blood flow in the brain cells that control your arm," Gene explains. "But the fact that it has been getting stronger each day means that this is just temporary. Your arm will come back." She is still worried, however, complaining that she sometimes feels that she is hallucinating in the hospital. "I've seen this hundreds of times," he reassures her. "It's because you've been confined for so long to this room. There have been studies done in which medical students are confined in beds like this for long periods of time, and guess what? They all start to have hallucinations like yours. Of course this assumes that medical students are 'normal'—perhaps a questionable assumption." She smiles for the first time since we came in. "These hallucinations will stop as soon as you are out of here," he continues. "Which should be soon!"

After many more patient visits and emergency "beeper" calls, evening approaches and Gene's day ends as it began, with a profound and tearful family meeting about treatment decisions for a seventy-three-year-old man who is unconscious from a heart attack and also suffering from the results of the last stages of a virulent and untreatable lung cancer. Earlier that morning, Gene had examined Mr. Harris in the intensive care unit. "I think he will die today or tomorrow," he tells me. "Six weeks ago, we performed an angioplasty to restore blood flow and reduce some of his chest pain. He was able to go home, enjoy the fall with his children and grandchildren, even rake the leaves in his yard—he's always been an active guy." But just last week, the blood vessel closed up again. It was surgically reopened with another angioplasty, but then closed up again, causing a massive heart attack and cardiac arrest. He was resuscitated and a breathing tube inserted. He remains in intensive care.

Last week, Gene had a long meeting with the family to talk about a treatment plan. They carefully read the living will that Mr. Harris had prepared earlier that year. This evening, Gene has arranged a second meeting with Mrs. Harris and two of their adult children. We are sitting in a small family waiting room near the intensive care unit. "As you know, we spent the past week trying to get Mr. Harris off the machines, without much success," Gene begins. "We have already resuscitated him once. The cancer doctor reports that his lungs are now bleed-ing, which obviously does not help. So we need to piece together what his wishes are for the next step."

Mrs. Harris, perched on the edge of a table, tearfully pulls a folded packet out of her purse—his living will. "I wish you could have seen him out in the yard last week," she says. Her daughter nods, sitting next to her husband, his arm around her, and takes up the story. "He was raking the leaves, trying to chase the squirrels away from the bird feeder. The kids were laughing and running around, trying to help him." Gene nods. "You know, I bet you'll never see a squirrel at that bird feeder without thinking of him," he says. "I know I'll always remember his energy."

He gently takes the living will from Mrs. Harris. "If his heart stops again, we need to think about what he would want us to do," he says. "We could try to start it beating with either drugs or a shock treatment." He waits for them to assimilate this information. "In my experience with patients who have the kind of lung problems that he has, such aggressive treatment of the heart may not have a good result." He waits again. "We don't want him to suffer," says Mrs. Harris. The daughter agrees. "He never would have wanted that. After all, he turned down a bypass operation last year because he didn't want to spend whatever time he had left from the lung cancer in recovery from heart surgery."

Gene begins an unhurried rumination. "We are at a kind of crossroads," he says. The family watches him attentively. "In this situation," he continues, "some people might choose to provide fluids and medication for his comfort, remove the breathing tube, and rely on either nature or the will of God. Others might want to do anything that might bring him back, even if only for a short while. And he might come back, but I think we need to prepare ourselves for the worst. The conflict is between not wanting to let go of him and not wanting him to have any more pain and suffering." They all nod, wiping tears from their eyes. Slowly, they begin to talk, gradually reaching the conclusion that the breathing tube should come out.

That evening, Gene writes orders in the chart to remove the tube, provide pain medication and intravenous fluids, but to take no aggressive measures should the heart stop beating. The next day, Mr. Harris did in fact regain some consciousness and spent several hours with his wife and children around his bed. Without the tube in his throat, he was even able to talk with them a little bit. Finally, and peacefully, he died.

"I was struggling with the family to find wisdom amid probabilities and uncertainties," Gene told me later. "As part of the struggle, it was important to me that the family knew that I didn't just see Mr. Harris as a sick old man with cancer and heart disease. I wanted them to understand that I appreciated him as the person he was."

It is after 7:00 P.M. The day is drawing to a close. On his way out of the hospital Gene stops at a telephone to call his wife and arrange dinner plans. Today is their seventeenth wedding anniversary.

An Agonizing Decision:
"If You Can't Be Yourself When Facing
Your Own Death, When Will You?"

One morning in 1988, Charlotte Harrington (not her real name) had stopped at a pay phone in the middle of a bustling downtown sidewalk to call her cardiologist. An earlier test of her heart rhythm had come back with a slightly abnormal result, so he had ordered a second one, just to be sure. Charlotte had worn a portable heart monitor for twenty-four hours, which had recorded every heartbeat. She was calling him this morning on her way to class to get the results.

She shifted her purse and briefcase full of papers and held the phone to her ear as she dialed the number. She reached him right away. "The results of your heart monitor test just came back," he said. "I want you to go to the hospital immediately. I've already called to tell them you'll be coming. You need to be admitted and start taking the anti-arrhythmia drug I told you about last week." (Anti-arrhythmia drugs are used to stabilize an irregular heartbeat.)

Charlotte felt a cold panic. "What are you talking about?" she stammered, oblivious to the crowds swirling past her. "I feel perfectly fine. Those irregular heartbeats only happen occasionally. You told me that this second test was just to make sure that the abnormality that you saw on the first test was not serious." Not giving him time to answer, she rushed on. "And what drug is that? Is it amiodarone? Is that the same drug that you told me last week was so toxic that you hoped I'd never have to take it?"

Even with the noise of people and cars around her, she could detect the urgent edge to the voice coming through the phone that she was by now clutching to her ear. He spoke deliberately: "We already know that you have cardiomyopathy (an abnormality of the heart muscle itself)," he said. "Now we also know that you also have nonsustained ventricular tachycardia—a very serious abnormal heart rhythm. Even if it happens only occasionally, people in your condition have a 75 percent chance of sudden death. *Do not go home first*. Just get in a cab and check yourself into the hospital now."

Charlotte took a deep breath. She knew that the type of cardiomyopathy she had—idiopathic hypertrophic subaortic stenosis (IHSS)—was a disease with potentially deadly consequences. Several people in her extended family were already ill or had died as the result of it. But she was thirty-six years old, feeling just fine, working on her doctoral dissertation in education and looking forward to a career of teaching, research, perhaps even marriage and children. By now she had edged herself as far as possible into the pay phone alcove. "You are telling me that I could very well die and my only hope is a highly toxic drug with serious side effects," she said. "I need to think about this. I need another opinion. I'm going to go home now." She hung up the receiver.

The memory of that phone call, along with the accompanying wave of terror and confusion that flooded her on that downtown street, are still vivid to Charlotte, even though the incident happened fifteen years ago. "I went home and yelled and screamed," she remembers. "I was in shock. I knew that I always had less stamina than other people, but I was also reasonably competitive and would push myself when I was out with friends, whether I was biking, canoeing, hiking or playing soccer. I never realized that there was an organic, physical limit to what I could do." In fact, she had only found out about her heart problem because of a persistent cough. "The doctor discovered I had asthma and wanted to put me on an inhaler," she says. "But he decided to do an EKG test of my heart first, to analyze my heartbeat. I had never had one before, and that is how they found out I also had cardiomyopathy."

By making the decision to go home instead of directly to the hospital, Charlotte knew that she was putting her life at risk, and it is not something she would recommend to others. But at the time, given the person she was, it seemed the only possible course of action. Throughout her life, she has always dealt with health problems, including serious back pain and allergies, by choosing alternative health-care methods—including acupuncture, herbal medicine, osteopathy, meditation and nutritional counseling—whenever possible. "I've never been terribly fond of doctors and prefer to try alternative methods if possible first. But at the same time I always listen carefully to the advice of conventional doctors, seek several opinions and think carefully about their recommendations," she says. "I'm also prone to allergies and extremely sensitive to the effects of medicines. I knew that amiodarone—the recommended drug to regulate my heart rhythm—would have helped to prevent sudden death, but I was also terrified about what the drug would do to the *quality* of my life, especially if I wanted to become pregnant. And I guess a part of me also wondered whether my risk level warranted such drastic measures."

It is generally acknowledged that many patients who take amiodarone experience some side effects, sometimes serious enough to stop the medication. These include potentially severe acute or chronic damage to the lungs. Less common side effects include liver toxicity as well as nerve damage. Despite these and other side effects, however, many of which can be controlled with changes in dosage, doctors who prescribe it feel that the life-saving benefits outweigh the disadvantages. Charlotte's situation is not an uncommon one: Doctors and patients often view the risks of treatment differently. While many doctors see low side effects as an acceptable risk, given the benefits of treatment, patients often see the same risks differently. "Even if there is a 1 percent chance of something happening," a patient might say, "if I happen to be in that 1 percent, the catastrophe happens to *me*, and all the statistics in the world don't mean a thing." It would be helpful for patients if doctors were to recognize and acknowledge these differing perceptions. Too often, however, that does not happen.

And in this agonizing decision lies the dilemma for the patient. If the philosophy of integrative medicine is based on the notion that patients are partners in their health care, what happens when a patient truly wants to "own her health"? When she makes a choice—based on her own experience, beliefs and life values—that the doctor believes seriously threatens her health, even her very life? "It would have gone against the very essence of who I am to immediately start taking a powerful, potentially toxic drug, when I was not entirely convinced that it was necessary, given the severity of my symptoms," says Charlotte. "I needed to explore further before I made any decision. I believe that the bridge between alternative and conventional medicine is the patient: I needed to find a doctor who would honor the person I was. After all, if you can't be yourself when faced with your own death, when will you do it?"

Exploring the Options

In Charlotte's continuing story, she sought second, third and even fourth opinions from different cardiologists. "One doctor thought the drug was unnecessary," she says. "Another wanted to implant a pacemaker/defibrillator. Another recommended a different drug with other undesirable sided effects. I decided to go to the National Institutes of Health (NIH) in Washington to be evaluated by experts who had been studying my particular disease for years. I just wanted a normal life." (For certain conditions, patients can request to be evaluated by specialists at the NIH.)

The advantage of going to the NIH, according to Charlotte, is that she learned almost everything there was to know about her disease, possible treatments and their side effects. "They did routine tests, stress tests, echocardiograms and two invasive studies: an electrophysiological study, during which they tried unsuccessfully to put me into heart failure, and a cardiac catheterization. Then they told me that even though my arrhythmia symptoms were sporadic and it was unclear how high a risk of death there was, they recommended medication as a precaution." Charlotte still was not convinced. "I wanted to have children and was worried about the effects during pregnancy," she says. "I also did not understand how you could know whether the drug was working if the symptoms happen so sporadically."

Charlotte went home, found a conventional cardiologist she felt she could work with ("someone who is open-minded," she says), and proposed using alternative methods to control the arrhythmia and to avoid medication, at least for the moment. They agreed that he would monitor her, and if the symptoms became more severe, she would begin the medication. It has now been fifteen years since that phone call on the sidewalk. Charlotte continues to be closely watched by her cardiologist, and she has developed a lifestyle that works for her, including Pilates workouts several times a week (a nonaerobic, nonstressful exercise method; see "A Closer Look at Pilates"), regular acupuncture and massage.

She also tries to control and manage her occasional heart symptoms with meditation. "The tachycardia (arrhythmia) does not happen very often," she says. "But when it does, I get a sense of dizziness, my peripheral vision narrows, my chest gets constricted, I feel like it is hard to breathe, even that I could pass out. I immediately drop my attention down to my heart and concentrate all of my energy there. I breathe very deeply and regularly, entering into a meditative state, to a slow count of two for each breath. As I count, I imagine my heart beating in rhythm with the counting. Biofeedback taught me that it is possible to center your attention on a part of your body and make physiological changes. I feel that I am 'teaching' my heart how I want it to behave. The arrythmia usually stops within about seven seconds. Of course, I have no way of knowing whether it would have stopped anyway, but I feel as if I am taking control of my health this way." (Please see chapter 6 for an explanation of biofeedback and data on its effectiveness.)

Charlotte knows that her methods of handling her heart problem are controversial. "For me, the question has never been about ignoring the recommendations of my doctors," she says. "It is about taking the time to sit with myself, think deeply about what I believe and what I want, and making an informed choice, rather than feeling victimized by my disease. That sense of power helps me to stay healthy."

She is also quick to say that she does not recommend rejecting effective medical treatments without carefully considering the risks. "I consulted with several experts, including the National Institutes of Health, and thought very carefully before deciding on my course of action. I also know that luck has played a big part in why I am still alive and doing well. For me, at least so far, this is the only way to live."

❖ ❖ ❖ ❖

Charlotte's story raises important questions in patient autonomy within the integrative medicine philosophy for which there are no easy answers. Cardiologist Eugene Lindsey, M.D., (whom we met in the "Day with a Cardiologist" story), has never met

Charlotte, but when asked for his opinion about her health-care choices, he has this to say:

"Charlotte's story underlines the discomfort we all have in dealing with medical uncertainty. Many doctors manage uncertainty (in her case the possibility of sudden death from arrhythmia)—and the accompanying fear of making an error that will hurt the patient—by being very conservative and directive. That is probably why her doctor insisted that she go immediately to the emergency room. He was responding to the material risk of sudden death.

"Charlotte chose to deal with her uncertainty by embracing it and assuming responsibility for her own health, along with the risks, which is one of the goals of integrative medicine," says Dr. Lindsey. "For her, the side effects of the proposed treatment were more real than the risk of sudden death. At the same time she proceeded with both wisdom and courage. She didn't get caught up in her doctor's fears, but neither did she discount his concerns: She sought several opinions, including one from the National Institutes of Health. She understood what she wanted for herself and made her decision not to take the drug on valid grounds. In fact, recent research indicates that many people with her form of cardiomyopathy and ventricular tachycardia may well be treated with less drastic methods.

"An important issue for me is how we as doctors continue to work with patients who do not accept the suggestions we make about their care. I would hope that we would say to the patient, 'Okay, that's your decision right now, but I would like to continue monitoring your condition closely, and for us to keep talking. Let's keep the options open and not burn the bridges to allopathic medicine. It is possible that your condition will change, and that we might want to rethink the treatment options.' As long as one is alive, there are very few decisions in life that cannot be reversed!"

A Closer Look at Meditation:
Taming the Elephant

The Vipassana (awareness) meditation practice described in chapter 4 is one of two major forms of meditation. It is also called "open" meditation. The other is called "concentration (or concentrative) meditation," according to psychotherapist and meditation instructor Andrea Lindsay, LICSW. (Please see box for a summary of meditation types.) "A dear friend and colleague of mine, Ben Brown, Ph.D., refers to the mind as if it were an elephant. In ancient Tibetan illustrations, the mind is usually drawn as an elephant," says Andrea. "The elephant has great power if it can be tamed, but left unchecked, it can also trample the ground and cause damage. The mind has the same potential." In her practice, Andrea works with patients whose physical illnesses are causing emotional difficulties, as well as people whose emotional states are expressed in physical illness, including gastrointestinal problems, hypertension and heart disease.

Andrea describes concentration meditation—which also has its roots in the Buddhist tradition—as a way to train the mind, to have it focus on one subject or idea, wherever you choose to put it, and hold it there. Using the elephant as an example, she says, "In concentration meditation you focus your mind on one thing: a candle, a flower, or simply the rising and falling of your breath, which is my preferred method. Compare it to tying an elephant to a stake. Every time your mind gets distracted and wanders away from the breath, you immediately bring it back. You do this without labeling where your mind has gone (as you might do in awareness meditation). You simply bring it back. In the elephant analogy, whenever the elephant wanders away from the stake, you gently guide it back. Eventually, the elephant learns to stay closer to home, just as you will learn to hold your mind exactly where you want it." The result of this transformation of your mind is deep relaxation, which has a number of health benefits.

The difference between concentration meditation and awareness meditation, says Andrea, is how much attention you pay to what has distracted the mind or where it has gone. "In awareness meditation, you label the distractions as 'thoughts,' 'feelings' or 'sensations,'" she says. "Or, in the elephant analogy, you keep track of where the elephant is wandering, and you watch it as it comes back."

By contrast, in concentration meditation, you do not label; you immediately bring the mind back without noticing where it has been, says Andrea. "This gives you the practice of catching the mind almost as soon as it wanders off. The eventual goal, which takes practice to achieve, is to be able to train and control your mind as you sit, focus on your breath and have no thoughts. Without this kind of training, it is sometimes difficult to even notice when your mind is wandering until it has been gone for some time!"

THE CONCENTRATIVE MEDITATION TECHNIQUE:
STABLE BODY, STABLE MIND

While a relaxed state is one result of meditation, Andrea points out that concentrative meditation, when you are doing it, is not about relaxation. "This is not done lying down, but in an erect, dignified, solidly seated posture," she says. "You say to yourself, 'I am going to consciously enter a state that will benefit my mind and body.'" In the workshops she gives for psychotherapists around the country and in Europe, Andrea spends a great deal of time on the proper meditation posture. "I show people a photo of a stone Buddha," she says. The image is of solid, balanced, unmoving stability:

- The legs can be resting on the floor or crossed on a pillow.
- The arms are not floppy, but are balanced on the knees or held with the left palm over the right just above the navel.
- The back is straight.
- The neck is slightly bent.
- The jaw is relaxed.
- The tongue is placed behind the front teeth.

This solid, balanced meditation posture has an effect on the mind, slowing down thought and constant reactions to outside stimuli and promoting controlled attention. The mind is then free to focus on the breath as it rises and falls within that solid body:

- Break down the breath into small points: the beginning in-breath, the slow rise up through the body, the slight pause, and then the beginning of the out-breath, the slow exhalation and the slight pause before the next in-breath.

Distractions will come, exactly as they do in awareness meditation, but do not label them. The moment you notice a thought, feeling, sensation or emotion, bring your mind immediately back to the details of the breath (as if you were firmly pulling that elephant back to its stake).

(continued)

The Nine-Round Breath

This is a quick form of concentration meditation that comes from Tibetan energy meditation practices. It has a profound calming effect, controls anxiety and is a powerful method of clearing the mind of everything except the present moment. This takes a few minutes and can be done anywhere, several times a day.

1. Close your eyes. Imagine that you are breathing in through the right nostril only and breathing out through the left, evenly, effortlessly and slowly. The more you imagine it, the deeper you go into a relaxed state. Do this for a total of three times. This completes the first round of three. (Do not worry if you can't actually breathe in only one nostril, just focusing and imagining is enough.)

2. Reverse the breathing. Imagine that you are you are breathing in through the left nostril and out the right. Do this three times. This completes the second round of three.

3. Breathe evenly and effortlessly through both nostrils, in and out. Do this three times. This completes the third round of three.

In the Tibetan tradition, this technique purifies and balances the energy on both sides of your body. Compare how you feel now to how you felt before the exercise.

Meditation for Mental Health and Physical Well-Being

Skill in either of the two major forms of meditation leads naturally to the other, says Andrea. "Although I prefer to teach concentration meditation first, as a formal sitting practice," she says. "Then people are more prepared to use the awareness meditation to become more focused and present as they move through their everyday lives." (Please see "Suggestions for Mindfulness in Everyday Life," to follow.) "Life becomes very rich if you are really paying attention to it, rather than merely going through the motions," says Andrea. "Concentration meditation will stabilize your body and mind, which then makes it easier to use awareness meditation to enrich your everyday life."

The by-product of all forms of meditation is relaxation and calmness and less "reactivity" to the ups and downs of life, says Andrea. "The way we react to stress is the basis of our suffering," she says. "By clinging to what we want and trying to get away from what we don't want, we are always reacting to something, and we are often not in control of this reacting state. Meditation can help slow that process and help us return to a state of equilibrium—to recognize and be aware, but not necessarily to react automatically. We know, for example, that meditation reduces blood pressure, changes brain waves, slows heart and breathing rate and has positive health benefits." (Please see research box for these findings.)

Meditation also benefits our mental health. "We learn that everything is impermanent, especially emotional pain and suffering," says Andrea. "For example, we know that depression and anxiety are characterized by negative thinking about yourself and your situation. Therapy attempts to change this kind of negative thinking and actively cultivate positive states of mind. Concentration meditation not only relaxes you, it teaches you how to put your mind somewhere and keep it there. If you are caught in worries about your illness or your pain, you can bring in something more positive, like visualization for health. If you hold your mind on that positive thought, it will change the way that you think. When you have control of your mind, you can choose to focus on the parts of yourself that are healthy, just like tending flowers in a garden, and focus less on the weeds. Even if something horrible and disappointing happens, you know that it will not crush you. You can use the power of your mind to nourish the beautiful flowers of your personality."

TYPES OF MEDITATION: A SUMMARY

There are so many different kinds of meditation that sorting them out can be confusing. In *Essentials of Complementary Medicine,* Lynda Freeman has a useful way of looking at the variations:

Two basic forms: concentrative meditation and open meditation. And within each form there are many types.

- **Concentrative meditation forms:** You focus your attention on one stimulus—a word or phrase, an object such as a candle, or your breath. If your attention strays, you gently bring it back to focus on the stimulus, over and over again. This form of meditation produces a "disciplined mind that can be still and at peace" with health benefits that include interrupting "repetitive and negative thought patterns that feed anxiety and depression . . ."

Types of concentrative meditation:

1. Transcendental meditation, founded by Maharishi Mahesh Yogi.
2. Formal Buddhist sitting meditation (see box for details of this type).
3. The Respiratory One Method (ROM) developed by Herbert Benson, M.D., who performed the original research on transcendental meditation and also developed the concept of the "relaxation response."

- **Open meditation forms:** You don't try to restrict your attention to only one stimulus (which is the concentrative method). Instead, you observe your thoughts, your bodily sensations and the sounds around you. The idea is to observe without judging them as good or bad, detaching your emotions and lowering your "reactivity" to what is going on. The goal is for negative thoughts and emotions to "lose their grip" and their power over your well-being.

The most widely used method of open meditation is Vipassana, also called "mindfulness" or "awareness" meditation, which is based on Buddhist practices and was developed for clinical use by Jon Kabat-Zinn, Ph.D. "This form of meditation seeks to observe what the concentrative methods seek to ignore (i.e., everyday life events and experiences). . . . The final goal is a state of continual nonjudgmental observation—of being totally 'awake' to the world, enlivened by life events, not overwhelmed by them." This is the form of meditation taught in the Duke SEARCH study, described in chapter 4.

Awareness Meditation: Don't Miss a Moment of Your Life

In 1984, Fern Ross Israel was thirty-three years old and the mother of three young children when her own mother was diagnosed with metastatic cancer of unknown origin. During the next two years, Fern traveled every other week (alternating with her sister) from her home in Boston to New York, where her mother was undergoing cancer treatment. "My first reaction was disbelief," says Fern. "This was my mother. My unconditional support in life. She had always been a strong woman, a schoolteacher in a rough section of New York. A tennis player. A loving parent, daughter, friend and wife. She had spent her life giving to others. Probably the only thing she did just for herself was to get her hair done on Fridays. I simply could not believe she had cancer."

The cancer was virulent and had already spread to the bones by the time of diagnosis. The treatments that were available in 1984 were not working. "I wanted to do more than fluff my mother's pillow and watch her die," says Fern, who at the time had some experience with alternative health methods. While she was a young mother, Fern had owned a home-based health-food cooking business. She had also been practicing yoga and meditation since 1979, and had gone abroad to Vienna to study spiritual philosophy, as well as alternative healing methods with masters, from different traditions.

So, when faced with her mother's cancer, Fern drew on all the knowledge she had at the time. "I did everything I could think of to stop the disease from spreading and reverse the cancer, from starting her on a macrobiotic diet to using compresses and having people pray for her," remembers Fern.

But even as Fern devoted her energies to stopping the disease, she realized that she was also missing what might well be the last precious moments of her mother's life. "I became aware that by focusing so much on the possibility of her death, I was losing my mother before I lost her," says Fern. "There is a poem by Mary Oliver that has always reminded me of the importance of staying fully aware and alive and not missing a moment of life. I realized that we don't die until we die and that I needed to be fully present with my mother—holding the space for her so that we would not miss a moment of whatever life she had left." This clear-seeing, focused awareness of what is happening *here and now* is for Fern the essence of her meditation practice. It allowed her to see and then let go of her fear of losing her mother in order to experience and enjoy her while she was still alive.

Fern's mother died on Valentine's Day, 1986, two years after her cancer diagnosis. "The last thing my mother said to me before she died was, 'Don't forget to take care of yourself, Fern, because no one else will.' Taking care of herself is one thing my mother had not done; she always put the needs of others first," says Fern. "I realized that even with all of the societal and cultural pressures on women, I needed to take the time to know myself and understand what I needed in order to be healthy. Meditation, for me, has been one of the most powerful tools to achieve that awareness and understanding."

❖ ❖ ❖ ❖

Her clients have described Fern, a petite, energetic woman with dark hair and a lively face, as a nurturing presence. In addition to serving as clinical director of the Mind/Body Stress Reduction program at Milton Hospital in Massachusetts, Fern also teaches yoga and Vipissana, or "mindfulness" meditation.

The essence of mindfulness meditation, according to Fern, is to develop a practice of awareness in everyday life, without the distractions of memories of the past (which is no longer here) or thoughts about the future (which has not yet arrived). This is most often done by focusing on the breathing; the movement of breath in and out of the body is a good way to remind yourself of the reality of the present moment. The benefit is freedom, calmness and inner peace. "You can bring this relaxed, centered presence to the chaos and ups and downs of life," says Fern. "When something happens, you don't have to react 'on automatic pilot'; you can stop. *See clearly* what is happening (instead of through the foggy lens of preconceived ideas). *Reflect* calmly. And then *choose* how you will react, rather than allowing yourself to succumb to your habitual reaction patterns."

Among its other benefits, mindfulness is a very good way to deal with physical pain, according to Fern. "With practice, patients can learn to observe the changing nature of the pain and hold their experience with compassion. When I meditate with patients, we often refer to these sensations as 'the' pain, or 'our' pain. This can change the experience of pain for some people, by allowing them to separate it from the essence of who they are." One of Fern's areas of expertise has become (not surprisingly) working with seriously ill and dying patients and their families. One of her patients was a young woman with a rare cancer that spread quickly through the fatty tissue of her body, causing great pain and eventually killing her within six months. "I taught her meditation and worked with her during her treatment and later in hospice," says Fern. "Her mother told me that the meditation practice helped her daughter more with the pain than the morphine drip she was given in hospice care."

Letting Go of Vietnam

After her mother died, Fern decided to enroll in a graduate program in mental health counseling. "I wanted to use mindfulness meditation to help others cope with difficult life transitions: grief, loss and death," says Fern. One of her internships was in a Veteran's Administration hospital, where she was assigned to work with a man who had fought in Vietnam. "He had classic post-traumatic stress," says Fern. "Even though he had fought in Vietnam twenty years earlier, he was still hypervigilant and was prone to angry outbursts and depression. Every time he heard a plane flying overhead he would experience rapid heartbeat, sweating and terrifying flashbacks. When he met with me, he would sit on the edge of his chair, facing the door, which we always had to leave open. He was constantly ready to bolt."

Fern found that meditation seemed to be one of the best ways to help this former soldier. "But first, of course, we talked," she says. "He did not understand why he had been having these symptoms for twenty years and had so much anxiety when he would go anywhere or do anything that reminded him of Vietnam. He told me heart-wrenching stories of being nineteen years old, of being afraid, and of watching his friends die. He trusted me with his story. Only then could we slowly begin to try to move into the present."

As she describes her approach to helping this patient, Fern quotes from Carl Jung: "Jung said that 'the only way out is through.' I felt that I did not need to 'fix' this patient so much as to sit with him and help him move through his powerful emotions, using the method of Stop. See. Understand. Choose. We used the focus on the breath to help him experience the reality of the present moment, here in this room, in this hospital, where he was safe," says Fern.

Ever so slowly, over the next year, Fern sat with her patient, sometimes talking, sometimes simply breathing, reminding him to let the fear go and to bring his mind back to the breath and to the present. "Within that year, he went from sitting bolt upright in his chair, with the door open, to relaxing back in the chair, closing his eyes, and allowing me to shut the door," says Fern. "Eventually, he was able to show me photographs and stories he had written about his Vietnam experience, and finally to cry about it. He could at last recognize and experience the grief and loss that belonged to the present; and to free himself from the terror, depression and rage that belonged to the past."

FERN'S SUGGESTIONS FOR
MINDFULNESS IN EVERYDAY LIFE

Practicing mindfulness does not necessarily mean that you sit for forty-five minutes each morning and focus on your breathing (although that is certainly one way to do it). We can learn to practice mindful awareness at chosen moments, within a day, to train ourselves to pay full attention to every moment. This sounds simple, but it is not always easy or remembered. Try to experiment with the following exercises in mindfulness:

- Choose a daily activity that you usually perform automatically and without any awareness. Bring relaxed, alert attention to:

  —Brushing your teeth
  —Taking a shower
  —Washing the dishes

- Try eating a meal slowly and mindfully without the distraction of thinking and the preoccupation with your surroundings. As soon as you feel the pull of the mind that plans, worries and judges, gently guide the mind back to the moment of tasting, smelling, feeling and swallowing the food. For example:

  —An apple
  —A piece of cake
  —A cup of tea
  —An entire meal

(Remember Mike Siddall in chapter 4, who said that this way of eating made him enjoy and appreciate food so much more?)

- Practice walking with full attention on the motion and feel of your body, without listening to music and without paying attention to thinking. Try to consciously follow the lifting, moving and placing of each step. For example:

  —Walk from the car to the front door of your home
  —Take a walk around the block
  —Walk from one room in your house to another room

(continued)

READER/CUSTOMER CARE SURVEY

BB1

We care about your opinions. Please take a moment to fill out this Reader Survey card and mail it back to us.
As a special **"thank you"** we'll send you exciting news about interesting books and a valuable **Gift Certificate.**

Please PRINT using ALL CAPS

First Name [ ] MI. [ ] Last Name [ ]

Address [ ]

City [ ] ST [ ] Zip [ ]

Phone # ([ ]) [ ] — [ ] Fax # ([ ]) [ ] — [ ]

Email [ ]

(1) Gender:
___ Female ___ Male

(2) Age:
___ 12 or under ___ 40-59
___ 13-19 ___ 60+
___ 20-39

(3) Marital Status
___ Married
___ Single
___ Divorced/Widowed

(4) Did you receive this book as a gift?
___ Yes ___ No

(5) How many Health Communications books have you bought or read?
___ 1 ___ 2-4 ___ 5+

(6) How did you find out about this book?
Please fill in ONE.
1) ___ Recommendation
2) ___ Store Display
3) ___ Bestseller List
4) ___ Online
5) ___ Advertisement
6) ___ Catalog/Mailing
7) ___ Interview/Review (TV, Radio, Print)

(7) Where do you usually buy books?
Please fill in your top TWO choices.
1) ___ Bookstore
2) ___ Religious Bookstore
3) ___ Online
4) ___ Book Club/Mail Order
5) ___ Price Club (Costco, Sam's Club, etc.)
6) ___ Retail Store (Target, Wal-Mart, etc.)

(9) What subjects do you enjoy reading about most? Rank only FIVE. Use 1 for your favorite, 2 for second favorite, etc.

	1	2	3	4	5
1) Parenting/Family	○	○	○	○	○
2) Relationships	○	○	○	○	○
3) Recovery/Addictions	○	○	○	○	○
4) Health/Nutrition	○	○	○	○	○
5) Christianity	○	○	○	○	○
6) Spirituality/Inspiration	○	○	○	○	○
7) Business Self-Help	○	○	○	○	○
8) Teen Issues	○	○	○	○	○
9) Sports	○	○	○	○	○

(14) What attracts you most to a book?
(Please rank 1-4 in order of preference.)

	1	2	3	4
1) Title	○	○	○	○
2) Cover Design	○	○	○	○
3) Author	○	○	○	○
4) Content	○	○	○	○

TAPE IN MIDDLE; DO NOT STAPLE

NO POSTAGE
NECESSARY
IF MAILED
IN THE
UNITED STATES

BUSINESS REPLY MAIL
FIRST-CLASS MAIL PERMIT NO 45 DEERFIELD BEACH, FL

POSTAGE WILL BE PAID BY ADDRESSEE

HEALTH COMMUNICATIONS, INC.
3201 SW 15TH STREET
DEERFIELD BEACH FL 33442-9875

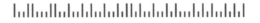

FOLD HERE

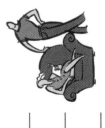

Comments:

- Experiment with mindful pauses throughout the day by stopping to observe your breathing. Choose to watch your breath, letting go of all moods, thoughts and distractions when you are:

—Stopped at a traffic light (with eyes open, please!)
—Waiting in line at the supermarket or movie theater

- Try answering the phone on the third or fourth ring. At the first ring, stop and become aware of your in-breaths and out-breaths.

- Drive to work without the radio, cell phone, coffee or other distractions. Why not try driving slowly, giving full attention to your moment in the car?

- Practice a ten-minute sitting meditation. Choose a comfortable and upright body position, close the eyes and relax into the breath. When the mind wanders and you notice you are lost in thoughts, simply guide your mind gently and decisively back to the breath. (This is a form of the concentration meditation described by Andrea Lindsay in the previous section.)

In addition to teaching yoga and meditation, Fern has a master's degree in mental health counseling and is also a Reiki master. In her private practice, she offers her clients mind/body therapy, which she describes as incorporating noninvasive body work with psychotherapy, helping patients access their stories and the source of their problems through the body. "I teach people how their emotional reactions are connected to the body," says Fern. Whether the work is meditation, Reiki, yoga or psychotherapy, Fern believes that people are helped through a connection to a greater life force. (Please see chapter 2.) "Whether we call it qi, prana or God, I believe that we are part of an energy field, and that our bodies can be helped by increasing the flow of healing energy within us," says Fern.

In her own life, Fern tries to follow her mother's advice and replenish herself. She has daily meditation and yoga practice, regularly receives acupuncture and bodywork, and walks for additional exercise. Once a year, she goes on a ten-day meditation retreat. "But we are all only human," says Fern with a laugh. "Once, I was filling up the bathtub, got distracted by a phone call, and the water overflowed onto the floor below. We had to clean up a huge, watery mess and repaint the whole room. This was a good reminder that I was not keeping a good balance between caring for myself and helping others. It is indeed a constant struggle to pay attention to the moments of our lives."

Meditation: What's the Evidence?

Ancient history, modern health benefits

The practice of meditation has been in use for thousands of years in many cultures, including Buddhist, Ayurvedic and Taoist traditions. In this country, there has been more than thirty years of research into various meditation practices, beginning with Herbert Benson, M.D., who performed the original research on the outcomes of transcendental meditation (a form of concentration meditation founded by Maharishi Mahesh Yogi.) Benson is perhaps best known for developing and researching what he has called "the relaxation response."

Meditation practices in various forms have shown health benefits: "In clinically controlled trials, mindfulness or awareness meditation has been demonstrated to effectively reduce anxiety and depression, including the condition known as post-traumatic stress; to significantly reduce chronic pain caused by a variety of medical conditions; to increase life functionality; and to reduce mood disturbance and psychiatric symptoms. Most of these outcomes were achieved with patients who had not improved with traditional medical care."[1]

Jon Kabat-Zinn, Ph.D., founded the Stress Reduction Clinic at the University of Massachusetts Medical Center in 1979. He is credited with adapting the Buddhist practice of Vipassana meditation into "mindfulness meditation" for clinical use. This form of meditation is now used throughout the United States in hospital-based stress management programs. (Please see, for example, chapter 4, for a description of such a program at Duke University Center for Integrative Medicine.)

Mindfulness meditation for anxiety and chronic pain

In 1992, Kabat-Zinn's clinical research in the Stress Reduction Program demonstrated the effectiveness of an outpatient group program based on mindfulness meditation in the treatment of anxiety. A follow-up study three years later "strongly suggests the long-term effectiveness" of the program although he notes that both studies "lacked a randomized control group for comparison and a control for concomitant treatment." In an earlier 1982 study, Kabat-Zinn demonstrated that a ten-week mindfulness meditation program was "an effective behavioral program in self-regulation for chronic pain patients."

---

[1] L. W. Freeman, *Best Practices in Complementary and Alternative Medicine: An Evidence-Based Approach* (Gaithersburg, MD: Aspen Publications, 2001), 8–11; 16.

Going to the heart of the matter

Kenneth R. Pelletier, Ph.D., M.D. (hc) in *The Best Alternative Medicine* highlights several important research findings on meditation and cardiovascular disease and hypertension, including the following:

Meditation significantly lowered both systolic (higher number) and diastolic (lower number) blood pressure in a randomized clinical trial conducted in Israel.[2]

Eight months of meditation improved circulation and exercise tolerance among twenty-one patients with coronary artery disease.[3]

Meditation lowered the blood pressure of African-Americans, a population at high risk for hypertension.[4]

(Please see chapter 4 for additional studies related to meditation and heart disease.)

And you don't even have to be sick

In addition to reducing pain, anxiety, depression and other symptoms of illness, Michael J. Baime reports that "Meditation also benefits individuals without acute medical illness or stress. People who meditate regularly report that they feel more confident and more in control of their lives. They say that their relationships with others are improved and that they experience more enjoyment and appreciation of life."

Can meditation be researched?

In the chapter on meditation that he wrote for *Essentials of Complementary and Alternative Medicine*, Michael J. Baime points out several problems confronting research into meditation as a medical therapy, including the difficulty of designing a convincing placebo: "Although the prospective, randomized, placebo-controlled double-blind study is the gold standard of clinical research, it may not be optimal for the investigation of meditation and similar mind-body therapies." Despite these problems, however, says Baine, "It can be argued that meditation works by the same mechanism as does the placebo effect. This point does not diminish the effect of meditation, but rather suggests that treatments that enhance the mind's capacity to heal the body (with low cost and little risk) may provide meaningful clinical benefits."

Despite any research problems, Lynda Freeman argues forcefully for the inclusion of meditation into clinical practice: "In medicine, there is a tendency to 'standardize'

---

[2] M. Cooper and M. Aygen, "Effect of Meditation on Blood Cholesterol and Blood Pressure," *Israel Medical Association Journal* 95 (1978), 1–2.

[3] J. Zamara et al., "Usefulness of the Transcendental Meditation Program in the Treatment of Patients with Coronary Artery Disease," *American Journal of Cardiology* 77, no. 10 (1996), 967–970.

[4] C. N. Alexander et al., "Trial of Stress Reduction for Hypertension for Older African Americans II, Sex and Risk Subgroup Analysis," *Hypertension* 28 (1996), 228–37.

a treatment, to strip that treatment of subjective as opposed to objective meaning, and to remove issues of consciousness from the outcome. If people have learned nothing else from consciousness and meditation research, it is that this approach is simplistic and ineffectual. Humans need to transform and grow just as they need food and water.... Consciousness and the need for transformation will not conform to medical opinion; medical thought is going to need to adapt to these critical issues of consciousness, as they relate to medical outcomes."

References

Alexander, C. N., et al. "Trial of Stress Reduction for Hypertension for Older African Americans II, Sex and Risk Subgroup Analysis." *Hypertension* 28 (1996): 228–37.

Baime, M. J. "Meditation and Mindfulness." Chapter 30 in *Essentials of Complementary and Alternative Medicine*, eds. W. B. Jonas and J. S. Levin. Baltimore, MD: Lippincott, Williams & Wilkins, 1999.

Baime, M. J. and R. V. Baime. "Stress Management Using Mindfulness Meditation in a Primary Care General Internal Medical Practice." *Journal of General Internal Medicine* 11, no. S1 (1996): 131.

Cooper, M. and M. Aygen. "Effect of Meditation on Blood Cholesterol and Blood Pressure." *Israel Medical Association Journal* 95 (1978): 1–2.

Freeman, L. W. *Best Practices in Complementary and Alternative Medicine: An Evidence-Based Approach*. Gaithersburg, MD: Aspen Publications, 2001.

Kabat-Zinn, J. "An Outpatient Program in Behavioral Medicine for Chronic Pain Patients Based on the Practice of Mindfulness Meditation." *General Hospital Psychiatry* 4 (1982): 33–47.

Kabat-Zinn, J., et al. "Effectiveness of a Meditation-Based Stress Reduction Program in the Treatment of Anxiety Disorders." *American Journal of Psychiatry* 149 (1992): 9336–9943.

Kabat-Zinn, J., et al. "Three-Year Follow-Up and Clinical Implications of a Mindfulness Meditation-Based Stress Reduction Intervention in the Treatment of Anxiety Disorders." *General Hospital Psychiatry* 17 (1995): 192–200.

Zamarra, J., et al. "Usefulness of the Transcendental Meditation Program in the Treatment of Patients with Coronary Artery Disease." *American Journal of Cardiology* 77, no. 10 (1996): 967–970.

Also see the bibliography for books on meditation and health by Jon Kabat-Zinn, Herbert Benson and others.

5

CANCER: A CONTINUOUS JOURNEY OF CHOICES

"I'm overwhelmed. I've become my own medical consultant without training!"

The theatre is dark. There is no curtain. When the lights come up on the stage, we see a woman with luminous blue eyes and high cheekbones. She is wearing wide linen pants that fall to midcalf and a matching top that looks like a cross between a sleeveless doctor's coat and a Nehru jacket. Her feet are bare. Her hair, growing back during a break from chemotherapy, frames her face in a blonde pixie cut.

She is motionless at first. One arm is straight up in the air, the other on the opposite breast. "One day in the shower I found a small lump in my breast," she says, looking out at the audience. "I called my gynecologist. He said I needed to get a mammogram. I find myself in a small, dark room with a large machine and a female technician."

For the next hour, the audience sits transfixed, witnessing the journey of dancer and performance artist BJ Goodwin after her diagnosis of breast cancer. Alone on the stage, she acts out her desperate search for alternatives to surgery and chemotherapy, and her eventual acceptance of the need to combine treatments from both worlds.

Keeping A Breast is a one-woman show, written and performed by BJ. Taking possession of the stage, she becomes, in turn, insensitive oncologists, single-minded alternative therapists, caring friends, and her own, scared self, using her hands to "talk" to her body: "How could my body do this to me? Was it growing up in the smog in L.A.? Was it because of my bad relationship with my mother?

Because I drank coffee with half and half in it? Was it the underwire bras, the chlorine in the tampons, chemicals in the food? It's my genes . . . they were too tight? (She hits her head) I forgot to have kids? I love sugar . . . I don't love enough? I HAVE REPRESSED ANGER!!!!"

Now 47, BJ began her career as a dancer right out of college. "It was either that or coach sports," she says in an interview. For several years she lived in New York City, dancing and performing in the downtown arts scene, gradually moving into "performance art," which she describes as the merging of visual art, theater, language and movement, incorporating the body by using it as a *part* of the art. "I was always completely comfortable in my body and always healthy," she says. "I didn't know what a doctor was." As early as the 1970s, she and her dance colleagues were studying and using such alternative movement techniques as Pilates, yoga, Feldenkreis and Alexander. "We lived on homeopathy, tofu, herbal medicine and dried weeds," says BJ. "We never went to doctors, because we couldn't afford them and they would tell us to stop dancing. And we'd say, 'Yeah. Right. Cut off your right arm.' Even before I got cancer, I hated the insensitivity of conventional medicine. That's what kept me away."

When she was thirty-eight, BJ left New York for the backwoods of Connecticut. "I was fried," she says. "And needed some quiet space. That's when I found my voice. I moved from dance to writing and performing autobiographical stories." She got married at thirty-nine and created a movement theater, combining music and dance, called "Seen and Heard" with her husband, a cellist.

Three years after her wedding, when she was forty-two, BJ's diagnosis of breast cancer thrust her into the world of conventional medicine. And she did not like it. "I had the lumpectomy, a second one to get clear margins (to find out if the cancer has spread), but what do I do now?"

Onstage, BJ continues her story: "After my lumpectomy, it was time to go back for my post-op consultation. I gathered together my husband, a well-researched list of questions and a tape recorder. It's amazing what I don't hear at doctors' appointments." She walks across the stage and pretends to enter a consultation room.

Suddenly, her demeanor changes from fearful timidity to an assured posture with a deep, projecting voice. BJ has become an oncologist before our eyes. She begins speaking: "You have an invasive ductal carcinoma, 1.7 centimeters in size," she pronounces, assuming the doctor's distant, slightly lecturing tone. "The question is how to predict the biological behavior of this tumor in you. What was it doing before it was removed? Was it just there or has it it spread to someplace else in your body?" Without giving the now-invisible BJ time to speak, BJ-as-the-doctor carries on: "We don't have a great test for systemic involvement. We do CAT scans, bone scans, liver/spleen scans, blood tests. But none of these are sensitive enough to find anything at the microscopic level."

BJ is herself again, wondering what the answer is. What are they recommending? "I finally understood what my options were," she says. "Remove most of my breast and use radiation and chemotherapy to kill any cells that might have spread elsewhere. That was my best chance of catching this cancer before it invaded my body." But there was a problem. "For me, at that time, slicing off my breast, or even a part of it, was not an option." She began reading voraciously about breast cancer and the treatment options.

"I had to be honest with myself; at that time I felt that the current options Western medicine had to offer, toxic doses of chemotherapy, lethal rays of radiation, and hormone-altering prescriptions of tamoxifen were not forms of healing. They frightened me." Onstage, BJ walks backwards, hands held protectively in front of her, until she is deep in the back of the stage, just the way she backed away from conventional medicine and its recommendations. "Friends began sending me articles from alternative periodicals, newsletters from clinics in Europe, books about people who are cancer free because. . . . And I find myself entering the world of alternative medicine."

Loud circus music now fills the theatre. BJ is suddenly a ringmaster: "Ladies and gentlemen, welcome to the land of healing! Where you can find your way back to complete health and you will probably feel better than you have ever felt in your entire life!" The circus music dies down, and BJ darts around the stage in desperation, acting out the next period of her life in quick vignettes, taking on the characters, complete with gestures and accents, of one alternative healer after another.

During the two years that followed, BJ tried dozens of alternative treatments, beginning with the healer who told her to go outside and walk in her bare feet to absorb the energy of mother earth. "I change my diet three times, eliminating almost everything at one time or another," she tells the audience. "Then there is bee sting therapy, home colonics (don't ask) and massive supplements (thirty pills a day). I rub my breasts with essential oils, collect weeds, dry them and make infusions. I take shamanic journeys, go to a sweat lodge, and even go to the woman in New York City for two hundred dollars an hour who works with angels and light. I apply pine tar poultices to my breasts for six weeks to draw the cancer out. I use Bach flower remedies, get a live red blood cell analysis and jump on a mini-trampoline to stimulate my immune system. Three times a day I sit quietly and visualize the cancer in my body. It appears to be a pile of black slime. Then I visualize something to eliminate the cancer." Now she is a Samurai warrior, brandishing an imaginary sword, uttering bloodcurdling war cries and hacking the cancer to pieces.

Onstage at this point, BJ stops in confusion: "Sometimes the alternatives are as difficult as what Western medicine asks you to do! I have an acupuncturist, a naturopath, homeopath, physical therapists—none of them agree on what kinds of supplements I should be taking." She circles the stage as she talks, seeming to search for answers she cannot find. "I am trying to stay on my diet (and I have never had to diet before in my life!), keep up with the latest drugs, treatments, doctors." She comes to center stage: "I'm so overwhelmed! I've become my own medical consultant without training."

A Second Lump and a "Hyphenated" Hospital

Then BJ finds a second lump. The alternative treatments are not working. Onstage, she suddenly becomes a swaggering John Wayne, thumbs hooked into her belt loops. "Weyell. . . ." She drawls. "Ah guess it's tahm to saddle up, little filly, and head on back to Western medicine. They can't *all* be wrong. Go on now. Go on and get yourself a *diagnosis*. It's tahm to go to a cancer treatment center, a medical industrial complex. (Pause) A *hah*fenated hospital."

"Whoa!" says BJ to John Wayne. "That's a huge paradigm shift!"

She then acts out what happens after John Wayne sent her back to Western medicine: Her first stop was a well-known cancer center for a day of tests and appointments. And yes, it did have a hyphenated name. BJ tells the audience how she had a needle biopsy and many tests, then wandered through the vast complex to find the oncologist's office: "They escort me to an examining room . . . There's a knock on the door. The doctor enters with three interns. 'Do you mind if they join us?' he says. 'It's a teaching hospital.' No . . . I mean yes. I feel intimidated with four men I do not know and me alone in this room. They interrogate me about my previous treatment choices, look at the results of the core needle biopsy and all the other tests, and make sure to show me the treatment center before I leave."

When it is time for BJ to return to find out the results of the tests, she comes prepared. She confides her plan to the audience with a conspiratorial wink: "I contact my friend Annie. She comes from a family of doctors. They do not intimidate her. On the day of the appointment we advance on the complex (she skulks around the stage), infiltrate the parking structure and find a strategic location for our vehicle. We don our protective gear—I am feeling a little scared—leather jackets, fluorescent punk rock wigs, sunglasses and big, red clown noses. We gain access to the elevator and secure a consultation room. The doctor enters with his back-up units."

The astonishing thing, according to BJ, is that the doctors do not laugh. They do not ask why they are wearing wigs and clown noses. *They pretend not to notice.* Instead, BJ-as-the-doctor says: "The cancer has metastasized to your lungs. You now have Stage IV cancer. At this point we can only recommend hormonal treatment. Because your tumor is estrogen-positive we need to stop your body from producing estrogen. You can do monthly injections of Lupron or Zoladex. Side effects: loss of sex drive, hot flashes and a dry vagina. Or, daily doses of tamoxifen. Side effects: doubles the risk of blood clots and increases the chances of liver cancer. Or, we can just remove your ovaries."

What happened next: "When I asked how long the drug treatment would be, the doctor gave me what I have come to recognize as 'the oncology look,' which means, 'it doesn't really matter, you don't have long to live.'" She backs up once more downstage. "Man, I get out of there fast. I need another opinion."

In an interview after her performance, BJ talks about the choices she made: "I realize now that I should not have ignored conventional treatment," she says. "Especially since none of these alternative practitioners advised me to have blood tests, X rays or scans done to see if the cancer was spreading, which, in fact, it was. After two years of alternative treatments, I found out that the cancer had spread to my lungs. Eventually, it also spread to my brain and pelvis. Now I advise people to use every tool available to fight the cancer, that nutrition, acupuncture, massage and physical therapy can help your body cope with the standard treatments, like surgery, radiation and chemotherapy.

"People should also make sure to have frequent tests, beginning with a baseline test, so they can monitor the progression of the disease. Medicine is not an exact science, the treatment protocols are constantly changing and individuals react differently both to the disease and various treatments. At the time of my diagnosis, I didn't understand the severity of what it meant when the cancer spreads, and I did not even have a relationship with a doctor who could explain it to me."

She now tells anyone who will listen: "Don't run away from conventional treatments, or you could end up like me, battling metastatic cancer."

A Visit to Cancer College

A friend then tells BJ about a doctor who runs an *integrative* cancer treatment program in Chicago that combines conventional treatment with complementary methods. "I go to Dr. Keith I. Block's Web site and download a twenty-five-page questionnaire. Are you right- or left-handed? How do you feel about each and every one of your personal relationships? How often and for how long do you brush your teeth?"

She visits the Block Medical Center, located in an office building, is warmly greeted by the staff, all of whom are wearing street clothes, and is delighted by the soft, rounded furniture, a kitchen filled with organic protein drinks, herbal teas and sesame seaweed crackers, the photographs of nature decorating the walls and the small water fountain. "I met with the doctor. He said, 'We consider cancer a chronic disease. As long as you stay alive the more treatment options will be available to you.' His eyes are filled with hope and a belief in my body's ability to heal."

BJ begins a conventional cancer protocol—Taxol and Herceptin—but that is only part of the treatment. She also meets a nutritionist who explains a complex diet and carefully considered supplement plan that is designed to support her body while she is receiving chemotherapy. She is back up to forty pills a day, but this time she does not mind so much. She also works with a personal trainer; learns yoga and qigong (Chinese energy exercises), meditation and biofeedback; has a full body massage while hooked up to the chemotherapy machine and learns EMDR (a type of eye movement therapy) to control anxiety. "This was more than a treatment facility; it's like going to cancer college," says BJ.

BJ still flies to Chicago once a month for her treatments, which, despite the supportive regimens, leave her exhausted and with digestion problems. It is now two years later. The tumor in her breast is larger, and the cancer that had already spread to her lungs during the period of alternative treatments is still there. There are also tumors in her brain and pelvis. She has temporarily discontinued the chemotherapy because of a terrible skin rash but is continuing with Integrative Manual Therapy (a form of bodywork that she calls "high-end but loving medicine"), acupuncture, yoga, swimming and mindfulness meditation. In a recent interview, she says, "Everyone heals in a different way, and it's a question of finding the way that suits you. When I realized that I wasn't having success with the alternatives, I turned to conventional medicine. Unfortunately, the cancer had spread during that time. But now I'm about to start taking a new drug, Anverzel, instead of chemotherapy. The doctors in Chicago also recommended Arimedex, a hormone drug, but I am choosing not to do hormone treatment at this time. I'm not giving up. There's hope in every moment."

In addition to trying to beat the cancer, BJ is focusing all of her energy on performing *Keeping A Breast* in communities and medical centers. It was recently made into a documentary and aired on public television. "I'd like to make it available to as many patients and medical professionals as possible," says BJ in an interview. Then her voice suddenly becomes very small. "I just hope I live long enough to see that happen."

As of this writing, BJ is still working with her doctors to control the spread of cancer. She describes her experience as a continuous journey of choices. "When the drugs do not work, a patient is thrown into a vast world of choices. And the doctors are not always very informed about options other than chemo and hormone therapy. It is up to the patient to sift through the incredible amount of treatments available, while trying to stay centered and not get desperate. During this process, I tried to listen to my own body and honor what I as a person could tolerate."

In one of the last scenes of *Keeping A Breast*, BJ describes a trip to Mexico that she took in the middle of her chemotherapy treatment. She comes upon a basilica in the center of the town: "I walk inside the basilica. It's dark and cool. At the very end in the apse is a large glass column. At the top is Our Lady of Health, the Virgin. She's made from corn stalks and orchid glue, painted beautifully; her dress is blue, and her skin is creamy white. Blue curtains surround her. If I come at the right time of day the sun shines in through the stained glass window and falls on her face. It's quiet except for the sound of the women praying in Spanish. . . .

"I sit down. Then I'm on my knees praying." (BJ gets down on her knees on the stage.) "This is not a usual practice of mine so it sounds more like begging. 'Look, I've had this cancer for a long time, could you please take it out of my body?' Then I remember all the other people I know who have cancer. 'And while you are at it, could you take the cancer out of their bodies, too?' Then I think of all the other people I don't know who have cancer, 'How about a miracle? Could you just eliminate cancer altogether?' Then I think about all the suffering everywhere, and I look up to God. 'Please, a lot of healing needs to go on down here.'

"And I'm on my knees for a really long time."

❖ ❖ ❖ ❖

Integrative Cancer Care: A Healing Synthesis

"You have one shot with cancer," says Barrie R. Cassileth, Ph.D., chief of the Integrative Medicine Service at Memorial Sloan-Kettering Cancer Center in New York City. "Take it out when it's small and hasn't spread, then kill any remaining malignant cells with radiation or chemotherapy. The key is to treat cancer early. The longer you wait, the more difficult it is to cure cancer." For more than twenty years, Barrie Cassileth has worked with cancer patients who combined mainstream medicine and other approaches. She has also taught, researched and written about complementary medicine. When she was associate director of the University of Pennsylvania Cancer Center, Cassileth developed programs in hospice, home care, counseling and research. She is the author of *The Alternative Medicine Handbook: The Complete Reference Guide to Alternative and Complementary Therapies*.

When she talks about cancer, Cassileth's voice takes on an edge of passion. "It's suicide to let a curable tumor sit there and grow," she says. "That is a disaster. The more people we can reach with that message, the better."

Cassileth came to Memorial Sloan-Kettering three years ago, when she was recruited to create a program in integrative medicine for cancer patients. "Memorial Sloan-Kettering is the oldest and largest private cancer treatment center in the world, and generally thought to be one of the best," she says. "So the challenge of creating an integrative cancer service there to help patients and family members was very appealing." Cassileth stresses that integrative medicine is not the same as alternative medicine: "It is a synthesis of mainstream cancer care and the best of complementary medicine. At Sloan-Kettering, the oncologists and surgeons take care of the tumors; we take care of the patients' bodies, minds and spirits. We calm them down, lift their spirits, teach them how to keep their bodies strong and help alleviate pain and reduce side effects of the disease and its therapies." The philosophy of treatment is that strengthening the body, mind and spirit helps patients battle the disease and use mainstream treatments more effectively. "Patients have told us that they could not have gone through their cancer treatments without our services," says Cassileth.

When asked about patients who choose to eschew conventional cancer treatment—whether surgery, radiation or chemotherapy—in favor of alterna-tive treatments, Cassileth points out what to her is obvious: "If alternative approaches to cancer treatment worked, they would not be alternative," she says. "They would be used in every hospital and cancer center in the world. But in fact, they are 'alternative' precisely because they are unproved, and some are harmful. Patients who rely only on alternative treatments for cancer do not do well."

In two Memorial Sloan-Kettering outpatient buildings, cancer patients and their family members can improve the quality of their lives while they or their loved ones are undergoing cancer treatment. The array of choices is abundant: massage, reflexology, Shiatsu and several other kinds of bodywork; spiritual healing; art and music therapy; acupuncture; hypnotherapy; several kinds of meditation; guided imagery and visualization; yoga, tai chi, Alexander Technique, nutritional counseling and many more healing regimens. (Please see Appendix I for descriptions of these and other complementary treatments.) The services are available to patients and families no matter what their hospital affiliation, points out Cassileth. And the Sloan-Kettering Integrative Medicine Service is open to family members and staff as well.

Inpatients at Sloan-Kettering can also take advantage of complementary ser-vices. On any given day, a visitor to an inpatient ward might encounter a medi-tation teacher, music therapists playing a live concert, massage therapists or a yoga class. All of these services are available at no cost for inpatients. Many of these practitioners might be working with patients alone or alongside chemo-therapy nurses, oncologists or pain experts. (Outpatients are charged a relatively low fee for these services.)

"We work in close collaboration with the Pain Service, the Psychiatry Unit, as well as the oncology treatment teams," says Cassileth. "We have found, for example, that complementary therapies can often reduce the amount of pain medication that patients require." (Please see chapter 7 for details about complementary therapies for pain.)

How do Cassileth and her colleagues choose what services to offer? "Our complementary services are all data-driven," she says. "The only modalities we use are those that have been shown to be effective. We do not offer interventions based on concepts that run contrary to our scientific understanding of the way the body works."

In fact, the Integrative Medicine Service, in addition to caring for patients, is heavily involved in research, conducting some twenty different studies to assess the value of various complementary interventions for specific problems of cancer patients. "We are also doing basic research on several anti-tumor botanicals (plant and herbal remedies) for their therapeutic effects," says Cassileth. "Our botanical research may one day yield a product that can be used in cancer treatment."

The service also teaches cancer patients who want to learn how to help themselves. "There are ways to eat, live and function that help make cancer treatment more effective," she says. Each patient receives a booklet and other materials with concrete suggestions of how to use nutrition, herbs, over-the-counter remedies and complementary therapies to "ease the way" during cancer treatment. The patient education booklets and classes help patients deal with anxiety and stress, backache or muscle aches, colds and flu, digestion problems, depression, headache, nausea, chronic pain and sleep problems. One booklet contains warnings about herbal products and supplements that have serious toxic effects, especially when combined with other medications, chemotherapy or radiation therapy.

"It is important for patients to know, for example, that high doses of certain vitamins can actually feed a tumor," says Cassileth. "The overall message is that, with correct information and mainstream and complementary therapies, patients can take responsibility for their own lives."

Cancer Treatment: What's the Evidence?

Much has been written about the effectiveness of complementary and alternative approaches to cancer treatment and prevention. However, most experts in the field seem to agree with Barrie Cassileth that conventional cancer treatment is still the best option for patients, and that complementary and alternative (CAM) therapies should be used *in addition*, rather than *instead of* conventional treatment.

With that view, it is useful to determine which CAM treatments best help cancer patients cope with chemotherapy, pain, radiation and surgery. In his 2001 review of the world's research literature in complementary medicine,[1] Edzard Ernst tells us that both acupuncture[2] and hypnotherapy[3] have been found useful in controlling the nausea caused by chemotherapy, as well as pain. Relaxation therapy (breathing exercises, muscle relaxation and imagery) helped women with breast cancer experience a "better quality of life."[4]

Ernst points out, however, that many CAM studies are "preliminary at best," although several may improve the well-being of patients with cancer. These include "mind-body programs for stress, acupuncture, acupressure or ginger for nausea, tai chi and other gentle exercise techniques for gaining strength, aromatherapy, therapeutic massage and relaxation techniques to reduce stress, herbal medicines for depression, anxiety, indigestion and other symptoms, as well as acupuncture for pain." Unfortunately for patients who are looking for answers, the evidence in these areas is, according to Ernst, "often anecdotal, inconsistent and collectively unconvincing." But, he goes on to say, "Collectively, these data suggest that CAM may gain an important role in palliative/supportive cancer care. . . . This area clearly deserves more research; in particular we need to know whether

[1] E. Ernst, ed., *The Desktop Guide to Complementary and Alternative Medicine: An Evidence-Based Approach* (London: Harcourt Publishers Limited, 2001).

[2] A. J. Vickers, "Can Acupuncture Have Specific Effects on Health—A Systematic Review of Acupuncture Trials," *Journal of the Royal Society of Medicine* 89DF (1996): 303–311.

[3] K. L. Syrjala, C. Cummings, and G. W. Donaldson, "Hypnosis or Cognitive Behavioral Training for the Reduction of Pain and Nausea During Cancer Treatment: A Controlled Clinical Trial," *Pain* 50 (1992): 237–238.

[4] L. G. Walker et al., "Psychological, Clinical and Pathological Effects of Relaxation Training and Guided Imagery During Primary Chemotherapy," *British Journal of Cancer* 801, 1–2 (1999): 262–268.

treatments are in any way superior to conventional methods of palliative/supportive cancer care."

Homeopathy helped patients tolerate radiation but did not reduce tumors

Eighty-two patients about to undergo radiotherapy treatment for cancer were randomly divided into three groups. One group was given a placebo, and the two other groups were given homeopathic remedies. All the patients were checked for radiation reaction in eighteen different tests each week during the course of radio-therapy. Both the groups taking homoeopathic medicines had 30 percent less severe reaction to the radiotherapy than the placebo group. No significant reduction in the tumor regression rates in the patients was observed.[5]

Massage and aromatherapy improved general well-being of cancer patients

This study, which used a small sample of cancer patients undergoing treatment, suggested that massage, especially when combined with aromatherapy (using essential oils) had a significant effect on anxiety, by helping patients relax and reducing physical and emotional symptoms of anxiety. For cancer patients under-going treatment, massage and aromatherapy are being used increasingly by nurses to enhance the well-being of patients in palliative care settings, yet little evaluation of these therapies has been undertaken. The authors call for more research to be conducted in this area with more patients.[6]

In cancer care, integration is preferable

An article by Milton suggests that therapies such as acupuncture, acupressure, homeopathy, herbal preparations, imagery, and Therapeutic Touch may help with cancer symptoms or treatment effects, and that the ideal healthcare system is one that integrates alternative and complementary healing therapies into conventional care.[7]

---

[5] A. Kulkarni and G. S. Burde, "Radiation Protection by Use of *Homeopathic Medicines*," *Hahnemannian Homeopathic Sandesh* 12, no. 1 (1988): 20–23.

[6] J. Corner and S. Hildebrand, "An Evaluation of the Use of Massage and Essential Oils on the Wellbeing of Cancer Patients," *International Journal of Palliative Nursing* 1 (1995): 67–73. Copies of the full research report for this study may be obtained from the Macmillan Practice Development Unit, Centre for Cancer and Palliative Care Studies, Institute of Cancer Research/Royal Marsden NHS Trust, Fulham Road, London SW3 6JJ, UK.

[7] D. Milton, "Alternative and Complementary Therapies: Integration into Cancer Care," *AAOHN* (American Association of Occupational Health Nurses) *Journal* 46, no. 9 (1998): 454–461; quiz: 462–463.

Bodywork After Cancer Surgery:
"My Arm Was Swollen to Three Times Its Size"

Marjorie Heffernan, who is eighty, had undergone a radical mastectomy for breast cancer in 1967, followed by radiation. She remained cancer free until 1989, when she had a lumpectomy in the other breast, with more radiation. Since then, there has been no further recurrence, but her right arm (on the same side as the mastectomy) began to swell after the surgery. "Starting at least fifteen years ago, my arm kept swelling, until it was three times the normal size," she remembers. "The only way I could wear turtlenecks—which I needed to wear to cover up the scarring from the mastectomy—pajamas or any tops with long sleeves was to actually cut the right sleeve off. And I could *never* wear nice dresses, only jumpers."

The cause of the swelling was lymphodema. Often, surgery for breast or prostate cancer involves damaging or removing the lymph nodes that are located under the arm or in the groin. These nodes are part of the body's immune system: They filter lymph fluid—a clear, watery liquid containing white blood cells—which circulates through tissues and organs, picking up bacteria, proteins and other debris that might be harmful. The lymph fluid then carries these "interlopers" back to the lymph nodes to be filtered out. For example, when coal miners inhale coal dust, or smokers inhale tar, the lymph system filters the dirt out of the lungs.

If your lymph nodes are missing or damaged, this lymph fluid can become blocked, so it builds up in nearby tissues, sometimes causing large, painful swelling in arms, chest wall, back, legs or groin. As the tissue becomes more swollen, it can become hard or "fibrotic," causing extreme pain.

One solution is "manual lymphatic drainage," which Cindy Stewart provides regularly to cancer patients who have had breast or prostate surgery. (Please see "Four Ways to Feel Better," for more about Cindy.) "I start at the neck, where the lymph system originates," says Cindy. "Beginning on the non-compromised side, I use light, rhythmical massage along the entire route of the lymph system. The goal is to get the fluid moving again, redirecting it and training the healthy part of the lymph system to take over the work in the area where the lymph node is missing or damaged."

"My doctors told me the swollen arm was just something I had to live with, and to be glad I had survived the cancer," says Marjorie. "But one day I read an article in the Sunday paper about lymphodema and realized that's exactly what I had." Through the article, Marjorie found and joined a support group for lymphodema patients and also learned that there were treatments for the condition in Europe. "When I first went to the support group, I was amazed at how many young women had lymphodema after breast cancer surgery," says Marjorie. "Through them, I found out about a lymphodema treatment here in Boston that had been started by a doctor who came over here from Europe, but it was frightfully expensive." Once again, a newspaper article helped. "My son saw an article in the local paper about Cindy. That was in 1997."

Cindy worked with Marjorie every day for four weeks. "At home, she needed to wrap the arm herself after each massage session and keep it wrapped for twenty-four hours," says Cindy. "This keeps the lymph fluid moving out of the arm." After four weeks, the arm was almost down to its normal size. "One day, after several weeks of treatment, Cindy put a stretchy pressure sleeve on my arm, and I realized that it was close to normal size," says Marjorie. "When I got into the car with my husband I burst out crying and cried all the way home. This was the first time in fifteen years that I could wear normal clothing with two sleeves." Marjorie still sees Cindy every three months for follow-up treatments. "I continue to wrap and massage the arm every night," says Marjorie. "It was a miracle the way Cindy changed my life. She's my angel."

Note that while Marjorie has to pay for the manual lymphatic drainage treatments herself, the therapy is offered routinely (and covered by insurance) in many European countries as part of standard medical care. In one study, the authors compared manual lymphatic drainage (i.e., Cindy Stewart's method) to pneumatic pressure methods (using inflatable sleeves pumped up with air) to treat lymphodema after mastectomy. They found that the manual method produced significantly better outcomes than the pressure therapy methods.[8]

---

[8] R. Zanolla et al., "Evaluation of the Results of Three Different Methods of Post-Mastectomy Lymphodema Treatment," *Journal of Surgical Oncology* 16 (1984): 210–213.

Tapping into the Immune Power of the Body

"Going one hundred miles an hour all the time," is how Marcelle Tennenbaum described her life before she was diagnosed with non-Hodgkins lymphoma. "I think that's what destroyed my immune system."

A native of Paris, Marcelle met her husband, Robert, an architect, while she was on holiday in the United States and he was a student at Yale. "We met at Christmas and were engaged by New Year's. We just clicked," says Marcelle, her impeccable English still carrying a slight Parisian accent. "That was forty-one years ago. Now we have two daughters and four grandsons."

Until she was fifty-five years old, Marcelle was energetic and healthy, rarely even catching colds. She worked full-time for a corporation that leased and managed retail space in shopping centers. "I was a typical corporate career woman," she says. "Dealing with stressful situations, traveling all over, negotiating contracts and managing properties."

But in that year she began to feel tired all the time. "I was *never* tired before," she says. "I couldn't figure out what was wrong with me." She decided to take advantage of her seniority and to retire from her job. Then I started walking every day for exercise. I thought that was all I needed." But the tiredness persisted. "Six months later, suddenly, out of nowhere, there was a severe pain in my ribcage. It hurt every time I breathed."

The next day, Marcelle's husband took her to the clinic of their health plan in Columbia, Maryland. "They did test after test, but six weeks later they still hadn't figured out what was wrong," says Marcelle. "They kept saying it was in my head, but I *knew* it was not in my head. Then my lung collapsed." Robert was rapidly losing patience. "He told them that he wanted a full body scan done, and he wanted it *today*," says Marcelle. "I was grateful that he was there to take charge. I was feeling too weak and ill to do much of anything."

The body scan revealed a spleen that weighed six pounds. (A normal spleen weighs eight to ten ounces.) "The doctors were shocked," remembers Marcelle. "They panicked, and they scared the wits out of me. They said I needed surgery. During a six-hour operation, the surgeon removed the enlarged spleen.

"But that wasn't the worst of it," says Marcelle. "Then they told me that I had non-Hodgkins lymphoma, and that's what had caused the spleen to get so large. The local oncologist at our health plan explained that this was a cancer of the lymphatic system and that in six months I'd be dead." Marcelle simply could not believe this. "I had recovered from the surgery quickly and had been able to resume my walking program within three weeks. I was finally feeling great again. And here was my doctor telling me I was going to die. It didn't make any sense."

Robert took action once again, arranging for Marcelle to be seen by experts at the National Institutes of Health in Washington, D.C. "Dr. Wilson examined me, looked at my tests, and then said to me, 'You look like a healthy woman. In your case, I'd like to see you watch and wait, and not jump into bone marrow transplants or chemotherapy just yet,'" says Marcelle. "By that time, Robert and I decided to switch my care to Dr. Aaron Rapoport at the Greenebaum Cancer Center in the University of Maryland."

Rapoport, a hematologist and stem-cell transplant physician, is an expert in cancers of the blood, including leukemia, lymphoma and myeloma. In addition to caring for patients, he does clinical research that investigates using the patient's own cells to boost the immune system and fight these cancers, as well as high-dose chemotherapy. "When I met Mrs. Tennenbaum, examined her and heard her history, I realized that she actually had a subtype of the cancer that is fairly slow-growing," says Rapoport. "In fact, people can often live with this type of lymphoma for years before requiring conventional cancer treatment."

The level of the disease is measured by the concentration of a certain protein "marker" in the blood, called IgM. These levels had dropped immediately after Marcelle's surgery, but then had slowly continued to rise. "When I met her, she had an IgM level of 941 milligrams (per deciliter of blood), and it was increasing," says Rapoport (A normal range would be approximately 200 or lower). "She also had an enlarged lymph node in her abdomen. Because of the indolent nature of this cancer and her open-mindedness to alternative methods, I decided that conventional cancer treatment was not indicated at this time." Marcelle read an article about Dr. Brian Berman, who directs the Complementary Medicine Program at the University of Maryland and decided to ask if he would see her.

"I had already begun to change my diet," says Marcelle, "but Dr. Berman inspired me even further. I eliminated all junk food and drank only bottled water. I went completely organic. I had increased my daily walks to about six miles, and he suggested that I also try qigong exercises to open my meridians and increase my energy. I took a class and now do it at home every day. I also received Reiki treatments, and even became a Reiki practitioner, and I did acupuncture once a week, which also helped with some unrelated back pain. Dr. Berman also started me on vitamin therapy as well as homeopathic medicines for the symptoms and to help reduce the IgM protein level in my blood." (Please see "A Closer Look at Energy Healing, Spirituality and Therapeutic Touch" for more about Reiki; and chapters 2 and 6 for descriptions and research about traditional Chinese medicine, including acupuncture and qigong energy work.)

Marcelle has kept up this regimen for nearly five years. "I am very diligent," she says. "When I start something, I do it. Especially since I knew that if the protein level reached 1,000, I would probably have to start chemotherapy and have a bone marrow transplant, both of which terrified me." Seven months into this complementary treatment combination, Marcelle's protein cancer marker levels began to drop for the first time. Between July of 1998 and February, 1999, the level dropped nearly 500 points, and the CAT scan showed that her lymph node had begun to shrink as well. Her most recent test showed a protein level of 275, barely above normal, and her lymph node has remained stable, only slightly enlarged. She is jubilant.

"It's like a miracle," she says. "I was able to strengthen my immune system and fight this cancer without medication. Both Dr. Rapoport and Dr. Berman believe that everybody's body has the ability to fight disease if you stimulate it properly. I also know I was lucky that the type of cancer that I had responded to this treatment.

Marcelle still has her protein level monitored regularly and if it remains stable, will only have to be checked once a year; the diet and lifestyle changes she has made seem to have become permanent. From his scientific perspective, Rapoport is cautious, although he is delighted with Marcelle's progress. "There is still no clear, scientific evidence that the complementary interventions she is using enhance immune function," he says. "Still, we must acknowledge that the immune system is complex, and does interact with the nervous system. Interventions that enhance emotion and general health may well have a beneficial effect on the immune system response to cancer. It is, however difficult to demonstrate immune system response in the laboratory—and even more difficult in real life."

Although he practices conventional oncology, Rapoport describes himself as open-minded to nonconventional and complementary interventions, especially for patients like Marcelle, who have a natural inclination toward such practices. He is careful to caution, however, that "Mrs. Tennenbaum's type of lymphoma, which is a low-grade, slow-moving cancer, is more likely to be amenable to complementary therapies, and there was no indication for conventional treatment at the time I saw her. However, I would not expect complementary treatment alone to work for more aggressive lymphomas."

❖ ❖ ❖ ❖

Fighting Breast Cancer with the Best of Both Worlds: "We Have Four Children. Going Home to Wait for Cancer to Recur Was Not an Option."

Julie Arredondo of Chandler, Arizona, was stunned when she woke up in the recovery room after her biopsy. "Babe, it was cancer," said her husband, Ralph, his face white. "I was still foggy from the anesthesia, but I could see how distraught he was," says Julie. "Behind him, the nurse was looking at me sympathetically. I couldn't believe what he was saying. All I could say was, 'What?' When we went home, I cried."

Julie was thirty-four years old and had four children. Her diet was healthy. She got plenty of exercise. "We had an active, full life; my husband had a successful business; I was getting a graduate degree in nutrition; life was good," she says. She was conscientious about her breast self-exams and had found the lump herself. She had even asked her doctor for more detailed instructions a few months earlier. ("I just had a strange feeling to be more vigilant," she says.) She followed the surgeon's advice and had a biopsy, although he had told her there was a 90 percent chance the lump was benign. "That's why I was so shocked at the diagnosis," she says. "But even more disturbing was the news that this was a very aggressive type of cancer, especially dangerous at my age."

The surgeon recommended a mastectomy as soon as possible, to be followed by chemotherapy. Julie decided to have the operation immediately. "I wanted to live," she says. Seven days after the biopsy, she was back in the hospital for the mastectomy. Six weeks after that, the chemotherapy was to begin.

Stunned as she was with the suddenness of her cancer diagnosis and mastectomy, Julie's real nightmare did not begin until June 1999, with the first chemotherapy treatment. "I was anxious about the chemotherapy," says Julie. "The nurse showed up with two *huge* syringes of bright red liquid. This was adriamycin. A second drug, cytoxin, was to go in through an intravenous drip."

Julie was concerned for two reasons: she is highly sensitive to drugs of any kind; and she has Type I (juvenile) diabetes, diagnosed after the birth of her second child. "After all of these years of protecting my body's health and specifically my circulation to *prevent* heart disease (a risk for diabetics), I was now about to take toxic drugs, one of which is associated with heart damage," she says. "But I felt like I had no choice but to agree to the recommended treatment. Even before my diagnosis, I had been following Dr. Andrew Weil's 8 *Weeks to Optimum Health*. After the diagnosis, I had tried to get seen at his integrative medicine clinic in Tucson, but there was a two-year waiting list. I knew I couldn't wait that long, so I decided to go ahead with the chemo."

The vomiting began almost as soon as Ralph pulled into their driveway after that first chemotherapy treatment. "I was opening the door and running into the house before he had even shifted into park," says Julie. The vomiting increased in intensity over the next few hours, so that soon there was not even a pause to catch her breath. "It became one continuous convulsion. I couldn't even straighten up to take a breath. None of the anti-vomiting drugs they had given me before the chemotherapy were working," says Julie.

The convulsive vomiting was to go on for the next twenty-four hours, but Ralph did not wait that long to call the oncologist. "Because I was dehydrated, we knew that I needed intravenous fluids to restore the correct balance of insulin and carbohydrates in my body, or I could go into a life-threatening diabetic coma," says Julie. "But the oncologist told Ralph that vomiting was to be expected. He did not address the diabetes at all. He said in twenty years he had never had to admit a chemotherapy patient and did not think it was necessary now. Ralph took one look at me convulsing, and said, 'I'm taking her to the hospital.'"

Ralph called 911 as soon as he had hung up from the doctor. "I was still vomiting in the ambulance, and they had trouble getting an IV into me because of the dehydration," says Julie. "And they could only use my left arm because of the mastectomy on my right side. I kept blowing the IV lines with the vomiting." Julie stayed in the hospital almost ten days. "By the second day, the violent vomiting had begun to slow down somewhat, but I almost passed out from weakness," says Julie. "Luckily, my insulin pump was the only thing working properly, and I used it to give myself insulin, but I knew that I also needed IV glucose to restore the proper balance in my body. My endocrinologist was on vacation, but I finally convinced the oncologist and the endocrinologist on call to order a glucose IV." To make matters worse, Julie had developed painful hive-like lesions on her face within a few days after the chemotherapy was given.

"My oncologist had no idea how to deal with a cancer patient with diabetes," says Julie. "We are a completely different species from the general population of cancer patients. If we don't address our special needs, the chemotherapy will kill us before the cancer does." After Julie's condition had stabilized and she was discharged, the surgeon and the oncologist decided to try again, this time with a different chemotherapy combination. "They administered two different drugs —methotrexate and 5FU—through an IV and sent me home with enough cytoxin pills to take three every day for seven days," says Julie. "I started vomiting after the second pill. I was so afraid that the uncontrollable vomiting would start again, that I just could not put another pill into my mouth."

She met with her oncologist once again, who told her that she appeared to have no tolerance for chemotherapy. "I said, 'What do I do now?' He told me to go home and wait for a recurrence. I said, 'We have four children. That is not an option.' And to top everything off, I was still trying to keep my diabetes under control." By this time, Julie's endocrinologist was back in town. "I told her that I wanted a new oncologist," says Julie. "From the beginning, the first oncologist had transformed me from an optimistic, energetic person into an emotional and physical wreck. For example, we had asked him, 'How do you know when you have cured cancer?' His answer was, 'When you die of something else.'"

A Ray of Hope

Julie's doctor referred her to a different oncologist, Dr. Ellen Gustafson. "She was my first ray of hope," says Julie. "She said, 'This cancer is treatable. There is no reason you can't be cured.' And she was the first person who ever asked Ralph how he was doing during all this. Dr. Gustafson was willing to work with me to figure out how I could tolerate chemotherapy. I decided to try Dr. Weil's clinic again." This time, Julie left a detailed message about her situation and got a phone call two days later, offering her a cancellation appointment that same week. "It is nearly a two-hour drive from my house to the clinic," says Julie. "So they were willing to arrange for me to see all of their specialists in one visit. I met with a clinical fellow, a nutritionist from the Arizona Cancer Center and a doctor of pharmacy on that first day. I told them everything that had happened, and that I had been following Dr. Weil's program on my own for the past year and a half."

Working closely with Julie and Dr. Gustafson, the staff at the clinic came up with a combined chemotherapy and complementary medicine program for Julie. The clinic is part of the University of Arizona Integrative Medicine Program, one of the nation's first academic programs in integrative medicine. In addition to caring for patients, the University of Arizona program, founded by Andrew Weil, M.D., also conducts research in complementary and integrative medicine and trains board-certified physicians through fellowship programs. "We are at an exciting time in the evolution of health care, as conventional and alternative medicine begin to coalesce," says Weil. "The speed with which medical institutions, including medical schools, are beginning to be open to integrative medicine is astonishing and very gratifying."

For Julie, the integrative program meant that she could have the best of both worlds: effective cancer treatment as well as complementary therapies to help her body cope with it. "The body responds to chemotherapy drugs as poison and tries to expel them as quickly as possible," says Ellen Gustafson, Julie's oncologist. "Julie is particularly sensitive to chemotherapy, and that is what caused the uncontrollable vomiting."

Julie knew she needed the chemotherapy, but she also knew that she needed help to tolerate the side effects. "We don't have an alternative cancer therapy," stresses Victoria Maizes, M.D., executive director of the Arizona Integrative Medicine Program. "We commonly urge people to do conventional cancer treatment, and we often see patients who have, in fact, completed the treatment. They are exhausted from the chemo. They're frightened that the cancer will recur, and they want to strengthen their immune system. They are looking for *adjuvant* therapies—to support and enhance the conventional treatment and mitigate the side effects. That is what we offer." The program serves not only cancer patients but also uses the same integrated approach to help patients with a wide variety of medical problems.

Dr. Weil describes Julie's situation, even with the diabetes, as fairly typical among cancer patients at his clinic. "Most cancer patients need and want advice about how to reduce toxicity and increase the efficacy of conventional treatments," he says. "They also want advice about how to reduce the risk of recurrences and improve general health."

✓ TAKE ACTION ✓

Best ways to cope with cancer treatment

Following are several suggestions from the University of Arizona Integrative Medicine Program to improve immune function and reduce side effects during and after chemotherapy:

During chemotherapy

What to avoid: "We do not advise antioxidants, such as green tea or vitamins E and C during chemotherapy, because there is potential risk that they interfere with the cancer-fighting properties of the chemo," says Victoria Maizes, M.D., executive director.

What works

To control nausea and exhaustion during chemo: Maizes recommends acupuncture; Chinese herbs; fresh ginger or ginger pills; small, frequent meals; and certain homeopathic remedies, such as ipecac and *nux vomica.*

For "anticipatory nausea": Guided imagery, considered a form of self-hypnosis, can be helpful. Maizes described one patient who used guided imagery in a different way, visualizing her cancer cells as being "misguided," and imagining that they were being retrained and redirected in "school." (Please see "What Is Guided Imagery?" in chapter 9.)

After chemotherapy

Maizes and her staff recommend several ways to build up the immune system:

Supplements and herbs, including coenzyme Q10; certain medicinal mushrooms; garlic; astragalus and green tea (for their antioxidant and anti-cancer properties); melatonin; vitamins E and C; selenium and mixed carotenes.

Immune-enhancing, anti-cancer diets that staff nutritionists develop according to the needs of each patient. Common recommendations for almost all cancer patients include:

Increasing the proportion of fruits and vegetables in your diet. Maizes suggests making a plant-based diet the bottom, largest section of your "food pyramid."

Eating more cruciferous vegetables, including broccoli, cauliflower, Brussels sprouts and cabbage, especially if you have a hormone-related cancer such as breast or prostate.

Eating fish for the beneficial omega-3 oils.

Eating organic food as much as possible, to give the immune system less work to do.

Julie began at the Integrative Medicine Clinic with a ninety-minute "intake interview" with one of the doctors. "Our goal is to fully understand the human being behind the symptoms and disease," says Maizes. "We teach our physician-fellows to delve into the context of the patient's life, to understand life-shaping events, strengths, intuitions, weaknesses and spiritual practices. We find it critical toward giving the patient advice. We try to reflect back to them a breadth of recommendations about how they might use the illness to transform their lives."

After meeting with Julie, the clinic staff worked with her and her oncologist to come up with a plan. Julie would be admitted to the hospital every three weeks, on a Monday, to start the chemotherapy. She would then spend the rest of the week in the hospital, so that her fluids and blood sugar could be tested regularly and modified, if necessary, with intravenous glucose and her insulin pump. "To control the vomiting, they gave me a combination of drugs which did help," says Julie.

In addition to the conventional medication, Julie followed a nutritionist's special diet to support her body during chemotherapy and address her needs as a diabetic. "I increased my intake of protein as well as plenty of fresh fruits and vegetables," she says. She also used weekly acupuncture—with "intense" sessions scheduled before and after each chemotherapy treatment—as well as Chinese herbs and dietary methods to control the nausea, both at home and in the hospital. According to a systematic review of the literature, acupuncture was found to have "a useful role" in reducing nausea induced by chemotherapy.[9]

"I juiced vegetables at home, mostly carrots combined with fresh ginger, and was surprised at how much that helped with the nausea between chemotherapy treatments," says Julie. "I also took ginger tablets when I felt a wave of nausea coming on." She kept up a regular routine of moderate physical exercise, which Maizes says is "invaluable" to good health during cancer treatment.

Using this combination of methods, Julie was able to tolerate the full course of seven chemotherapy treatments, delivered over a period of twenty-one weeks. "I was discharged from the hospital for the last time on November 6, 1999," says

---

[9] Vickers, "Can Acupuncture Have Specific Effects on Health?"

Julie. "It was the day I turned thirty-five and my daughter, our youngest, turned five. We had the most incredible feeling as a whole family that day, and an amazing celebration. We had made it!"

It has been more than two years since that day. While Julie did find one other breast lump, it was benign, and her scans and blood tests have shown no further recurrence of the cancer. Her hair has grown back, curly, thick and shiny, and she looks tall, slim and healthy. "People cannot believe I was ever sick," she says. She is now working full-time for the One Hundred Club of Arizona, a non-profit organization that provides financial benefits to the families of public safety personnel who have been killed or injured in the line of duty.

Victoria Maizes has many success stories like Julie's, but she is quick to caution against "blaming the patient" when things do not go as well. "It is impossible to detect all of the environmental, genetic or psychological influences on disease, especially cancer," she says. "We believe that there are multiple reasons why people get sick, and while mind-body therapies are very potent, people should realize that the causes of disease are complex."

In discussing the philosophy of integrative medicine, Maizes also talks about the importance of the healing process in both living and dying. "Whether or not people will survive their cancer, we believe that there can be growth and healing in the experience," she says. "As Michael Lerner teaches us so eloquently, the process of healing into dying can be a powerful opportunity for coming to peace in the journey of life."

SOY AND BREAST CANCER

Researchers at the University of Illinois at Chicago have found that soy may actually enhance the cancer-fighting effects of one breast cancer drug, tamoxifen. In an animal study, it was found that tamoxifen alone reduced the number of carcinogen-induced tumors by 29 percent. Soy alone reduced the number of tumors by 37 percent. But the two in combination reduced the number of tumors by 62 percent. Andreas Constantinou, Ph.D., associate professor of surgical oncology and associate director of research in the university's Functional Foods for Health Program, reported these findings in March 2001 at an annual meeting of the American Association of Cancer Research in New Orleans.

In a more recent study, Constantinou and his colleagues investigated whether the tumor-fighting effects of soy are due to soy compounds known as isoflavones. They found in animal studies that soy protein isolate—*whether or not it contained isoflavones*—prevented chemically induced breast tumors in rats, when compared to a diet that did not contain any soy. In fact, the diet that contained soy alone, without isoflavones, seemed to be slightly more beneficial. This study, published in May 2002 was the first to demonstrate these results. "Our findings are somewhat controversial," said Constantinou shortly after the study was published. "Up until now, there has been the general belief that soy isoflavones are beneficial in preventing breast cancer. In this particular study, in rats, it was shown that soy itself is beneficial, with or without isoflavones, and that isoflavones may even reduce the benefits slightly. Our research is continuing."

In an ongoing study with Northwestern University, Constantinou and other researchers are investigating soy protein isolate in human clinical trials of women who are at high risk for breast cancer. "We are evaluating whether women who are given soy protein isolate lower their cancer risk by measuring 'molecular cancer markers' (changes in cells or molecules that show a predisposition to cancer), when compared to women whose diets do not include soy protein isolate," says Constantinou. Cancer markers include cells that have damaged DNA, oncogenes (cancer-causing genes) that become "switched on," as well as specialized cells that suddenly becoming unspecialized. "If a cell that is specialized becomes

(continued)

unspecialized, there is potential for a tumor," explains Constantinou. "Unspecialized cells divide much more quickly and therefore have the potential to become cancerous." Results from this study should be available late in 2002 or early 2003. "Our preliminary animal studies indicate that soy is beneficial in preventing breast cancer," says Constantinou. "We do not yet know the optimal dosage of soy protein isolate, but if women are looking for guidelines, twenty-five grams of soy protein has already been recommended as beneficial to prevent cardiovascular disease."

Constantinou is familiar with recent controversial studies that link soy to the *promotion* of breast cancer. He notes that these studies used mouse models that he feels "were not appropriate" to provide data for cancer prevention in humans. "These studies used purified 'genistein,' an isoflavone or plant-derived estrogen (also called a phytoestrogen)," he points out. "It is important to realize that purified genistein is not the same as soybeans and that soybeans are a lot more than genistein. With supplements such as genistein and soy isoflavones, there are simply not enough data yet to determine whether they are harmful or helpful," he says. Within the next year, Constantinou will be publishing research further exploring the relationship between soy and the anti-cancer drug tamoxifen.

The University of Illinois at Chicago/National Institutes of Health Center for Botanical Dietary Supplement Research in Women's Health can be reached at 312-996-7253, or *www.uic.edu/pharmacy/research/diet.*

(Please see also chapter 10 for more about botanical research for women's health, particularly menopause.)

INTEGRATIVE MEDICINE TREATMENT CENTERS AND INFORMATIONAL WEB SITES

The University of Arizona Program in Integrative Medicine, Patient Care Services: 520-626-7599 or 520-626-9355 or e-mail questions to *imclinic@ahsc.arizona.edu*. Web site: *www.integrativemedicine.arizona.edu/clinic.html*.

Memorial Sloan-Kettering Integrative Cancer Service, New York City. Outpatient Center: 212-639-4700. Inpatient Services: 212-639-8629. Web site: *www.mskcc.org/integrativemedicine*.

Dana-Farber Cancer Institute, Leonard P. Zakim Center for Integrated Therapies, Boston. 617-632-3322. Web site: *www.danafarber.org/patient/zakim.shtml*.

Block Medical Center for Integrative Cancer Care, Evanston, Illinois. 847-492-3040. Web site: *www.blockmedical.com*.

Cancer information Web sites:

www.cancerdecisions.com (Ralph Moss, Ph.D.)

www.annieappleseedproject.org (contains information about alternative and conventional treatments as well as relevant research summaries.)

References

Constantinou, A., et al. "Soy Protein Isolate Prevents Chemically Induced Rat Mammary Tumors." *Pharmaceutical Biology* 40 (2002): 24–34.

Ernst, E., ed. *The Desktop Guide to Complementary and Alternative Medicine: An Evidence-Based Approach*. London: Harcourt Publishers Limited, 2001.

Lerner, M. *Choices in Healing: Integrating the Best of Conventional and Complementary Approaches to Cancer*. Cambridge: MIT Press, 1994.

Syrjala, K. L., C. Cummings, and G. W. Donaldson. "Hypnosis or Cognitive Behavioral Training for the Reduction of Pain and Nausea During Cancer Treatment: A Controlled Clinical Trial." *Pain* 50 (1992): 237–238.

Vickers, A. J. "Can Acupuncture Have Specific Effects on Health?—A Systematic Review of Acupuncture Trials." *Journal of the Royal Society of Medicine* 89DF (1996): 303–311.

Walker, L. G., et al. "Psychological, Clinical and Pathological Effects of Relaxation

Training and Guided Imagery During Primary Chemotherapy." *British Journal of Cancer* 801, 1–2 (1999): 262–268.

Zanolla, R., et al. "Evaluation of the Results of Three Different Methods of Post-Mastectomy Lymphodema Treatment." *Journal of Surgical Oncology* 16 (1984): 210–213.

 Integrative Cancer Care: What's the Evidence?

A large body of literature supports the use of complementary therapies in cancer care particularly in the area of diet, nutrition and guided imagery. (Please see Appendix II, under "Cancer," for a select listing of research studies in these areas, compiled by the University of Arizona Program in Integrative Medicine.)

Eating fruits and vegetables, for example, has been consistently related to a reduction in cancer risk. Antioxidant nutrients, including vitamin C, vitamin E, carotenoids and selenium, have been shown to inhibit cancer cell growth individually and in combination, although in some studies a worsened clinical course has been shown.

Guided imagery has a long history of popular use among cancer patients. Most studies are small, and survival benefit has not been shown, although cancer killer-cell activity has been shown to increase. The strongest evidence for guided imagery relates to mitigation of anticipatory nausea related to chemotherapy.

The anti-cancer properties of medicinal mushrooms have also been studied. Clinical trials show increases in natural killer-cell activity, reduction in tumor markers and increased survival. Different anti-cancer mechanisms have been postulated. In several studies, the suspected anti-tumor compound in the mushrooms—arabinoxylane—was synthesized in rice bran.

Please note that these therapies are in addition to, and not meant to replace, conventional cancer treatment and should only be used under medical supervision.

FOUR WAYS TO FEEL BETTER

1. A Closer Look at Muscular Therapy: Melting Away Pain

When massage therapist Cindy Stewart presses on a muscle that is in spasm with just the right amount of pressure, she can actually feel it give way. "It is as if the hard muscle melts under my fingers," she says. "Muscles go into spasm for a good reason: usually to protect an injured ligament by restricting any motion that might cause further damage. But over time, even after the ligament heals, that tight muscle can create chronic pain."

Tight muscles are only one cause of pain, says Cindy. Scar tissue is another. "When ligaments or muscles are injured, even by tiny 'micro-tears,' scar tissue begins to form in six to eight days to repair the damage," she explains. "Normally, this scar tissue—made of collagen—gets laid down over the injury like a tangled jumble of spaghetti, going in all directions. Often, this tangled collagen restricts the lengthwise movement of the tissue, so people experience pain when they try to regain their full range of motion."

Most of Cindy's clients come to her because of chronic pain in the lower back and neck, usually caused by motor vehicle accidents or some other physical trauma. "Their pain has restricted their lives," says Cindy. "It affects the way they walk, what activities they can do, how they move their bodies in daily activity. They don't want to live on pain medications for the rest of their lives. So they turn to massage."

Cindy, forty-six, is an athletic-looking woman with short blonde hair and a ready smile. A swimmer and biker, she has always been attracted to the idea of helping people reach their full physical potential. One of her favorite college jobs was working with disabled children in a summer camp, under the direction of a physical therapist. "I was majoring in health and physical education and just loved helping these kids learn and achieve new athletic goals," says Cindy. "It was so rewarding to see their excitement when they accomplished something that I wanted to be with them all the time. So I drove the bus to pick them up in the morning and even started teaching them swimming and art. I did it all." After college, Cindy spent twelve years coaching women's college basketball at Brown, Keene and Harvard Universities. "But those seventy-hour work weeks started to burn me out," says Cindy. She first considered becoming a physical therapist but finally settled on massage therapy. "I wanted the direct, hands-on contact with people and their rehabilitation," she says. After graduating from the Muscular Therapy Institute in Cambridge, Massachussetts, Cindy did advanced training focusing on the treatment of injuries. "I had had a lot of experience with athletic injuries as a coach, so this seemed the natural path for me," she says.

Cindy uses what she calls a "frictioning" technique to break up the tangled mass of collagen scar tissue that restricts movement and causes pain. The technique involves using her fingers to probe deeply into the area of the pain. "I use my fingers to massage across the width of the injured ligament, rather than the length," says Cindy. "This is called cross-fiber frictioning and it also helps release the fascia." (The fascia is a like a "sleeve" of tissue that overlays all muscles and organs and can become restricted by scar tissue after an injury.) "By going *across* the ligament, I can begin to break up the collagen fibers of the scar tissue and encourage the body to lay down new *lengthwise* collagen that follows the line of the ligament and will not restrict movement." If this work is begun within a few days after the injury—within pain tolerance—Cindy says she can often avoid the buildup of restrictive scar tissue in the first place.

Cindy describes one client who had such severe neck pain after a car accident that she could not turn her head. She also had some numbness in her arm. "She had tried physical therapy, but it did not give her permanent relief," says Cindy. "And she didn't want to do these exercises for the rest of her life." Cindy used the frictioning technique to break up the restrictive scar tissue, and also gave her client "homework" that included icing the area and stretching exercises to keep the new scar tissue long and supple. After several weeks, the client regained more range of motion and the numbness disappeared. As an added bonus, her long-standing headaches became less intense and less frequent.

In addition to reducing scar tissue, the frictioning technique also works on tight muscles, Cindy points out. "But because muscles cover a larger area, I might use all my fingers, or even my elbow, to go across the muscle and break up the tight fibers. By contrast, breaking up scar tissue on a ligament might take just one finger frictioning across the fibers.

(Please see the previous chapter for a special massage technique, called "manual lymphatic drainage," that Cindy uses to reduce swelling after breast and prostate cancer surgery.)

No matter what part of the body Cindy is working on, she describes an almost "instinctive" feeling that guides her. "You need just the right amount of pressure to break up scar tissue working within the client's pain tolerance; and if a muscle is in spasm, too much pressure might make it worse. You need to coax it to release," she says. "After so many years, I have learned to trust what I feel is going on under my fingers."

WHAT IS MASSAGE?

Massage involves touch and movement. It is "the systematic manipulation of the soft tissues of the body to enhance health and healing," according to Lynda W. Freeman, Ph.D., author of *Best Practices in Complementary and Alternative Medicine: An Evidence-Based Approach with Nursing CE/CME.* Freeman credits a researcher's determination to help her own infant with the beginning of therapeutic massage—also known as touch therapy—as a medical treatment in this country. With the birth of her premature daughter, Tiffany Field, Ph.D., looked for ways to help her thrive and gain weight, according to Freeman. "She massaged her daughter daily and found that this practice reduced the infant's anxiety, encouraged her to take more formula and helped her gain the weight. This led Dr. Field to hypothesize that similar and additional improvements might be observed in other premature infants if they were massaged in a similar manner."

Dr. Field tested her hypothesis in several clinical trials, finding that premature infants who were massaged grew and developed better than those who were not massaged. She has since gone on to perform massage therapy research for other conditions and is now director of the Touch Research Institute at the University of Miami School of Medicine. Of course, the practice of massage in this country was going on long before Dr. Field began her research. Freeman summarizes the highlights:

In the nineteenth century, two physicians and brothers brought the "Swedish Movement Cure" to the United States, using their techniques to stimulate skin, muscle, blood vessels, the lymph system, nerves and some internal organs. The first massage therapy clinics in the United States were opened by the Swedes after the Civil War. During the first part of the twentieth century, Swedish massage became popular at private health clubs, hospitals and with professional sports teams. The practice declined during the 1940s and 1950s, coming back into prominence during the holistic health and healing movements of the sixties, and the wellness movement that began in the seventies.

(continued)

"This led health professionals to reevaluate the therapeutic value of touch and massage," writes Freeman. The American Nurses Association recognized massage therapy as an official nursing subspecialty, and therapeutic touch, an energy form of healing, was warmly embraced by nursing professionals." (Please see "A Closer Look at Energy Healing, Spirituality and Therapeutic Touch.") "Of greatest impact was the growing number of massage therapists performing massage and body work full-time." In some European countries, such as Germany, massage is considered part of conventional medicine.

2. A Closer Look at Trager Movement Education: Easing Mind and Body

The woman was in her mid-thirties and no one could explain the constant, excruciating pain emanating from her lower back. She had seen doctors and tried many alternative treatments, all of which gave her only temporary relief. Her physician had finally referred her to Martin R. Anderson, a Trager practitioner.

"My colleague brought her to see me," remembers Martin. "She could barely walk into the office. She was hysterical crying, and said she was going to vomit. I had been practicing for nearly seventeen years, but at that moment my professional confidence nearly dropped to the floor. How could I possibly help her?"

Trager Movement Education, developed by the late Milton Trager, M.D., is an approach to the body that encourages mental and physical release, along with a feeling of openness, spaciousness and ease within the body. Practitioners learn to "hook-up" with the client, who lies fully clothed on a padded, comfortable table. "Hooking up," Martin explains, brings him into an almost meditative state. "I try to connect—with compassion and understanding—with what the client is feeling at that moment, and allow her to direct what I do next," he says. During a typical session, Martin rhythmically moves the client's arms, legs and trunk with small, gentle rocking, or "floppy," motions. At times he might also cradle the head, trying to sense where there might be potential release of tension. "While I work, I ask the client to tell me her response to the movements: Does this feel tighter? Looser? More or less painful?" says Martin. "At the same time I try to project a feeling of peace and calmness from deep within myself."

A typical session begins away from the table, with playful mental gymnastics, which Trager called Mentastics. First, the practitioner asks, "What does this movement feel like? Is there a softness, an ease, an openness in your shoulder or hip?" When the client is ready, the work continues on the table. The next step is a deepening of the positive feeling: "Could it feel even lighter? Don't force it, just notice the feeling and see how your body answers." At this point, the practitioner might suggest a gentle modification of the movement and ask the client to notice the result. "Trager is an exploration," says Martin. "I might take a limb and play with it, move it in a different way, explore a new feeling of release. We do not 'work' tight muscles; we try to project a sense of lightness. The idea behind the practice is to help nerves send new messages to the brain—messages that communicate pathways to ease and freedom of movement, rather than the messages of tightness and pain that might have become a habit. Milton Trager used to say, 'There are no tight muscles, only tight minds.'"

[*Author's note:* This, of course, is a different view of the body from that of muscular therapists, such as Cindy Stewart, who focus on the actual physical structure of the tissue. Most experts advise you to trust your instincts about what your body needs and talk to a variety of practitioners about their approach. ("Closer Look" sections such as this one will also give you the perspectives of individual practitioners.) I have found that I get the best results when I choose practitioners with whom I feel comfortable and with whom I can "connect."]

Martin is well-suited to the Trager style of therapy. He was a professional actor before becoming certified as a Trager practitioner. He helped to found The Next Move theatre company in Boston and acted in a number of ongoing productions, including *Shear Madness* and *Sister Mary Ignatius Explains It All For You.* "I am trained in improvisational theatre, and Trager is all about improvising," he says. "If something unexpected happens onstage, you have two choices: You can either get rattled and freeze up, or you can dive down deeper inside yourself to find your own inner resources, which help you decide what to do. The second method has served me well both on stage and in my work now."

When faced with his sobbing patient, Martin needed to look very deep within himself. "I got into a meditative state as I helped her get onto the table and propped her up with pillows," he says. "I then started a very gentle, rocking motion of her legs, not going anywhere near the painful back area, trying to send messages of peaceful, quiet movement to her back from my own mind and from the leg motions. I kept talking with her the whole time, asking, 'Does this movement feel okay? How about this?'"

The woman began to relax, even taking a few deep breaths. "Every time she took a breath, I would say, 'That looks like a lovely, deep breath.' Eventually, she stopped crying. Then I came up to her head and did a gentle massage of her temples, face and jaw; her breathing slowed and her body began to release tension. She said, 'You have very healing hands. I feel safe.' When that starts to happen, when the guard is let down, I can begin to send subtle messages of a new way of being in the body, trying to get around the fortress that was keeping her muscles so tight. I did a little rocking of the belly, then back to the legs."

After two hours, the woman got up from the table. "Before she did, I showed her a small lower back movement that she could do by herself at home to relieve pain," says Martin. "When she stood up, she said she had no pain for the first time in weeks, but she was afraid to move. Then she walked across the room and burst into tears because she felt no pain. I said to her, 'Your body knows how to organize itself like this, to move without pain and with deep relaxation. It came from your mind, and you can do it again. When you feel pain coming on, remember how it felt to be on this table.' Milton Trager called this phenomenon 'recall.' Other people call it 'kinesthetic hypnosis.' But whatever we call it, I know that the only thing I did was help her gain access to the deeper part of her mind that was causing the holding of tension in the muscles."

Martin called his client the next day and kept in touch with his colleague, who is also a Trager practitioner. "The no-pain situation lasted for a day and a half," says Martin. "Then it started to come back, but not so intensely. My colleague is still treating her with the Trager approach and the pain is becoming more manageable. She is not using any medication to control it."

Martin points out that the rhythmic Trager motions have helped several of his clients with diseases that induce muscle spasticity, including Parkinson's, multiple sclerosis and cerebral palsy. "When used along with conventional drugs and medical treatment, Trager can offer patients a balancing rhythm that counteracts the tremors and spastic movements," he says. "For example, I used the technique with a forty-five-year-old man, a psychiatrist, with severe Parkinson's: He had uncontrollable swinging motions of his arms. I got him on the table, and the rocking rhythm of my hands counteracted the spasticity, at least temporarily. He got off the table, his swinging motions stopped, and he said, 'I don't get it. It's too simple.'"

At the end of his life, when he was in his eighties, Milton Trager himself suffered from severe Parkinson's disease. Martin attended one of the last classes that he ever gave. "Word had it that he was very depressed and not well," says Martin. "So we were astonished when the classroom door flew open and in came Milton with his wife, Emily. He was holding a tape of Herb Alpert and the Tijuana Brass Band and insisted that we play it. He had discovered that strong musical rhythms helped to counteract his own tremors and spasticity. So we all danced around to the music, led by Milton, finding his own inner rhythm."

3. A Closer Look at Oriental
Bodywork Therapy: Tending the Garden

The first thing you see when you walk into Adele Strauss's waiting room is the almost full-size tiger under the coffee table. It is a very large toy, of course, but artistically constructed and almost startling in its realism. "He comes alive at night," says Adele with a smile. And indeed he looks like he might. He sits in regal repose, paws crossed, head held high, benignly surveying his small kingdom. He seems to fit in perfectly among the Chinese rosewood furniture, some of it antique, and the Oriental tapestry designs on the wall coverings and upholstery. Adele's office occupies several rooms on the first floor of a cozy Victorian house she shares with her husband, Hector Hambides, a musician and massage therapist.

The tiger seems an appropriate symbol for Adele, who practices a combination of massage methods, as well as acupuncture and herbal therapy. She is a small woman but appears anything but fragile. Her arms, hands and legs seem filled with wiry muscle, and she gives the impression of being able to gather up surprising amounts of strength into that small frame. One wouldn't be surprised to see her flip a two-hundred-pound man over her head with ease. (Something she has never even come *close* to doing!) Instead, she uses her strength to massage the tight muscles of her clients, coaxing them to release their tension so that healing energy can flow through them once again.

Adele grew up In South Africa, where she worked as a professional photographer and studied psychotherapy. "But for most of my life I felt like an artist without an art," she says. "Something powerful wanted to be expressed, but I didn't know what it was." Knowing that they could not live any longer under the apartheid regime, she and her husband moved to the United States. During their first New England winter, Hector became very sick with asthmatic bronchitis. "He was bedridden for three months with the worst cough I had ever heard in my life," says Adele. "Then a friend suggested that he try acupuncture. After just one treatment, he began to get better. I was astounded and had to learn more about Chinese medicine. When I discovered that world, I felt like I had finally found the art I had been yearning for all my life."

Adele began with the study of Oriental massage techniques. "Shiatsu is a Japanese massage method based on the principles of Chinese medicine," says Adele. "It is designed to move qi energy that is stagnant by pressing with the hands on specific points on the body that lie along the energy pathways or meridians. I combine that pressure with stretching muscles, ligaments, sinews and tendons. This combination of pressure and stretching helps to move the 'stuck' qi and restores the flow of vital energy in the body. (Please see chapters 2 and 6 for descriptions of Chinese medicine and qi.)

Over time, Adele began to combine Shiatsu massage with *tui na*—a Chinese deep tissue massage that incorporates similar pressure and stretching techniques along the energy pathways of the body. "I developed my own combination of massage techniques that I call 'Oriental bodywork therapy,'" says Adele. "I feel like a gardener, tending the bodies of my patients, strengthening their vital energy so that they can begin to heal themselves." Nine years ago, Adele added acupuncture and herbal medicine to her "gardening" tools. She uses her combination of methods to treat conditions that include chronic pain, allergies, upper-respiratory weakness and infections, chronic bronchitis, sinusitis, lung disorders, migraines and gastrointestinal problems. She also treats a full range of gynecological disorders. "I've had a 100 percent success rate in infertility treatments this year!" she says proudly. "Five out of five women who came to me with fertility problems are now pregnant." If they are interested, she also offers counseling to her clients about lifestyle and nutrition.

"When my clients become discouraged, I sometimes say to them, 'You are not to blame for your pain or illness. For years, your body has responded to stress by tensing the muscles and secreting the fight-or-flight hormones. These responses are only meant to happen for a few moments, when, for example, a tiger is chasing you. But when it happens every day, over a period of years, it may cause chronic pain. The stress hormones may also erode or break down your immune system and your ability to fight off disease.'"

Adele is committed to her clients. "My work is much more than a job. It reflects my spiritual path and my deepest understanding of life," she says. "Ultimately, we are all looking for peace and harmony within our bodies, to let go of all that is hindering us and to understand how we are connected to all that is in the universe."

4. A Closer Look at Ayurvedic Massage: Rebalancing Body, Mind and Spirit

In India, Ayurvedic massage is a way of life. Geeta Sharma, whose story about fibromyalgia is in chapter 6, remembers Ayurvedic massage experts visiting the homes in her village in India every week to treat family members. Parents in India learn to massage their children to relieve the discomfort of illness, or simply for relaxation. As we saw in chapter 2, Ayurvedic medicine is based on the principle that disease is caused when the body is out of balance. There are three basic body constitutions (or *doshas*) according to Ayurveda: *Vata, Pitta and Kapha.* Together, these *doshas* represent every element in the universe—air, water, fire, earth and space (ether). These elements are thought to be represented in the body. Each person has all three constitutional types, but usually one or two predominate. And when any of these is out of balance, disease or discomfort results. Ayurvedic massage is one way to correct the imbalance. (Details about Ayurvedic medicine, as well as research studies of the practice, are in chapter 2. In addition to Geeta Sharma's story about fibromyalgia, chapter 6 also includes the perspective of an Ayurvedic practitioner.)

Chandan Rugenius has been an Ayurvedic massage therapist for nine years. He specializes in *Abhyanga* or deep tissue massage. "The difference between Ayurvedic and other forms of massage lies in both the technique and the length of time," he says. "I work with the patient for anywhere from three to five hours, using special oils as well as magnet and light therapy. The goal is to rebalance the *doshas* of the body." (Please see chapter 2 for fuller explanations of the *doshas* and their related diseases.)

The *Vata dosha,* explains Chandan, is represented by the air and "ether" (space) elements and governs the mind and the nervous system. People who are predominantly *Vata* are imaginative, full of ideas, creative and fast-moving. But when *Vata* is out of balance, people can become overstimulated, anxious and have disorders related to the nervous system and digestion.

People who are predominantly *Pitta*—which is represented by fire—are intelligent, perceptive and visionary, but their perfectionist nature may cause them to become too critical and demanding, and consequently easily upset. They must guard against "flying off the handle."

A predominance of *Kapha,* which is represented by water and earth, means a person is reliable and patient. However, when *Kapha* is out of balance, these people may feel slow and bogged down in their own inertia, which can lead to weight problems.

How does Ayurvedic massage help to rebalance the body constitutions? First, the deep tissue massage removes blockages to the flow of prana, or life force, which helps to normalize the *doshas* that are overactive. "Also, we choose special oils, depending on the nature of the problem, each of which has different properties," says Chandan. "Oils prevent dryness, increase the suppleness of the skin, and prevent many of the effects of premature aging. Mustard oil, which is commonly used, relieves stiffness of muscles and helps reduce pain and swellings. It opens the pores of the skin and acts to purify the blood."

If you want to devote a few more hours to your massage, Chandan will apply a special paste called *Ubtan,* which is made up of a combination of oils and medicinal herbs, which are left to dry and then removed through vigorous massage—itself considered therapeutic. "It is customary in India for brides-to-be to have this treatment before the wedding," says Chandan. "It cleanses, lubricates, softens and adds a healthy luster to the skin. The paste also helps to stimulate the body to remove excess mucous. And turmeric, one of the ingredients in the paste, provides iodine in a form that can be absorbed by the body. This stimulates the nerves throughout the body and enhances strength and stamina."

Chandan emphasizes that massage alone may not be enough to rebalance the body. "We use diet, herbs, meditation, yoga and special breathing exercises, as well as cleansing techniques, magnets, light and sound," he points out. "Ayurveda is a total system, designed to treat body, mind and spirit."

ANCIENT TRADITIONS FOR MODERN TIMES

Massage therapy has been a health practice of most ancient cultures, including China, India, Persia, Arabia and Greece. Hippocrates used massage to treat sprains and dislocations; Aristotle treated exhaustion by massaging the body with oil and water; and oil massage was used in Sparta and Athens in preparation for vigorous exercise. Descriptions of *tui na* and acupressure (used by Adele Strauss in this section) appeared in the pages of *The Yellow Emperor's Classic of Internal Medicine,* written twenty-five hundred years ago and believed to be the first book of Chinese medicine. Indian Ayurvedic practices (used by Chandan Rugenius in this section) date back to the fifth century B.C. The recent revival of infant massage in this country has been patterned on the ancient practice of Indian baby massage.

 Massage: What's the Evidence?

One of the first researchers to test the benefits of massage, Dr. Tiffany Field, found that "premature newborns who received massage therapy showed greater growth, weight gain and improved cognitive and motor development at eight months than non-massaged infants."

Since that time, research from randomized controlled studies reviewed by Edzard Ernst suggested positive effects for anxiety, premenstrual syndrome and for elderly institutionalized patients. For patients with fibromyalgia, it has been suggested to relieve pain and depression and improve the quality of life. It also was found to have potential for the treatment of both low back pain and chronic constipation.

A Cochrane review of massage therapy reported that "evidence to support massage as a treatment to promote development in preterm and/or low birth-weight infants is weak." (Chapter 1 describes the research of the Cochrane Collaboration.)

Massage for pain

In her own review of the literature, Lynda Freeman cites several studies finding that massage benefits not only patients with fibromyalgia, premenstrual and low back pain, as described above, but also patients with other kinds of pain. These include:

Cancer: Male (but not female) cancer patients experienced significant short-term pain relief immediately after massage. Cancer patients also experienced increased mental clarity, general feelings of well-being, the release of unexpressed emotions and decreases in anxiety as a result of massage.

Surgical pain: Patients admitted for abdominal surgery were matched with a control group. The massaged group had significantly lower perceptions of pain twenty-four hours after surgery. Patients forty-one to sixty years old benefited the most.

Arthritis pain: Children with juvenile rheumatoid arthritis (one of the most common chronic diseases of childhood) were massaged by their parents for fifteen minutes each night. Another group practiced relaxation with their parents for the same amount of time. At the end of thirty days, both the parents and children in the massage group experienced lower anxiety (determined by behavioral observation and levels of cortisol, a stress hormone, in the saliva). The massaged children reported significantly less pain after massage and fewer pain episodes than the relaxation group.

Migraine: Massage therapy decreased the number of migraine headaches and reduced sleep disturbances and related distress symptoms.

Labor pain: Women recruited from prenatal classes were assigned to massage in addition to Lamaze training. A control group had only Lamaze training. Laboring women received massage during the first fifteen minutes of each hour of childbirth. The massage group had less anxiety and pain, less need for medication, a significantly shorter labor period, a shorter hospital stay and less postpartum depression than the control group.

Burn pain: Massage therapy for burn patients reduced anxiety, anger, depression, pain and itching.

References

Brattberg, G. "Connective Tissue Massage in the Treatment of Fibromyalgia." *European Journal of Pain* (London) 3 (1999): 235–245.

Ernst, E. "Abdominal Massage Therapy for Chronic Constipation: A Systematic Review of Controlled Clinical Trials." *Forschende Komplementarmedizin* 6 (1999): 149–151.

Ernst, E. "Massage Therapy for Low Back Pain: A Systematic Review." *Journal of Pain and Symptom Management* 17 (1999): 65–69.

Ernst, E., ed. *The Desktop Guide to Complementary and Alternative Medicine: An Evidence-Based Approach.* London: Harcourt Publishers Limited, 2001.

Field, T., et al. "Massage of Preterm Newborns to Improve Growth and Development." *Pediatric Nursing* 13 (1987): 385–387.

Field, T., et al. "Massage Therapies' Effects on Depressed Adolescent Mothers." *Adolescence* 31 (1996): 903–911.

Field, T., et al. "Labor Pain Is Reduced by Massage Therapy." *Journal of Psychosomatic Obstetrics and Gynecology* 18 (1997): 286–291.

Field, T., et al. "Juvenile Rheumatoid Arthritis Benefits from Massage Therapy." *Journal of Pediatric Psychology* 22 (1997): 607–617.

Field, T., et al. "Massage Therapy Effects on Postburn Scar." *Journal of Burn Care and Rehabilitation* (in review).

Fraser, J., et al. "Psychophysiological Effects of Back Massage on Elderly Institutionalized Patients." *Nursing* 18 (1993): 238–245.

Freeman, L. W. *Best Practices in Complementary and Alternative Medicine: An Evidence-Based Approach*. Gaithersburg, MD: Aspen Publications, 2001.

Hernandez-Reif, M., et al. "Migraine Headaches Are Reduced by Massage Therapy." *International Journal of Neuroscience* 96 (1998): 1–11.

Hernandez-Reif, M., et al. "Premenstrual Symptoms Are Relieved by Massage Therapy." *Journal of Psychosomatic Obstetrics and Gynecology* 21 (2000): 9–15.

Malkin, K. "Use of Massage in Clinical Practice." *British Journal of Nursing* 3, no. 6 (1994): 292–294.

Nixon, M., et al. "Expanding the Nursing Repertoire: The Effect of Massage on Post-Operative Pain." *Australian Journal of Advanced Nursing* 14, no. 3 (1997): 21–29.

Rubik, B., et al. "Manual Healing Methods" in *Alternative Medicine: Expanding Medical Horizons. A Report to the National Institutes of Health on Alternative Medicine Systems and Practices in the United States*. Bethesda, MD: National Institutes of Health, 1992.

Sims, S. "Slow Stroke Back Massage for Cancer Patients." *Nursing Times* 82, no. 13 (1986): 47–50.

Vickers, A., et al. "Massage Therapy for Premature and/or Low Birth Weight Infants to Improve Weight Gain and/or Decrease Hospital Length of Stay" (Cochrane Review). In *The Cochrane Library*. Oxford: Update Software, 1998.

Weinrich, S. P. "The Effect of Massage on Pain in Cancer Patients." *Applied Nursing Research* 3, no. 4 (1990): 140–145.

6

LIVING WITH ILLNESS: WEIGHING THE OPTIONS

"I felt like my body had shut down."

From Financial Warrior to Defender of Health

Paul Fraser thought he had it all figured out: It was during the late 1980s; he was nineteen years old and studying business in college. He and his friends had the same idea. They were going to become investment bankers, make millions by the time they were thirty, then retire and have fun. For Paul, that meant writing novels and practicing martial arts, two of his passions. In fact, in addition to going to college, Paul trained six nights a week in a martial arts studio. "I felt at the pinnacle of strength and vitality. I was also well on the way to becoming the biggest jerk you can imagine," says Paul. "When I got into the business world, I was going to crush people."

Then he had a bone scan.

Six years earlier, when Paul was thirteen, he had been diagnosed with a rare disease that penetrates bones and joints, turning the interior into a gel-like substance. With enough accumulation of this substance, the bone can collapse under pressure, even from a minor trauma. Paul's condition was discovered accidentally during a routine lung X ray for pneumonia. "They found a significant amount of the disease in my right shoulder, and a smaller amount in a few other places in my body, including my right pelvis," says Paul. "For unknown reasons, this disease only attacks one side of the body."

Surgeons reconstructed the shoulder, using bone from the Paul's left hip joint. The doctor recommended an X ray every six months. "I had been told that once

I stopped growing, there would be little chance of a recurrence of this disease," says Paul. Six years passed, with no further evidence of bone deterioration. "I figured I was more or less out of the woods as I neared my twenties," says Paul. In the meantime, he had become a high school athlete and developed his passion for martial arts. At nineteen, he went to the doctor to have what he thought would be his final MRI bone scan.

The test was easy and painless, and afterwards Paul went back to class completely unconcerned. A few days later he got a phone call. "The mass of diseased cells in my right pelvis had nearly doubled in size in the six months since the last scan," says Paul. "The doctor told me I now had a tumor that was large enough to cause the pelvis to collapse with one trauma. I was told to suspend all physical activity immediately, including, of course, martial arts." Paul's doctor scheduled surgery to remove the tumor and reconstruct the pelvis with healthy bone, the same procedure that successfully repaired his shoulder six years earlier.

"I wasn't too concerned," says Paul. "Even though they had raised the possibility of a malignancy, I had recovered so well from the first surgery that I thought of this as a temporary setback. I would work hard to regain my strength." However, things did not work out quite as he expected. The tumor—by then the size of a softball—along with margins of bone around it were successfully removed and sent for biopsy, and the pelvis was reconstructed with healthy bone, which was expected to grow together with the remaining bone. "My surgeon came to see me a few days later and asked me to stand for the first time, which I did," says Paul. "I asked him for the results of the biopsy, and he said, 'Let's get you lying down first, then we'll talk.'" The tumor was malignant, but there was some good news, the surgeon told him. The margins around the tumor were clear and the malignancy was of a low grade. "He said not to worry. He'd be checking me every few months, but he felt I'd be just fine."

Paul is not sure whether it was the news that his body was suddenly producing cancer cells or whether the surgery had taken more out of him than he thought, but he was not recovering. "I had no strength, no energy to do anything," he says. "It seemed as if my body had shut down. The bone wasn't healing; I would vomit every time I tried to eat. I lost weight, developed high blood pressure and became very weak. I felt as if my body had given up and gone on strike." Paul's family and friends were becoming concerned. They told him that he did not look well. Tests uncovered no explanation for his lack of progress.

Finally, someone suggested depression. "The suggestion seemed reasonable enough," says Paul. "But I wondered: Was I weaker because I was depressed? Or was I depressed because I was getting weaker?" The hospital sent a psychiatrist to see Paul. "He asked me if I wanted to talk about my physical condition. I said, 'No, I don't want to talk about it. I want to do something about it. I'm a results kind of person.' The psychiatrist said, 'Often a refusal to talk means you're feeling hostile and angry.' So I kicked him out."

After that, Paul was discharged home to his parents. "My doctor said to me, 'Gain some weight, get some rest and we'll start you on physical therapy. And let us know if you want to see a psychiatrist.'" By this time Paul was managing to keep some food down, and could walk with some difficulty, but only with crutches. "I never knew what food I'd be able to eat on any given day," says Paul. "It drove my mother crazy. She's Italian. Food is love." He spent three months at home, rarely going out. "I was not improving and did not understand why," says Paul. "But I was realizing that I could not live like this. I had to do something."

One day, Paul was feeling well enough to meet a friend for lunch. "I was waiting for the bus," he remembers. "And I saw a sign across the street that said Acupuncture Clinic. I had heard of acupuncture but hardly knew what it was. I had always made fun of 'New Age' things. I was a concrete, cause-and-effect person. Things needed to be grounded in evidence for me to take them seriously. But, for some strange reason, which I still don't understand, I felt it was imperative that I go into this shabby-looking building and talk to whomever was in there. I felt that I would find an answer there." The bus came, but Paul did not get on it. Instead, he hobbled across the street on his crutches.

A Double Life: Money by Day, Life Force by Night

In the shabby-looking building, Paul met the man who would change his life. Fei Tam is a practitioner of Chinese medicine who took one look at Paul and seemed to know just what was wrong with him, despite the fact that he spoke very little English, making communication difficult. "I got on the treatment table, fully dressed, and he passed his hand over my body, touching two places near the incision. 'Pain here and here,' he said. He was right of course. Those two places hadn't stopped hurting since the surgery. Then he said, 'Sometimes the whole leg feels like only half a leg, and your digestion, no good . . . so nervous . . . you don't sleep. No energy either.' Everything he said was true. How could he have known?"

Fei Tam inserted some acupuncture needles and passed his hand over Paul in a rhythmic motion, then told him to take a nap. "After about a minute, I felt as if warm water was flowing just beneath the surface of my skin," says Paul. "My right leg grew warmer, and there was a tingling sensation in my back. . . . I felt very peaceful and relaxed for the first time in months. And then the areas where there was pain began to pulse, and I had the sensation of the pain around the surgical site being slowly drained out of my heel." When Paul stood up, he felt stronger, "as if an internal pillar was supporting me," he says. But then the weakness returned. "Fei handed me my crutches and said, 'Don't worry. That was the first treatment. A few more, and no more crutches.'"

Paul went back to Fei Tam every week after that and started buying books about Chinese medicine. "After six weeks, I had graduated from two crutches to a single crutch," says Paul. "Three more treatments, I went to a cane. Three more after that, no more cane." Paul's digestion became normal (much to the delight of his mother), and the scans revealed that the bone had started filling in (much to the delight of the surgeon). "My surgeon said to me, 'We don't understand it, but if it works for you, keep doing whatever it is.' When I explained to him and his medical students about the acupuncture treatments, one of the students said to me, 'You don't really believe that stuff, do you?' I said, 'No,' and got up and walked out. Here was this wonderful thing that had helped me, and they made me feel like an idiot for believing in it."

Paul was developing an insatiable curiosity to learn more about Chinese medicine, and Fei Tam became a combination teacher, mentor and second father to him. "I learned that all of Chinese medicine is based on the concept of qi, the life force," says Paul. (Please see chapter 2 for a discussion of how different cultures and medical traditions interpret this life force.) "Inserting acupuncture needles is only one way to strengthen the life force within our bodies. Some people can actually cultivate qi within themselves, using special breathing, meditation and exercises (called qigong) to accumulate large amounts. They can then 'transfuse' their abundant energy to help others who are ill. This is what Fei was doing every time he passed his hands over my body, and I felt that warmth, tingling and strength, even without the use of needles."

Feeling stronger meant that Paul could go back to school. He changed his major from business to literature, with a concentration in poetry. When he graduated, he came back to get a job and also to study qigong and acupuncture with Fei Tam. "I wanted to learn to do this—to cultivate and use this life force called qi, so that I could take care of myself and everyone I loved," says Paul. "At the time, I never realized that healing others would become my life's work." To support himself, he used his business background to become a stockbroker in a large downtown firm. Nights and weekends he would study with Fei.

"I was leading a double life," says Paul. "Money by day and life force by night. I would arrive at Fei's office in my business suit, completely stressed from the frenetic pace of a stockbroker's life. Fei would ask me what I had been doing. One day, I said that I had been rushing around, trying to save time. He said to me, 'What do you do with the time you save, put it in a jar? You cannot save time, you can only spend it.'" Paul took a month off to travel to China with Fei to study with one of his teachers. About a month after he got back, the company laid him off. "It was like being paroled," he says. He had applied to graduate school in literature, thinking he would be a professor, but then Fei invited him to work with him.

"I started treating patients with *tui na*, a combination of acupressure, deep tissue massage and qigong." (Please see box, "Some Theories About Qi".) Paul worked with Fei for three years, treating patients and observing and training with Fei in acupuncture. "I had more work than I could handle," says Paul. "I never finished graduate school. I really liked this new work. It was the first job I ever had where people were happy to see me!" In 1992, Fei rented a new space, paid the rent for a year, and told Paul to move into it alone. "He told me I was ready to go out on my own," says Paul. "About six months later, I asked Fei if I could pay him back for the year's rent. He refused to let me. He said, 'Someday, find a student and do the same thing.'

"Fei Tam gave me my life back and then showed me how to live it," says Paul. "I felt as if my life had been lost and restored in a matter of months." Paul still studies and practices qigong with another teacher (Fei Tam is trying to retire). A few years ago, he opened his own practice, in Norwell, Massachusetts, called Integrative Physical Therapy, in partnership with his sister and his best friend, who had also decided to study with Fei after seeing how Paul's life was changing. They provide *tui na* massage, acupuncture, qigong energy treatments and qigong classes.

The offices of Integrative Physical Therapy are peaceful, airy and harmonious. There is herbal tea, plants thrive on windowsills, and the walls are adorned with photographs of Paul's teachers and beautiful Chinese calligraphy. Although he designed the space, Paul himself seems almost an anomaly. Dressed in a sky-blue designer sweater, khakis and loafers, he looks like he just stepped off the golf course after a corporate foursome. At thirty-four, his dark hair and boyish good looks seem reminiscent of his earlier life as a stockbroker and athlete. But the true essence of Paul lies in his eyes. Deep and penetrating, they observe a visitor unflinchingly, and they are filled with warmth and compassion for what he sees.

When asked about the contrast, Paul laughs. "I've always been a scrapper," he says. "But now, instead of being a financial killer, I go after people's illnesses. My nature hasn't changed, but it has grown softer, more refined. I want everyone to experience the power of qi—the life force—and the strength, joy and vitality that saved my life."

SOME THEORIES ABOUT QI—THE LIFE FORCE THAT IS
THE FOUNDATION OF CHINESE MEDICINE
(Based on the Teachings of Fei Tam)

- The natural world is overflowing with this life force. It is in plants, trees, water and minerals. Our bodies contain a great deal of it. It is what we feel when we breathe and eat and when we are rested after sleeping.
- Qi is "magnetic." When it enters and flows through a body it draws more from the abundance of nature.
- Qi is energy that is in perfect balance, and it seeks to bring everything that it comes into contact with into harmony, wholeness and balance as well.
- Disease is defined as the body being "out of balance," because the flow of qi is weak or blocked. Removing the blockage and freeing or increasing the flow of qi within a person's body can help restore the balance and lead to health.
- Thousands of years ago, people learned about qi from observing the human body as it interacted with nature. Wise ones discovered that different movements and changes in breathing affected how qi moved and was accumulated in a person. This was the birth of qigong, which includes forms as diverse as the slow, meditative movements of tai chi and the vigorous and potentially destructive movements of self-defense. (There is good research evidence that tai chi improves balance and reduces falls in the elderly. Please see chapter 11.)
- Over thousands of years of observation, these movement and breathing techniques were also developed into systems designed to restore health and vitality when people became ill.
- Certain people, called "adepts," became so skilled at cultivating qi that they could pass on their abundance to people who were ill, almost like a "transfusion." They did this by using their hands or even the energy of their own positive intentions, visualizing a healthy heart or digestive system.
- Over time, the technique of *tui na*—a combination of acupressure, deep tissue massage and qigong—evolved as a more direct way to move energy and send qi into the body.
- The adepts became so sensitive that they could hold a plant in their hands, feel its life force and understand how it would interact with the life force of a human being. This was the birth of Chinese herbalism.

(continued)

- Eventually, the adepts recognized that qi travels in the human body along invisible pathways, called "meridians." Hundreds of points along these meridians are "gateways" into the body's energetic flow. The practice of acupuncture uses needles as "antennae" to attract qi energy into the body, remove blockages and stimulate the flow of qi.

 ## Acupuncture and Qigong: What's the Evidence?

Traditional Chinese medicine (TCM), which includes acupuncture, qigong, *tui na* massage, nutrition and herbal therapies, has a history of at least three thousand years. "Presently, about one-quarter of the world's population uses TCM. In various forms, TCM has spread to Japan, Korea, Southeast Asia, Europe and the Americas. In the United States, some twelve million people currently go to TCM practitioners. Out of the estimated $14 billion a year that Americans spend on alternative medicine, TCM accounts for $1 billion, 75 percent of which goes for acupuncture."[1]

Many of the practices of TCM have been incorporated into mainstream medicine, in addition to settings that offer mind/body medicine. In Children's Hospital in Boston, for example, there is a Medical Acupuncture Service, directed by anesthesiologist and pediatrician Yuan-chi Lin, M.D., M.P.H. The service treats headaches, abdominal discomfort, chronic pelvic pain, teenage endometriosis, urological disorders, bedwetting, chronic musculoskeletal pain and cystic fibrosis.

In the operating room and postoperatively, acupuncture has been used successfully on patients who have bad reactions or allergies to anesthesia and to prevent side effects. This is called "acupuncture-assisted anesthesia."[2]

At Massachusetts General Hospital (MGH), a study is currently underway to study the effectiveness of acupuncture in treating the one-sided paralysis of stroke called

---

[1] K. R. Pelletier, *The Best Alternative Medicine: What Works? What Does Not?* (New York: Simon & Schuster, 2000).
[2] Y. Lin, "Acupuncture Anesthesia for a Patient with Complex Congenital Anomalies," *Medical Acupuncture* 13, no. 2 (2001): 50–51.

hemiplegia. "There are many research studies in the Chinese literature about the effectiveness of acupuncture for hemiplegia, but they do not meet Western research standards of randomized control trials," says David E. Krebs, Ph.D., P.T., who is director of the MGH Biomotion research laboratory. "A research grant from the National Institutes of Health is also funding a study on the use of tai chi in neurological disorders." Results from these studies are not yet available.

Other data about the effectiveness of acupuncture are located throughout this book (for example, see chapter 7 on pain, chapter 2 on the vital force and acupuncture and chapter 8 on trauma), but here is a summary:

In systematic reviews of its effectiveness, acupuncture has been found to be an effective treatment for several kinds of pain, chemotherapy-induced or postoperative nausea, and recovery from stroke or traumatic brain injury. There is less conclusive evidence that it is helpful for conditions that include asthma, back pain, fibromyalgia, migraine, neck pain and osteoarthritis. It was not found to be helpful for weight loss or smoking.

Qigong

This form of Chinese energy work, involving physical movements and breathing exercises, is described in the story about Paul Fraser in this chapter. Qigong is intended to promote health by directing and increasing the internal flow of qi, or life force.

Qigong lowered blood pressure

The research evidence is positive, according to Pelletier. In his book, Pelletier cites studies showing that qigong lowered blood pressure and reduced death and illness from stroke.

Qigong helped cancer patients improve strength and appetite

According to another study at a hospital in Beijing, Pelletier reports that "Ninety-three patients with advanced cancer were treated with a combination of drugs and qigong exercises, while a control group was treated with drugs alone. Eighty-one percent of the qigong group showed an improvement in strength, 63 percent in appetite, and 33 percent were free from diarrhea, compared to improvements of 10 percent, 10 percent, and 6 percent, respectively, in the other group."

Qigong lowered cholesterol

In a study in China, one hundred men with hypertension and elevated cholesterol were divided into two groups. One group practiced qigong for a year, the
other did not. The qigong group was found to have significantly lowered measurements of "bad"cholesterol and higher levels of "good" cholesterol.

References

Ernst, E., ed. *The Desktop Guide to Complementary and Alternative Medicine: An Evidence-Based Approach.* London: Harcourt Publishers Limited, 2001.

Lin, Y. "Acupuncture Anesthesia for a Patient with Complex Congenital Anomalies." *Medical Acupuncture* 13, no. 2 (2001): 50–51.

Pelletier, K. R. *The Best Alternative Medicine: What Works? What Does Not?* New York: Simon & Schuster, 2000.

Wang, C. X. "Effects of Qigong on Preventing Stroke and Alleviating the Multiple Cerebro-Cardiovascular Risk Factors: A Follow-Up Report on 242 Hypertensive Cases Over 30 Years." Proceedings, Second World Conference for Academic Exchange of Medical Qigong, Beijing, China (1993): 123–124.

Wang, C. X. "Influence of Qigong Therapy upon Serum HDL-C in Hypertensive Patients." *Chinese Journal of Modern Developments in Traditional Medicine (Chung Hsi i Chieh Ho Tsa Chih)* 9 (1989): 516, 543–544.

❖ ❖ ❖ ❖

Antibiotics and Qi:
The Evolution of an Integrative Physician

Glenn Rothfeld's eyes are large and dark, accented with thick, dark eyebrows.
They are penetrating, taking in and analyzing information about the patient sitting in front of him. As he listens to her words, he is noticing the color of her skin,
the condition of her hair, whether she is restless or relaxed and the quality and
timbre of her voice. When he talks to her, he notices her response: Does she argue
with his suggestions or meekly accept them? Does she need a sympathetic listener
or is she impatient for a quick solution to her problem? Will she feel insecure
about her health unless there are tests done, even if she does not really need them?

It is immediately clear that Glenn is not a conventional physician. Not only does he have a degree in acupuncture (M.Ac.) after the M.D. that follows his name, but he does not practice in the usual doctor's office. From the small fountain that greets you at the door to the warm colors and fabrics, the space is both soothing and beautiful—designed, in fact, in consultation with a feng shui master (using Oriental principles of energy and balance). Glenn is the founder and medical director of one of the oldest complementary/integrative medical practices in the country, now known as Whole Health New England. While he treats patients with a wide variety of illnesses, his medical practice is particularly used for the treatment of chronic and degenerative diseases, including arthritis and other conditions of chronic pain, women's health, allergies, chronic bowel problems, heart disease, multiple sclerosis and Parkinson's disease.

A former clinical fellow of the Harvard University School of Medicine, Glenn is currently assistant clinical professor of family medicine at Tufts University School of Medicine. In addition to his conventional medical degree, Glenn studied acupuncture at the Traditional Acupuncture Institute in Columbia, Maryland, with advanced work at the College of Traditional Chinese Acupuncture in Leamington Spa, England. He is the author of seven books on complementary medicine topics, which include advice to patients and analysis of relevant research on alternative methods of treatment.

"I look at my patient from several perspectives," says Glenn, describing a recent patient visit as an example. "I watch her closely as she complains of her bowel and digestive problems, and several possible diagnoses and treatments run through my mind. She might have ulcerative colitis, which would require a barium enema or colonoscopy. She might have a parasite or an infection, which would call for laboratory cultures or antibody testing. Or perhaps she has a yeast overgrowth or bacterial imbalance in her digestive tract caused by antibiotics, steroids or birth control pills."

Glenn also focuses on his patient's lifestyle and personality. "What kind of person is she? What is her life like at home and at work? Is she happy? Where does her stress come from? Is she having a deficiency in her spleen energy qi?" (Please see the box: "Some Theories About Qi.")

"In Chinese medicine," explains Glenn, "spleen qi deficiency does not necessarily mean that there is something wrong with the spleen itself (although there might be). It means that the energy pathway—the meridian—that runs through the spleen may be weakened or blocked, not generating enough 'heat' to control fluids in her digestive tract. This deficiency could cause diarrhea and bloating. If that is the case, all she might have to do is take certain warming digestive herbs and stop eating cold foods and drinking soda."

Glenn sees integrative medicine as a continuum: "At one end are conventional interventions, such as surgery, drugs and antibiotics; chemotherapy and radiation treatments for cancer; and procedures and tests, including colonoscopy, angioplasty and magnetic resonance imaging. On the other end of the continuum are complementary diagnostic and treatment practices, including Chinese pulse and tongue analysis, massage, herbal treatments, chiropractic treatment and acupuncture. My job as an integrative physician is to determine where on that continuum I should intervene diagnostically and therapeutically. And I have to continually be aware of my patient's lifestyle, preferences and beliefs."

It turned out that the woman with the bowel problem was grabbing food at business meetings and eating breakfast in her car while she talked on her cell phone on her way to work. (Can't you just feel your stomach tightening as you read this?) Conventional testing revealed that she also had a severe dairy allergy. "The digestive tract is the biggest immune organ in the body, twenty-eight feet in length, the size of a football field if you calculate its surface of fingerlike tiny protrusions, and lined with antibodies," says Glenn. "The digestion is a large part of the barrier that protects us from toxins in our environment. In addition to eating foods that she was allergic to, this patient was not giving her body a calm environment in which to digest properly, thereby depleting her body's energy."

We are connected to the cycles of nature

As he tries to determine what is interfering with his patients' health, Glenn draws upon everything he knows from the worlds of both conventional and complementary medicine. "One of the strongest complementary tools I have is the Chinese Five Element theory," he says. (Please see the box for details about the Five Element theory.) The cycle of nature—as well as our bodies—depends on the harmonious balance of two types of energy yin and yang. (Please also refer to chapter 2.) In the time when people were always aware of and part of nature, says Glenn, they were also aware of these two energy forces. "When they looked up, they saw something that was hot, light and dry. It was dynamic, active and expansive. It was transcendent; it couldn't be grasped, measured, quantified. It was the sun; it was heaven. The ancient Chinese described this as yang energy. When they looked down, they saw something that was cooling, moist, solid, dark and immobile. It held and nourished things; it grew things when given heat and light from above. It wasn't transcendent. It was manifest. It could be held, measured and quantified. It was earth, and the Chinese called it yin."[3]

BRIEF SUMMARY OF THE CHINESE FIVE ELEMENT THEORY
[Source: Glenn S. Rothfeld, M.D., M.Ac.]

The ancient Chinese Five Element theory is one of the integrative medicine diagnostic tools that Glenn Rothfeld uses. The theory is that while each of us is unique, our bodies, minds and spirits usually tend to correspond to one of the five elements that exist in our world: wood, fire, earth, metal and water, which are in turn related to five seasons in the cycle of nature: spring, summer, late summer (harvest time), fall and winter.

- Spring: birth, rebirth and rapid growth; symbolized by the wood element (a tree sprouting from the ground), followed by . . .
- Summer: continued rapid growth, heat; symbolized by fire (which is fed by wood). When the crops are mature, it is time for the . . .
- Late summer harvest: heavy, still air; a full, satisfied feeling in nature; symbolized by the earth element, which is created by fire, and in turn gives rise to
- Autumn: symbolized by the metal element; an emotional quality of grief, of letting go; increased coolness, dryness, less activity. Cold, quiet metal loses what is non-essential, preparing the world for . . .

(continued)

---

[3] G. S. Rothfeld and S. Levert, *The Acupuncture Response: Balance Energy and Restore Health—A Western Doctor Tells You How* (New York: McGraw-Hill/Contemporary Books, 2002), 21.

- Winter: minimal activity on the surface symbolized by water. The surface quietness hides the hidden activity of seeds building their reserves underground in preparation for the spring, and the bursting forth of new growth.

Each type of energy has physical manifestations of health and illness, according to Glenn Rothfeld. For example:

- **Wood energy** (Spring) requires flexibility and clarity of thought and vision. Examples of wood health problems would be a gnarled, stiff arthritis, or tight neck muscles that lead to tension headaches, or visual problems.
- **Fire energy** (Summer) relates to the heart, and thus to intimacy and communication with others. Because it has to do with communicating between the heart and the rest of the body, cold hands and feet (e.g., Raynaud's disease) might be a fire problem. Also, the type of depression that is associated with flat emotional affect can be seen as a lack of fire.
- **Earth energy** (Harvest) is all about nourishment. Abdominal bloating, irritable bowel syndrome and nausea are all examples of Earth energy problems. Other problems include dizziness (lack of connection to the earth) and aching of the earth (flesh) of our bodies—that is, muscle aching.
- **Metal energy** organs include the large intestine (which lets go) and the lung (which receives pure air, giving the aspect of holy quietness that is associated with the autumn). Asthma, constipation and eczema (the skin is considered part of the lung energy, since it breathes) are all metal problems.
- **Water energy** has to do with reserves, the ability to get through hard times. Lack of energy, fearfulness (lack of courage), low blood sugar and blood pressure are all water problems.

❖ ❖ ❖ ❖

After twenty years of practice, Glenn can look at each one of us, and from the color of our skin, the type of body we have, the way we interact with the world, the sound of our voice and many other clues determine what "season" we fall into, and what is our predominant "element." He combines this information with conventional medical diagnostic techniques to understand not only our symptoms, any internal imbalance of our *yin* and *yang* energy that might be causing disease, but also our relationship to illness and health—the *meaning* we ascribe to our physical condition. This combined knowledge helps to guide his treatment choices.

Smoking is a good example of how the Five Element theory is useful, according to Glenn. "Just about everyone knows that smoking is bad for you, but people still smoke, because information alone is not what motivates most people," he explains. "Some people smoke because their friends do and the social aspect is most important to them (the influence of "fire" energy–seeking intimacy); some people need the oral gratification, something in their mouths ("earth" energy–seeking nourishment); some people feel empty inside and need to feel something warm filling their chests (an influence of "metal" energy, which has the emotional quality of grief); some people need to clutch something or they will shake with anxiety and fear ("water" energy); and some people have such frustration and rage that if they don't occupy their hands, they might strike someone ("wood" energy). Addressing these issues would address more reasons why people smoke."

Glenn also uses the Five Element theory to sense the neediness or emptiness in people, almost without thinking. "Sometimes, it is clear, for example that a patient thinks she needs an MRI in order to be able to let go of her symptoms—even if it is not necessary. This might reflect a water energy problem—a need for reassurance, or an earth energy problem—a need to have acknowledgement that she is really suffering with her illness, or a need to have someone pay attention to her medical problems. Sometimes, a person whose imbalance is metal requires a sophisticated test because of the need for the 'best' of everything," says Glenn. "If I can fill this neediness in other ways, through acupuncture or herbs to build up her energy and her life force, think of all the money to be saved in unnecessary medical tests!"

The Five Element theory is all about the individual, not the condition, according to Glenn. "The question is, who is this person who has depleted his or her reserves, hormones or energy? Has the depletion come from the constant vulnerability of fire, the driving, pushing, never-stopping quality of wood, the inability to get nourished by anything (earth), the backing up of toxins, or lack of fresh air and inspiration that accompanies it (metal), or are they fundamentally lacking in reserves (water)?" (Remember Sir William Osler's quote in the Introduction? This renowned Victorian-era physician and teacher said, "It is more important to know what sort of patient has a disease than what sort of disease a patient has.")

For example, points out Glenn, "Some people are driven, they have to have an order, they need something to push against. That is springtime energy—the energy it takes for a sprout to push up through the ground. If it gets thwarted—if something stops this person from achieving a goal in life, there is a gnarledness, which may be reflected in headaches, lack of structural flexibility and vision. This person needs to have his energy softened and moved. One popular herbal mixture that we use is known as 'free and easy wanderer' or 'gentle rambler.'"

Fire energy, by contrast, needs to be warmed and circulated, says Glenn. "We might use moxa, an herb that is burned over the skin or needle to heat up an area, and we would use acupuncture points that solidify the internal sense of protection, allowing someone to 'come out of his shell.'" And when earth energy doesn't move, it's like food that's undigested, says Glenn. "This turns to something called 'dampness.' It needs to be moved, warmed up (no eating cold foods!). We also encourage walking and movement generally. Similarly, when metal gets brittle and cold, we usually want to warm it (moxa again), and promote the letting go process in the colon, and the body/mind generally. And since water energy has to do with reserves, we build the reserves using acupuncture, moxa, increasing fluids, herbs and proper sleep. Unless we understand all of this in our patients, we don't address their needs."

One patient, for example, was having trouble sleeping. She would wake up frequently during the night. "She was also having the early symptoms of menopause (perimenopause), had a tight upper back and neck and was prone to anxiety and constipation," says Glenn. "Why does she wake up a lot? Maybe she is anxious, under stress or depressed." He shakes his head impatiently. "My two *least* favorite diagnoses are stress and depression," he says. "What does that mean? Many people are under stress and don't wake up all night. And even though insomnia often occurs as a menopausal symptom, I wanted to look deeper by focusing on where her energy is depleted. I did this by measuring the levels of several hormones through assays (blood and urine tests) at different times of the day and night.

"We found that she was not producing enough of several hormones and proteins, including tryptophan, serotonin and melatonin, which, when deficient, are linked to sleep problems. Because she was under stress, her adrenal glands were putting out excessive amounts of adrenaline and epinephrine and other hormones that promote alertness. She also had low blood sugar, caused by a combination of stress and diet, which was making it more difficult for her to cope with her other problems.

"When she lay down at night, pressure from her tight neck and back muscles irritated the nerve endings of the sympathetic nervous system (which activates the alert flight-or-fight response to stress), further exacerbating the insomnia," says Glenn. The treatment? "I gave her supplements to bring her hormone deficiencies back up to normal levels, and magnesium to help relax the tight neck and back muscles. As an added benefit, magnesium, when given orally, also helps ease constipation. I also recommended a glass of warm milk at night: The extra protein helps prevent an adrenaline surge, and the milk also contains tryptophan, a sleep-promoting hormone."

Glenn also frequently uses Chinese herbs to address perimenopausal or menopausal symptoms. He explains how these symptoms can be diagnosed in relation to Five Element theory (see also chapter 10 for more about women at midlife). These symptoms can manifest "with heat abnormalities, such as hot flashes, which relates to the fire element, particularly what the Chinese call the 'triple warmer,'" says Glenn. "Agitation and depression relate to wood energy in the liver; eating binges, sweets cravings, feeling 'puffy' and 'logy' relate to earth energy imbalance; constipation, sadness and sense of loss all relate to metal energy; and, most frequently, the symptoms of depleted water energy can lead to dryness, restless insomnia, hot flashes, night sweats and fatigue."

A Fervor to Push Beyond Conventional Medicine

Glenn Rothfeld went to medical school during the early 1970s—a tumultuous time in this country, and describes himself as a product of those times: "I entered medical school filled with a fervor to practice a different kind of medicine from the one being taught. I was deeply suspicious of the prevailing medical establishment, which I saw as too reliant on technology and drugs."

As a second-year medical student, Glenn lived in a rural house with other medical students. "We started reading books by Adele Davis, a biochemist and nutritional writer," he says. "We began stir-frying vegetables in woks and eating brown rice. I even started putting brewer's yeast on my popcorn!" In 1973, Glenn and his fellow students brought Davis to lecture at their medical school. "We cooked a big meal with her and she talked about how vitamins and nutrition affected health. I began to understand that I, as a doctor, could prescribe B-vitamins, for example, to help my patients with specific health problems. I date my first understanding of the role of nutrition in health to that time."

Glenn and the other students also began reading about stress as a cause of disease. "Hans Selye, M.D., was the first to describe a stress response and the ways that stress can cause disease," he says. "Then the Beatles went to India, started meditating and put out the *White Album*. Shortly after that, we all started meditating and noticing how the practice reduced our own stress levels. Herbert Benson, M.D., and Keith Wallace, M.D., both of Harvard Medical School, published studies about what Benson called 'the relaxation response' and how a practice of meditation could actually modify blood circulation, reduce blood pressure and improve health and healing. We brought Dr. Wallace to speak to the medical class about meditation and health."

A third formative influence for Glenn was journalist James Reston's account in the *New York Times* of his appendicitis surgery in China in 1972. "Reston was accompanying President Richard Nixon to China when the journalist suffered an attack of appendicitis and needed surgery," says Glenn. "Doctors there used acupuncture to control Reston's pain, and he later wrote about the experience, introducing the practice to many Americans for the first time." When he began his own medical practice, Glenn began to study nutritional and herbal medicine and to apprentice himself to acupuncture masters, eventually enrolling in an acupuncture training program for physicians and continuing his studies in England.

As his practice grew, Glenn expanded his services to include homeopathy, energy and massage work, acupuncture and biofeedback therapy, in addition to conventional medical treatment, including physical therapy. He hired an expert in herbal medicine from Europe and began developing vitamin and supplement formulas, eventually opening his own retail pharmacy, called The Natural Apothecary. He also began to practice one of his signature treatments: the infusion of vitamins and supplements intravenously. "Many patients, particularly those with chronic diseases, take pills and other medications orally," says Glenn. "In some cases, these interfere with the absorption of vitamins and nutrients, preventing them from getting to the cells where they are most needed. Also, certain nutrients, like magnesium, can cause diarrhea when given orally. (Of course, this is useful if the patient is constipated!) By contrast, when we infuse vitamins and minerals intravenously, we are putting them directly into the bloodstream. From there, they can be delivered to the cells that need them without interference from the digestion process."

In addition to treating patients, Glenn also does a fair amount of writing and teaching. "I have trained many doctors and nurse practitioners in integrative medical practice; I believe in it completely," he says. "But it does not come easily to everyone."

✓ TAKE ACTION ✓

Best ways to cope with chronic illness
Suggestions from Glenn Rothfeld, M.D.

1. **Massage:** Studies show that massage is not just for feeling good, but can boost immunity, lessen pain, improve sleep and enhance your mood. And remember, it takes energy to keep a muscle in spasm, and massage makes that energy more available. (Please see "Four Ways to Feel Better" for more about massage.)

2. **Homeopathy:** This system of medicine, which is used by billions of the world's population, relies on the idea that the body has an innate ability to heal, if given the right energy "message." It is gentle to the point of being almost risk-free. (Note: There is scientific controversy about the effectiveness of homeopathy, although there are studies that suggest that it is useful as a treatment for some conditions. Please see "A Closer Look at Homeopathy.")

3. **Antioxidant nutrients:** All chronic disease, whether it is cancer, heart disease or autoimmune conditions, have in common the oxidation of tissue, with resulting damage. Oxidation is the process whereby a cell ages by coming into contact with oxygen. The fatty part of cells (called the lipid membrane) becomes rancid when in contact with oxygen for long periods, just as oils do in the air. Vitamin E is the main antioxidant that protects lipid membranes; this is why some people associate vitamin E with anti-aging. Metals in the body also become oxidized, just like iron rusts and copper tarnishes. These oxidation reactions can prevent our cells from doing their jobs (i.e., encouraging enzymes to function). Our tissues protect against this damage and can reverse oxidation by containing adequate levels of antioxidant substances like vitamins A, C and E, minerals selenium and zinc, and accessory nutrients n-acetyl-cysteine and alpha lipoic acid. The antioxidant enzyme glutathione peroxidase is also an important protector. Supplementing these nutrients, in consultation with your doctor, may be a good idea.

4. **Movement:** There are barely any situations in which movement and exercise are contraindicated. If you can, exercise regularly. Even a simple daily walk will help. If you can't walk, then seated exercises or even moving in bed can be accomplished. Movement brings blood, energy and oxygen to tissues, oxygenates us and lifts our spirits.

5. **Colorful fruits and vegetables:** Bright colors and tasty flavors are the result of powerful substances in nature called flavonoids. These substances improve circulation and function of our body tissues. Some, like lycopene from tomatoes,

(continued)

have anti-cancer properties. Others have been shown to improve heart function. There are hundreds of flavonoids in foods, and these "medicines" are available in your salad bowl. (Please see "A Closer Look at Healing Herbs" as well as the research on diet and cancer in chapter 5; and diet and heart disease in chapter 4.)

6. **Acupressure:** Similar to acupuncture, which uses needles to move "qi" (life force) and promote healing, acupressure is also derived from Chinese medicine. Shiatsu is a similar Japanese system. Practitioners use finger pressure instead of acupuncture needles to remove blockages in the qi. (Adele Strauss, described in "Four Ways to Feel Better," uses acupressure and Shiatsu bodywork.)

7. **Breathing:** Yes, we all breathe without thinking. But frequently, circumstances keep us from breathing deeply and taking fresh oxygen into our bodies. Anxiety might make our breath shallow, or pain might limit our chest motion. Remembering to breathe slowly, deeply and fully can increase the oxygen in our bodies, and therefore our energy and vitality.

8. **Yoga:** For centuries, yoga has been an integral part of Ayurveda, the native healing system of India. Now we know from modern studies that yoga promotes healing and lessens pain. And not all yoga involves twisting yourself in knots like the pictures; simple yoga postures are doable by nearly everyone. (For more on breathing exercises and yoga, please see "A Closer Look at Yoga.")

9. **Adaptogenic herbs:** Certain herbs have been studied for their ability to make the body more resilient and able to cope better with stress. These herbs are called "adaptogens." Common and well-studied adaptogens include eleutherococcus (formerly known as Siberian ginseng), rhodiola and astragalus. These are also known for their safety, although you should always check first with your doctor. (Please see "A Closer Look at Healing Herbs.")

10. **Gather a support group:** Going it alone is never a good way to cope with chronic illness, and it can lead to depression and diminishing function. Having the support of others is a powerful antidote to the worst effects of illness and is associated in studies with increased life expectancy. (Please see "A Closer Look at Energy Healing, Spirituality and Therapeutic Touch.")

Rebelling into Health

Marin has long, curly hair, expressive eyes and a perpetually inquisitive look. She arches her eyebrows and peers through her glasses as if trying to grasp every nuance of meaning in a conversation. She uses only one name, she explains, with a wink, "like Cher, Madonna, Liberace, Moses and God." The motorized, wheeled "scooter" that she uses to get around the house (she has another one for outdoors) is rarely still, even when she is talking or listening. She moves forward to emphasize a point, swivels around to ask her visiting aide for a glass of water, or turns slightly to explain a piece of artwork on her wall or the sculpture and flower arrangements on her low, Japanese-style dining table surrounded by large floor cushions. Because her left hand is weakened from multiple sclerosis (MS), she deftly uses her right hand to move the scooter, hold the cordless phone and field a near-constant stream of phone calls. Today, she is arguing with the car dealer who overcharged her for repairs to her disability-adapted van. (Yes, she drives herself wherever she needs to go.) As she talks about her life, her stories are sprinkled with salty language and a quick wit.

In addition to a degenerative form of multiple sclerosis, she has had a hip fracture caused by osteoporosis; she has survived breast cancer; a cancerous polyp in her colon and rectum that required a partial colon resection; a ruptured ovarian cyst and bowel surgery. "Actually, the MS is the least of my problems right now," she says. "The hardest part of life this year has been regaining my strength and getting my life back."

Glenn Rothfeld, M.D., is Marin's doctor. "I found him after some disastrous forays into allopathic medicine, beginning from childhood, when a doctor lost a skin biopsy," she says. "Growing up, I had no idea about nutrition. I believed that all vegetables came out of a frozen package. I guess I rebelled against all of that as an adult. I started eating macrobiotically, became a massage therapist in Greenwich Village, and eventually moved to Oregon, which was then the 'mecca' for alternative therapies, to become a chiropractor."

In 1982, while she was in chiropractic school in Oregon, she began to notice a persistent weakness in her left leg. A neurologist in Oregon diagnosed multiple sclerosis. "At that time, a spinal tap was the accepted way to confirm this disease," she says. "I refused. I also refused the only treatment given in the early eighties: steroids or prednisone for big flare-ups of symptoms. One famous neurologist told me that if I were his daughter, he'd put me in the hospital and start me on chemotherapy. I said, 'Thank God I'm not your daughter.'"

In addition to macrobiotics, Marin explored many other alternative treatment options for MS. "I went to the Edgar Cayce Clinic, got hooked up to a gold synthesizer, used castor oil packs, megavitamins and even tried 'psychic surgery' with healers from the Philippines who used energy from their hands to perform 'knifeless operations' on the body. I also got all the silver amalgam fillings taken out of my mouth, because they contain mercury, which is toxic. While none of these methods was a cure, they helped me to get to a place where I could accept that it's not about a cure, it's about the process of healing. Going after a 'quick fix' is not a realistic goal for chronic disease."

In the 1960s, Michio Kushi brought the macrobiotic nutrition movement to the United States, setting up the Kushi Institute in Brookline, Masschusettes. In 1985, Marin left chiropractic school to immerse herself in the macrobiotic lifestyle. "I had had a consultation with Michio in California," she says. "By then I was walking with a cane and was still looking for that elusive cure. He told me that if I followed his very strict macrobiotic diet for nine months, I would be cured. So in Brookline, I shared a house with two macrobiotic room-mates and devoted myself to this very time-consuming method of eating."

The diet did not help. "I got significantly worse," says Marin. "I went from one cane to two canes. And eating the same food every single day caused me to develop food allergies that I had never had before. I was miserable: afraid and depressed at having left my life in Oregon to do this. I realized that Michio's statement that a diet would cure MS was absurd. Out of my depression, I began to understand that healing cannot focus only on the physical. It needs to involve the spirit and mind as well as the body."

It was at this low point in her life that a yoga teacher told Marin about Glenn Rothfeld and his integrative medicine practice. At the time, she was enrolled in two master's degree programs in two different states: studying social work in Boston, where she now lives, and psychospiritual psychology in Philadelphia. "I went to Glenn expecting either some mumbo jumbo about qi, or that he was going to give me this allopathic thing," says Marin. "Instead, he gave me a full Western and Eastern exam, and then actually sat, looked into my eyes and really talked to me. He told me that my kidney energy showed him that I was a person with a strong will, which is my big strength, but also my undoing. I felt as if he was uncovering the real me. For the first time, I felt seen." After she began seeing Glenn regularly, Marin says, she realized that she needed to slow down a bit. "Glenn helped me to see that I should not push so much, and I should listen to my body more," she says. "I am still learning to balance the reality of my body with my very strong will."

❖ ❖ ❖ ❖

When he talks about Marin, whom he has known now for fifteen years, Glenn Rothfeld continues to marvel at her courage, strength and vitality. "She is one of the most strong-willed people I know," he says. "I believe that she would not be alive today if not for her *will* to live. Chinese medicine helps me to understand her more fully.

"My treatment of her combines elements of both Eastern and Western medicine," says Glenn. "Marin's strong kidney energy means, according to the Five Element theory, that she is strongly influenced by the 'water' element and 'winter' energy. Everything is in reserve, the way the earth stores up its energy reserves during the winter in preparation for spring. But there is a price to pay for this kind of energy: What happens when you exhaust the reserves?" (Please see box for details about Five Element theory.)

In Marin's case, her reserves of vitamins, minerals and antioxidant enzymes were very low. This happens often with chronic disease, as well as with many elderly people, according to Glenn. "Chronic diseases such as rheumatoid arthritis, ulcerative colitis, lupus, multiple sclerosis, chronic fatigue syndrome, Parkinson's and fibromyalgia all stimulate the cells of the body to produce oxidizing compounds, such as hydrogen peroxide, in an attempt to destroy the abnormal or diseased cells. The oxidation process triggers the body to produce *antioxidants*, in order to cool down and balance this reaction. Remember that the body is always seeking to restore the proper *homeostasis* (balance) or, in Chinese terms, the proper balance between *yin* and *yang* energy."

The main antioxidant produced by the body, according to Glenn, is an enzyme called glutathione peroxidase. This enzyme requires selenium to perform its function of scavenging and dismantling the products of inflammation and oxidation, called free radicals, that are deadly to the body's cells. The oxidation process, as well as toxins, drugs and stress, can all deplete the supply of this necessary enzyme, causing unchecked damage to cells. In a condition like MS where any damage to nerve cells can lead to further dysfunction, the antioxidant function of glutathione is critical.

"So we need to find ways of replenishing the reserves of this antioxidant enzyme for patients like Marin," says Glenn. "The problem is that glutathione, the main component of glutathione peroxidase, is not easily absorbable through the gut, especially if people are taking other medications in pills, as most people with chronic disease do. In addition, the medications prescribed for people with chronic diseases, particularly the elderly, often interfere with the absorption of nutrients. The result is that many of these people are nutrient deficient. Marin's blood tests, for example, showed very low levels of magnesium, as well as several vitamins and nutrients. But if we gave magnesium to her orally, it would cause diarrhea, something she, with her bowel problems, certainly did not need."

The problem of absorption of glutathione, as well as other vitamins, minerals and enzymes that his patients need, led Glenn to the practice of using intravenous infusion, bypassing the digestive system altogether and going directly to the bloodstream, which carries it to the cells that need it. "We know, for example, that calcium tightens muscle tone, and magnesium softens tone," says Glenn. "We have found that intravenous magnesium helps patients with the characteristic spasticity of multiple sclerosis by almost instantly relaxing the muscle spasm." ("It's very effective in relaxing the intense spasticity in my legs and left arm," says Marin.) Unlike most MS medications for spasticity, this does not cause fatigue. Glenn has also found that intravenous magnesium is beneficial for patients with migraines, asthma, chronic back pain and some symptoms of Parkinson's. "It is also the best treatment for fibromyalgia that I know," he says.

In addition to intravenous magnesium and the antioxidant glutathione, Glenn also gives Marin regular intravenous infusions of vitamins and minerals. "She needs to keep her fluids and nutrients up to help her body cope with all of its health challenges," he says. Marin also has regular acupuncture, and her allopathic treatments include regular follow-ups for the recent surgeries and breast cancer. To date, despite the MS and the bowel surgeries, she still has full control over her bladder and bowel function. "I feel that Glenn's acupuncture treatments that focus on balancing my kidney meridian are responsible for this," says Marin.

Marin Today: Weaving a Tapestry of Personal Growth

The past fifteen years have been a significant journey for Marin. "For the first few years after my MS diagnosis, my focus and point of reference was *outside* of my body," says Marin. "While I don't reject much of what I tried, including macrobiotics, it was really the inner work that has transformed me and helped me find peace." Through her ongoing involvement in deep psychospiritual therapy, Marin discovered what she refers to as "right use of will . . . Glenn has always said that I am a strong-willed person," she says. "I am learning through psychospiritual therapy to use that will to build my *inner* strength: to listen to my body when it tells me when to surrender and when to persevere. Instead of always striving for that elusive external cure for my problems, I am learning to listen to my own truth."

In addition to her therapy, she also sees a physical therapist/osteopath. "He works on my body, but with a deep connection to my energy as well," she says. "He can tell, for example, simply by touching my feet, what part of my body needs his attention, and where my emotional blocks are." (Please see "A Closer Look at Osteopathy.") The third part of Marin's ongoing work is with Glenn. "He doesn't merely relieve symptoms," she says. "His treatments work on a profound level—healing mind as well as body. I am a very informed consumer, and a doctor like Glenn supports me in making my own decisions about my health. Nobody, no matter how brilliant, knows my body better than I do. I can't work with anyone who doesn't respect my sense of what I need and my own body-mind intelligence."

These healers—the psychotherapist, the physical therapist/osteopath and the integrative physician—are three threads of what Marin calls her tapestry of growth. "They form a pattern of healing," she says. "Through working with these people, I am now able to stay more in the present."

In the past few years, Marin has faced more than a dozen traumatic events. "I am learning that when I become involved in a crisis, whether it is a cancer diagnosis, a broken hip or totaling my van, I can become paralyzed by fear if I allow myself to be re-traumatized by *past* crises or traumatic events. But when I can keep myself HERE and NOW, naked with the feeling of what is actually happening in this moment, life is more bearable." Marin also has a deep faith in a higher spiritual power, which she says makes her feel safe. "I used to have fear in every cell of my body. Now, I know that I will be able to cope with whatever comes. Even if I were to lose the use of all my limbs because of MS, I would still be able to create by holding a paintbrush between my teeth. I will still be *me,* inside."

✦ ✦ ✦ ✦

Fibromyalgia—Finding Answers from Ayurveda

Geeta Sharma, M.D., M.P.H., became a psychiatrist because she wanted to challenge herself. "In India, where I grew up and went to medical school, there was hardly any training provided in psychiatry," she says. "So after I graduated, I came to the U.S. and decided to do a residency in psychiatry at the University of Connecticut Medical School and its affiliated Health Center. Being a psychiatrist gives me the opportunity to understand and analyze complex problems, and that is what I love to do."

For the next twenty years, however, Geeta could not figure out what was wrong with *her.* She began to feel exhausted all the time. "I had hardly any energy, but at the same time had difficulty sleeping," she says. "I had pain in my whole body and felt, at varying times, cold, dizzy and anxious. I had chronic sinus infections and allergies and a feeling that was close to hypoglycemia (when the blood sugar is low)."

Despite these problems, Geeta was determined to live a normal life. She got a second degree—a master's in public health—from Johns Hopkins, married and had children. In 1998 she began her current position as director of the Acute

Inpatient Psychiatric Unit at the Walter P. Carter Center, which is affiliated with the University of Maryland Medical School and Medical System, where she is also assistant clinical professor of psychiatry.

But her symptoms persisted. "There were days when I had to drag myself out of bed to go to work," she remembers. "My husband was the one who took our children to parties and on outings. On weekends, all I wanted to do was stay home, rest and try to deal with the pain and lack of energy." Despite extensive testing, her allopathic doctors could not diagnose her problem, although they did prescribe medications for the pain and insomnia. "I also tried acupuncture, Chinese herbal medicine and homeopathy, but nothing helped," says Geeta. "Now, thanks to my own research, I know that I was suffering from fibromyalgia—a chronic disease that is characterized by chronic pain as well as chronic fatigue—which is difficult to diagnose and treat. But before I knew that, I was discouraged and disappointed. I looked the same, so it was hard for my family and friends to realize that I was sick, and that made it worse."

Then, one Saturday morning in 1998, a colleague called Geeta to tell her about a "Whole Life Expo" that was happening that day. "I told her that, as usual, I was too tired and uncomfortable to go anywhere," says Geeta. "But she insisted on reading me the list of exhibitors—she's a good friend who works with me, and is very persistent! When she got to a listing about Ayurvedic astrology and palmistry, something clicked in my mind."

Having grown up in India, Geeta has many childhood memories of the Ayurvedic medicines and healing practices that were part of everyday life there. (Please see chapter 2 for a description of Ayurveda.) "Ayurvedic medicine is something that most people in India know automatically, because we grow up using the herbs and natural remedies in our homes," says Geeta. "When my friend mentioned Ayurvedic astrology, it touched off a powerful series of child-hood memories: My mother would give us turmeric powder and honey in hot milk for any internal injury or infections. If we had muscle or joint pain, we would make a 'dough' of turmeric powder, whole wheat flour and a little salt, heat it in a flat pan, wrap it in a cloth and apply it as a poultice to the affected area to speed healing. Turmeric powder is used for minor cuts because it has a kind of 'antiseptic' property."

For skin problems, including eczema, pimples and dermatitis, Geeta remembers garlic—lots of it. "My mother would serve us a clove of garlic with meals, and put crushed fresh garlic on our skin. This would heal the problem," she says. "And always, during cold weather, we would have extra ginger in our food, as well as ginger powder in hot milk. It helps to keep the whole body system warm."

One of Geeta's best memories—one that might sound particularly wonderful to Westerners—were the people who came to the houses in her neighborhood each week to give Ayurvedic massages to everyone in the family. "The Ayurvedic belief is that the whole body needs to be massaged regularly with certain oils to help keep the mind grounded in the body. I was always the kind of person who lived very much in my head, for example, without an awareness of my body, so I would trip and bump into things. But when someone massages your whole body, it helps to integrate and connect your mind with your body. And besides, it feels absolutely wonderful!" (For more about Ayurvedic and other forms of massage, please see "Four Ways to Feel Better.")

With her move to the United States and the all-enveloping experience of her postgraduate work and a professional life based on Western medicine, Geeta lost touch with the Ayurvedic traditions of her past. But the mention of Ayurveda by her friend brought it all flooding back. "I suddenly decided that I needed to go to this health exposition," says Geeta. "I wanted to meet the Ayurvedic practitioner. I just had a feeling that I might find an answer there."

That day, Geeta met Ghanshyam Singh Birla, who was giving an introductory lecture on Vedic palmistry and astrology. "After the lecture, I made an appointment to see him. We talked for a long time about my symptoms, and he reminded me about the Ayurvedic belief that many illnesses are the result of imbalances within the body. I felt immediately that this was the answer for me."

Ghanshyam offered to treat Geeta with Ayurvedic methods. "He said, 'I promise that if you come to see me once a month for three days, I will guarantee that you will get better, and I won't leave you alone until you do get better,'" remembers Geeta. "No one had ever said anything like that to me before, so I agreed. I traveled to his clinic in Canada once a month. He began treating me with deep Ayurvedic massage, using a combination of warmed oils, including mustard oil and sandalwood oil, focusing particularly on the very tight, painful muscles of my shoulders, neck and back. On my scalp, he used almond oil. He taught me special yoga positions, such as the sun salutation, and yogic deep-breathing exercises (called *pranayama*) to do every day. I was also told to do the deep-breathing exercises during the massage sessions, during which time I listened to recordings of two mantras (Sanskrit phrases that are thought to be healing) for sound therapy to reduce stress."

Part of Geeta's treatment included dietary changes, the addition of certain Ayurvedic herbs, and the use of Ayurvedic astrology and palmistry as diagnostic tools. Unlike the Western concept of "magical" astrology and palm reading that predict the future, the Ayurvedic sciences of astrology and palmistry, based on practices that are thousands of years old, are used to understand body types, personality characteristics and the diseases to which we are prone. (Remember that in chapter 2, Dr. Vasant D. Lad, one of the country's leading authorities in Ayurvedic medicine, tells us that the Sanskrit word for Vedic medical astrology means 'light': "We use Vedic astrology, as well as palmistry, as 'the light of life,' to guide us and to understand our physical and emotional strengths and weaknesses," says Dr. Lad.)

However, as we also saw in chapter 2, scientific research on Ayurvedic medicine in general is minimal, and studies on Ayurvedic medical astrology and palmistry are virtually nonexistent. Although these latter practices have been in use for thousands of years, it will be impossible to scientifically evaluate their effects on health until there is research.

Geeta Gets Better

Over a period of several months, Geeta noticed improvements in her health and general outlook on life for the first time in twenty years. "The massages and yoga caused the pain to lessen; the breathing and meditation calmed my mind and lowered the level of anxiety, and my energy level came up with the dietary changes and herbs. I am sleeping better and have a more positive outlook on life. Now, the only time I have pain is when I am under stress, but even then it doesn't last that long."

Ghanshyam worked on several levels to help Geeta: "When I met her, she was able to do her job but had little energy left to function in the rest of her life," he says. "Some days, she felt as if she could not get out of bed. The first challenge for her was to establish and stick to a daily routine that included regular exercise and meditation, yoga and deep-breathing exercises.

The Ayurvedic massage was a key part of Geeta's treatment, according to Ghanshyam. "She would look quiet while she was lying on the massage table, but I could tell that her mind was going one hundred miles an hour," he says. "We needed to get that *Vata* energy under control or the massage would be of little value." With instruction, Geeta learned to do deep-breathing exercises during the massage, visualizing the *prana* (life force described in chapter 2) traveling up her spine as she inhaled and then back down again as she exhaled. "Many Ayurvedic practices are based on awakening the *chakras*, or invisible energy centers in the body, which are located at various points along the spine, in the throat and in the area between the eyebrows," says Ghanshyam. "We also used a combination of heated oils, including mustard seed, sesame and sandalwood oils to rekindle her *Pitta* (or fire) energy, which had grown sluggish. The deep-tissue massage also helped the problem of tight muscles in her back, neck and shoulders, increasing circulation and allowing them to *breathe* again." (See chapter 2 for a description of the *Vata* and *Pitta* body types.)

In addition to the massage, yoga, breathing, meditation and dietary changes, Ghanshyam recommended the purifying treatment called *panchakarma*. "Her symptoms and our Ayurvedic analyses indicated that both her small and large intestines were filled with toxins," says Ghanshyam. "Before she started to change her diet, we used special herbs and intestinal cleansing methods to eliminate these toxins, and we recommended that she fast on certain days. After this, she began a special *Vata*-pacifying diet, which eliminated red meat, but included plenty of stews with cooked vegetables, soups, cooked grains and other warm, comforting foods. She needed calming and warming food—along with certain *Vata*-pacifying herbs, in order to reduce the imbalance that was producing anxiety, insomnia, muscle tension and other symptoms."

As Geeta began to feel better in her body, she also began to notice a change in her personality: "I had always been a fairly rigid person, thinking that there was only one way of doing things, and it was my way," she says. "But now that I was making a commitment to get better, I began to look at how my rigid attitudes might have contributed to my rigid, painful body. I began to consciously make an effort to understand the point of view of others. This made my life more harmonious. The very interesting thing that was also happening was a change in my handprints. When I compared the handprints that Ghanshyam had taken when I first met him to prints taken a year later, there were actually significant visible changes in the lines of my hands."

During this time, Geeta also noticed that she was relating to her patients in a different way. "I realized from my own experiences that change can only happen if the pain or suffering is so unbearable that the person has no other choice. I used to get frustrated when patients didn't follow my treatment recommendations. But now, it is easier for me to accept people as they are and to accept that they will change when they are ready. I understand on a deeper level than I ever did before that this is *their* suffering and in the end, the treatment will only be effective if it is *their* choice. Interestingly, when I can expand my own point of view to accept their resistance to treatment, I find that they are often more willing to make the choice to get better."

❖ ❖ ❖ ❖

✓ TAKE ACTION ✓

An Ayurvedic Prescription for Health

The main goal of Ayurveda is to heal the person, rather than the disease or the symptoms. The following recommendations are general categories of Ayurvedic practices. Ayurvedic practitioners adapt them for individual constitutional (*dosha*) imbalances—for the particular body, mind and spirit of each patient, whether primarily *Vata, Pitta* or *Kapha,* or some combination. (See chapter 2 for details of these *doshas.) It is important to see an Ayurvedic physician for a correct diagnosis of your particular dosha type before undertaking any treatment plan.*

1. Daily exercise. About thirty minutes a day of brisk walking or other aerobic exercise to strengthen muscles and invigorate the cardiovascular system.
2. A daily practice of reflection and meditation, preferably with the use of Sanskrit mantras (phrases or affirmations).
3. Yogic deep-breathing exercises twice a day to harmonize and calm the unbalanced *dosha* energy from the inside. These breathing exercises incorporate deep concentration and visualization, calming the mind while oxygenating the cells of the body. They are also used to activate the energy centers of the body, called *chakras.*
4. Daily yoga exercises to stretch and strengthen the body, and to unite body and mind.
5. Regular massage with warmed oils (some combination of mustard seed, sesame, camphor, sandalwood, jasmine, or other oils appropriate to the unbalanced *dosha*). Massages can also include application of special herbs onto the skin, magnets, aromatherapy, visual therapy, using colored lights and sound therapy using musical tones or recorded mantras. (Please see "Four Ways to Feel Better," for more about Ayurvedic massage.)
6. Adjust diet and Ayurvedic herbs to the particular *dosha* type.
7. If necessary, intensive cleansing of the intestines using *panchakarma,* herbs and other techniques.

In Search of Balance and Joy

Ghanshyam Singh Birla's fascination with healing began more than sixty years ago, with his grandfather in India. "My grandfather was a contractor by trade, a builder of bricks and mortar," says Ghanshyam, "but his true passion was building healthy bodies and minds. In all of his spare time, he would study ancient Ayurvedic texts, concoct herbs, create mixtures of oils, teach meditation mantras and distribute his healing knowledge to all who came to our house. He did it with love, never charging anything. There was a constant flow of Ayurvedic experts as well as people needing help in and out of our house. The patients would arrive crying and leave smiling, and I would wonder to myself, 'What is my grandpa doing?'"

Determined to find out, Ghanshyam attached himself to his grandfather, watching, asking questions, learning from his grandfather's friends and helping whenever he could. "I grew up with all of the richness of his knowledge," says Ghanshyam. "My biggest interest was in the connections between human morphology (body structure), emotions, thoughts, spiritual beliefs and individual predispositions to disease. All of these interrelationships can be seen in the Ayurvedic physical exam, as well as in Ayurvedic astrological and palm analysis. Both the astrological chart and the very palms of the hands reflect past experiences as well as patterns of thought and emotion."

And Ghanshyam emphasizes, "We absolutely do not use the ancient wisdom of astrology and palmistry to predict the future, only to understand the past and the present, and to guide us in the prevention of disease. The goal is to achieve and maintain health so that we can live in happiness and joy."

For the past forty-five years, Ghanshyam has collected thousands of handprints to demonstrate how the patterns of lines in the hand change in reaction to changes in deep-seated personality and behavior patterns. "I deeply believe that we can use the hands to help us better understand why someone is ill or unhappy," says Ghanshyam. "When one's thinking or emotions change, so do the hands. My hope is that research will one day demonstrate this fundamental connection between the brain and the lines of the hands."

When Ghanshyam first met Dr. Geeta Sharma, he examined her by using Ayurvedic analysis of her body type, including the shape and condition of her face, hair, eyes, teeth, gums and tongue, as well as the condition of pulses at different points on the body. He watched the way that she breathed, moved and spoke. "Then I went even deeper to understand her psyche," he says. "Each finger on the hand represents one of the five senses and its corresponding element, and different parts of the hand represent the planetary configurations at the time of birth. Ayurvedic medicine is based on the belief that humans are microcosms of the universe."

Ghanshyam used all of the information that he gathered about Geeta to arrive at a diagnosis: "Her *Vata dosha* was highly aggravated, which explained her anxiety, sleeplessness and tense, tight muscles," he says. "It became clear that balancing her *Vata dosha* would help with the insomnia, anxiety, fatigue syndrome, chronic muscle pain and her fears. An unbalanced *Vata* can even create hallucinations." As we saw in chapter 2, the *Vata* energy affects the nervous system, heart, large intestine, skin and lungs. "Everything I did for Geeta was focused on balancing and calming her overactive *Vata* energy," says Ghanshyam.

Geeta has kept up her regular visits to Ghanshyam for the past three years, although she goes less often now. In addition to the massage therapy, she continues to have occasional Vedic astrology and palmistry consultations. "It has been astounding to me to see how different my handprints look now when compared to the prints I had done three years ago," she says. She has also kept up her yoga and meditation practice, as well as her dietary changes. As she described above, her symptoms have lessened dramatically. "Her skin now has a luminous glow," says Ghanshyam. "And her hands have lost the bluish tinge they had when I first met her. Now, they shine like brilliant stars."

❖ ❖ ❖ ❖

Toxic Injury—When the Environment Makes You Sick

Before you visit Anna Olivera (not her real name), she needs to ask you some questions: What will you be wearing? Were the clothes washed in laundry detergent? What kind? Were they dry-cleaned? What kind of shampoo and soap do you use? Do you wear perfume or hairspray? If you answer even one of these questions by mentioning a product that you found on the shelf of a supermarket or pharmacy, Anna will have a severe headache, neck ache, breathing problems, body pain and a burning sensation in her chest almost as soon as you walk into her house.

Anna—a forty-one-year-old former computer engineer and professor of computer science—has a permanent toxic injury called multiple chemical sensitivity (MCS). Although there are ways to minimize some of the symptoms, there is no known cure. She did not get this injury because of a chemical spill or a dangerous occupation. She became permanently injured at the age of thirty-six when the company she worked for moved to a newly renovated office building. Grace Ziem, M.D., M.P.H., Dr.P.H., knows why.

An Expert on Toxic Injury

Grace Ziem has never met Anna Olivera, but she has seen thousands of patients like her. "About 80 percent of my patients who are chronically ill because of exposure to chemicals were injured in the workplace," says Ziem. "A common cause is working in what have come to be called 'sick buildings.' Other causes include exposure to pesticides, solvents, combustion products and other irritants and neurotoxins." Ziem is a national authority on toxic injury—which is defined as damage to the body, often the central nervous system, caused either by prolonged—or shorter and more intense—exposure to toxic chemicals. She has been practicing environmental and occupational medicine since 1979, when she was a physician for the Health Effects Unit of the Maryland Occupational Safety and Health Administration. In that year, she also won a National Science Foundation fellowship to provide education and technical assistance on occupational hazard recognition and control to workers and supervisors.

Since then, she has consulted, testified and lectured on toxic and chemical injury—including toxic injuries to Gulf War veterans—in medical schools, for the U.S. Congress, the U.S. Environmental Protection Agency, the National Academy of Sciences and the World Health Organization. She has published several research studies on the subject. Along with her M.D. and M.P.H. from Johns Hopkins, where she taught in the School of Public Health for twenty-five years, she also has a doctorate in public health from Harvard. Now, she is teaching occupational medicine (which focuses on illnesses that derive from the workplace) at the University of Maryland School of Medicine.

❖ ❖ ❖ ❖

Anna Olivera's story is typical of many of Grace Ziem's patients. Before Anna became ill, she had a full, active life. She enjoyed the physical challenges of hiking, tennis and outdoor sports, as well as both modern and jazz dance. She had traveled to South America and Africa, backpacked through Europe and driven cross-country in a van. Both before and after they had children, she and her husband enjoyed a rich cultural life, including theater, concerts and dance performances. They loved dining out. She was committed to her career but was able to balance her professional ambition with her family.

"I had been with my company for several years, and was thrilled with a recent promotion to manage a design team," says Anna. "I was also teaching computer science part time at a nearby university. My youngest daughter had just started kindergarten, and the older one was in third grade. I was respected in my field, happy in my family life and had never had any serious health problems. All that changed when I moved into my office in the newly renovated building."

The basement office had several high transom windows to the outdoors, but they were kept shut because it was January when the company moved. "The office felt damp and musty, despite the new carpets, computer and furniture," says Anna. "The rugs had been shampooed and treated for stain resistance and the walls had been freshly painted." Within a few weeks, Anna began noticing symptoms of what she thought was a cold or flu. "I had a tight, sore throat, hoarseness, dry cough, pain in my sinuses, joint stiffness, a tightness in my chest and general fatigue," she says. "I also found that I was having trouble concentrating on my work, as well as with writing, which had always come easily to me." When Anna also developed what she describes as a "stabbing pain" in the right side of her chest, she went to the emergency room of her local hospital.

The diagnosis was viral pleuritis, an inflammation of the lining of the lungs. "They said it was probably due to the flu that I seemed to have at the time," says Anna. "They sent me home with medication and told me I needed bed rest." After a few weeks at home, Anna felt better, although she still had some chest pain. "The sore throat and headache were gone, and my energy was back, so I went back to work," she says.

By the end of Anna's first day back in the office, all of her previous symptoms had returned. "My doctor said I must have gone back too soon," says Anna. "I stayed home for another week and, feeling better once again, went back to work. After a couple of days this time, all of the symptoms were back. I felt like I had a severe sinus and throat infection." Anna's doctor referred her to an ear-nose-throat specialist and an infectious disease specialist. "They evaluated me for lupus, rheumatoid arthritis, Lyme disease, connective tissue and autoimmune disorders," says Anna. "We tried to figure out if I could have picked up anything in my travels. I did, in fact have a sinus and throat infection, but that did not explain the body pain and difficulty concentrating."

All the tests were negative. Her doctors had no explanation for her symptoms. "At that point, I was concerned but not panic-stricken," says Anna. "I had no history of serious illness in my family and had always been very healthy. I figured that whatever this was would work itself out." In the meantime, Anna was told to stay home, this time for longer. After a couple of months, she was feeling better. "The infections and headache were gone, I had more energy and the muscle pain was gone, although I did still have chest pain," she says.

"It Suddenly Hit Me.
Is My Office Making Me Sick?"

So one morning in May, Anna went back to work. "After just a few hours—it wasn't even lunchtime yet, all of my symptoms were back, as bad as ever," says Anna. "Suddenly, it hit me like a ton of bricks. It had all started when I moved into my new office. Was my office making me sick? Then I thought, *This is crazy.* I went home that afternoon, felt better and came back to work the next day. I immediately felt sick again and had to go home." Anna kept this up for several more days. "By the end of the week, it was clear that I felt sick in my office, and better anywhere outside my office," she says.

She called her doctor. "He told me to stay out of the office, so I called my supervisor. She said that a colleague down the hall was retiring and I could move into that office. It was spring. We could open windows. But by then I was afraid to stay in that building. I had been talking to friends and had heard about someone who had become permanently ill from a 'sick building,' so I refused to stay in that building. They agreed that I could move into another building nearby that the company also owned, and they sent experts to check out my old office."

The experts discovered, according to Anna, that during the remodeling the ventilation shafts leading to her office had been boarded over by mistake. "There was virtually no air exchange or air cleaning in that room," says Anna. "To make matters worse, I discovered that my office was next to a storeroom where they kept chemicals for cleaning. I was also in the habit of keeping my door closed as I worked, so I was spending eight hours a day breathing unventilated air, including the chemical gases coming off of the treated rugs and freshly painted walls—I had been in a 'chemical soup.'"

In the new building, Anna's condition stabilized. "I was not getting worse, although the symptoms were not yet gone," she says. Then Anna's supervisor told her she could not do her old job—managing a software team—from a different building. She needed to be in the same building as her staff. She could use a different room. "We tried conference rooms, other offices, opening windows, using air conditioning, but frighteningly, the symptoms were beginning to come back," says Anna. "I was desperate not to lose my job and the career I had worked so many years to build, so I tried every way I could think of to make it work. Nothing helped."

Than an even more frightening thing began to happen: "I found I was having headaches, breathing problems, chest pain, fatigue and poor concentration even when I was home, or when I went to the mall or a restaurant, or a movie theater," says Anna. "I felt like I was in the middle of a nightmare and I couldn't wake up."

✦ ✦ ✦ ✦

This nightmare was permanent, but it could have been prevented if Anna had been told by her doctors to heed the early warning signals of toxic injury and immediately remove herself from the office environment that was causing them. But neither she nor her doctors had any idea of the cause of her symptoms. And by the time they found out, permanent damage had been done to her nervous system. "When people are exposed in the workplace, even if they know that the environment is making them sick, they often have to choose between their health and their paychecks," says Dr. Grace Ziem, the toxic injury expert. "So they try to 'tough it out,' since they are often powerless to change their environment. Whether they are working on an assembly line or in a sick office building, they can't afford to leave their jobs." To make matters worse, points out Ziem, chemicals in the workplace are usually at higher intensities than in the home, and people are exposed to them for long periods during the day. The situation becomes particularly dangerous if, as in Anna's office, there is poor or nonexistent air ventilation and cleaning.

"All petrochemicals and many chemicals—such as ammonia, chloride and other chemicals that are found in everyday products—cleaning solutions, stain prevention compounds, fresh paint, solvents and scented products—can cause irritation when they are inhaled or touched," says Ziem. "With the initial exposure, people may have some warning symptoms, which include respiratory (breathing) distress, sinus pain, sore throat, nasal irritation, chest tightness, coughing, wheezing and neurologic symptoms, such as confusion, and concentration and memory problems." Sometimes, there is not even a warning smell, says Ziem, as many of these chemicals (especially pesticides) have little or no odor at levels that can induce illness. People may not even be aware that they are taking them into their lungs with every breath.

If people recognize and take action at the first symptoms of toxic exposure, they can avoid permanent damage, according to Ziem. "There are now five different studies, all of which confirm that the most effective intervention is reduced exposure to irritants," she says. (Please see research section.) "The patients I have who changed jobs, relocated or made their homes nontoxic and avoided exposure to pesticides become more mildly affected, and I don't need to intervene nearly as often." She still, however, has a yearlong waiting list of chemically injured patients waiting to see her for the first time.

✓ TAKE ACTION ✓

Preventing Permanent Toxic Injury

1. **Pay attention** to the early warning signs, especially if you have recently changed your work or home environment. These include: respiratory (breathing) distress, sinus pain, headache, sore throat, nasal irritation, chest tightness, coughing, wheezing and neurologic symptoms, such as confusion and concentration and memory problems. You may or may not notice any odor in the air you breathe.
2. **Investigate** the potential cause, along with your employer and your doctor.
3. The most effective intervention at this stage is to **reduce your exposure to the irritants,** to allow the brain cells and respiratory tract to heal. This should be done both in the workplace (often extremely difficult) and in the home. You can request "reasonable accommodation" to reduce exposure at work, school, apartments and condominiums. Many states have consumer organizations for patients with "Multiple Chemical Sensitivity (MCS)" that provide books, names of experts and information about lifestyle changes to eliminate irritating chemicals in the home. Even if you have no symptoms, it is always a good idea to try to reduce toxic cleaning products in your home, and, if you remodel, consider using nontoxic paints, building materials and fabrics.

   If you develop a permanent injury: (NOTE: It is important to consult carefully with your doctor before trying any of these treatments. Some may be harmful for certain patients.)

   If, even after changing your work and home environment, you still have symptoms, there are several treatment options. The most promising, according to Dr. Ziem, is the "hyperbaric oxygen chamber," an enclosed chamber in which oxygen is introduced at increased pressures to help repair damage to brain and nerve cells.

Other treatments that have been helpful to some patients:

1. Individualized dietary changes to assist healing of toxic injury.
2. A nebulized (broken up into a fine mist for inhalation) form of glutathione, the most important antioxidant occurring naturally in the body.
3. Gentle exercise and activity that does not exacerbate fatigue.
4. Nutritional and hormonal supplements (including thyroid, adrenal, estrogen, progesterone and melatonin). *NOTE: Hormonal supplements are usually more effective when deficiencies exist.*
5. Natural substances or, if needed, medications to balance neurotransmitters in the brain.

(continued)

6. Allergy desensitization treatments if allergy is present and symptomatic.
7. Anticandida (yeast infection) and antiparasite treatments.
8. Detoxification treatments.
9. Alternative therapies, including homeopathy, acupuncture, naturopathy, osteopathy, chiropractic treatment, bodywork, herbs, macrobiotics, Ayurvedic medicine, visualization and meditation. (Please see Appendix I for descriptions of alternative practices.)

Crossing Over—How Permanent Injury Happens

All too often, says Ziem with some frustration, manufacturers do a poor job of providing accurate safety sheets on the chemicals they sell, so that employers and consumers may not be aware of the potential hazards. "This results in an extremely dangerous situation," she says. "By trying to 'tough out' these symptoms in the workplace, people run the risk of crossing the line from chemical irritation to permanent toxic injury." Depending on the intensity of exposure and the length of exposure time, people may develop a chronic inflammation of the respiratory tract (lungs) with neurologic inflammation, according to Ziem. "The primary target of toxic injury is neurologic: the brain and central nervous system," she says. "The brain is the organ that commands every system in the body. If its cells are permanently damaged, so are the messages that it sends to the lungs, digestive system, hormone-producing glands such as the thyroid and adrenals and, tragically, the reproductive system: Affected women have tremendous difficulty becoming pregnant, and if they do deliver successfully, the babies may have some impaired function."

A "spreading effect" is a common reaction among severely injured patients, according to Ziem. "When the nervous system is permanently damaged, it begins to communicate with the person's immune system, causing it to react to lesser and lesser irritants," she says. "In effect, the damaged brain cells are telling the body, 'even this small irritant is too much for the permanent inflammation in your lungs.' This 'crossing over' into permanent damage can happen in weeks or months, but once it happens, there is little we can do, although the anti-oxidant glutathione has reduced symptoms significantly for patients. In addition, treatments in a hyperbaric oxygen chamber—at 1.5 ATM and without germicides in the chamber and other less toxic precautions in the facility—properly done, can permanently improve brain function." (Please see box for other conventional and complementary treatments.)

❖ ❖ ❖ ❖

Looking back on her experience now, Anna Olivera can analyze what happened to her. "I never understood—and none of the many doctors I saw warned me—that repeated exposure to the irritating chemicals over a period of months could result in a permanent injury," she says. "When I was finally diagnosed with multiple chemical sensitivity (MCS) by an occupational physician, it was too late. I had become a victim of the 'spreading phenomenon' of MCS." She began having severe headaches, breathing problems, chest burning and body pain symptoms when she was near shampoos or body lotions that were fragranced, clothes that had been washed in commercial detergents, most household cleaning products, newspapers, book print, some plastics, smoke, fumes from the computer and TV, pesticides, fertilizers, mulch, paint, makeup, any public transportation, any kind of treated rugs or upholstery . . . and the list goes on.

What does this mean for her life now? "The most painful thing for me—both financially and emotionally—was leaving my job and giving up my career," says Anna. "I can *still* no longer be near a computer without discomfort. We had to give away most of our family's clothes—once clothes have been washed in detergent, there was no way to remove the fragrance. I drive a seven-year-old car, but I can never drive in my husband's car, because it is relatively new and the carpet and upholstery treatments are still sending off gases. I can't go on vacation and sleep in a hotel. I can no longer go to the theater, church, movies, the mall or out to dinner in a restaurant."

Even after completely changing her life and environment, Anna still gets symptoms every day that include headache, neck pain, sore throat and fatigue, that come on within a few minutes of exposure. "If my neighbor uses fabric softener sheets in her dryer, and my windows are open, I have a reaction," she says. "Or it might happen if I walk my kids to the bus and there is car exhaust, or if I eat certain foods. Even opening the mail can be a problem because of printing inks."

However, Anna is basically a positive and emotionally strong person, and these attributes have helped her adjust. "I realized early on that I needed to find ways to enjoy life," she says. She has, for example, developed a passion for outdoor figure skating. "There are few irritants at an outdoor rink and it gives me great exercise." She also enjoys hiking, biking, picnics and other outdoor activities with her family. Instead of going out to dinner, she invites friends over. "Many of my friends are careful with their clothes, and they don't use fragranced personal care products," she says. But just in case, she keeps a large supply of sweatshirts and sweatpants for people to change into if necessary. She has also managed to find a way to enjoy dining out: outdoor restaurants. "I know all of the best cafés for miles around," she says.

Hard as it was to lose her professional identity, she still rejoices in her parent role. "The difficulty there is that I can only volunteer at school for outdoor activities," she says. "And it is hard not to be able to see my kids perform in school plays and concerts."

She has adjusted her medical care as well. "I found a primary care doctor whose specialty is occupational medicine," she says. "My last doctor wanted to put me on psychiatric drugs. I had to face real ignorance about this illness. It is most certainly not a psychiatric illness or a phobia!" Anna uses a range of complementary therapies to cope with the frequent head and neck pain, including acupuncture, craniosacral therapy, and neuromuscular massage. She also has regular intravenous infusions of vitamins and minerals. "These therapies have helped me decrease my overall level of sensitivity," she says. "My life feels more stable now, and while I miss much of what I was able to do before, I have found some measure of joy and peace with the people I love," she pauses before continuing. "I guess I'm lucky. I'm an optimist."

Toxic Injury and Multiple Chemical Sensitivity: What's the Evidence?

The term multiple chemical sensitivity (MCS) was first used by Dr. Mark Cullen of Yale to refer to "a chronic illness acquired in relation to an environmental exposure affecting more than one organ system, with symptoms aggravated by exposures to chemicals at levels orders of magnitude below those that cause noticeable illness in the healthy population."

MCS is being increasingly recognized as a growing health problem. A paper published in 1999 and signed by thirty-four physicians from around the country stated that "The millions of civilians and tens of thousands of Gulf War veterans who suffer from chemical sensitivity should not be kept waiting any longer for a standardized diagnosis while medical research continues to investigate the etiology of their signs and symptoms." The paper also reports on state health department surveys in New Mexico and California that found that two to four percent of respondents had already been diagnosed with MCS, while 16 percent reported "unusual sensitivity" to common, everyday chemicals. In addition, government studies in the United States, United Kingdom and Canada revealed two to four times as many cases of chemical sensitivity among Gulf War veterans than among an undeployed control group.[4]

In a 1989 study, Nicholas Ashford of MIT and Claudia Miller, M.D., of the University of Texas Health Science Center in San Antonio, concluded "chemical sensitivity exists as a serious and widespread public health problem warranting action by medical and governmental agencies."

In its 1993 position paper, the American College of Occupational and Environmental Medicine stated, "Increasingly, MCS has become a troublesome medical concern of individuals and their physicians. The impact of this condition on the well-being, productivity, and lifestyle of those affected can be dramatic."

Grace Ziem, M.D., M.P.H., Dr. P.H., (please see related story) has been researching toxic injury and treating patients for more than thirty years. Among her findings on diagnosis and treatment:

---

[4] "Multiple Chemical Sensitivity: A 1999 Consensus." *Archives of Environmental Health* 54, no. 3 (May–June 1999): 147–149. Signed by thirty-four physicians.

- **Chemical sensitivity "commonly occurs following prolonged or too-intense exposure** to pesticides, other petrochemicals, and coal-derived chemicals or combustion products. . . . Thus, social efforts to avoid unnecessary exposure of workers and the public to these substances could have significant beneficial effects for primary prevention as well as for reducing illness in persons who are already chemically sensitive."

- **Overlap of MCS with chronic fatigue syndrome and fibromyalgia syndrome:** In one of the first studies to assess the overlap of all three of these illnesses, Ziem and Albert Donnay evaluated one hundred consecutive patients in a private practice specializing in occupational and environmental health. They found that almost all (88 percent) of the MCS patients also met current diagnostic criteria for chronic fatigue syndrome, and almost half (49 percent) also met fibromyalgia diagnostic criteria. MCS was also found to overlap with allergy by 50 percent and vice versa. The authors recommend that patients in all categories be routinely screened for the other related disorders to improve early detection, treatment and prevention. The authors postulate that in many cases the three syndromes may in fact be the same disease, aggravated by exposure to petrochemicals.

- In a survey of patients, as well as a review of the literature, Ziem concludes that "exposures which can induce chemical sensitivity involve symptomatic, usually repeated, exposures to pesticides, solvents, combustion products, remodeling, sick buildings, carbonless copy paper (occupational heavy use) and other irritants and petrochemicals. Accompanying toxic injury often involves the immune, endocrine and nervous systems as well as impairments in detoxification, energy and neurotransmitter metabolism, protein, mineral and other nutrient deficiencies and gastrointestinal changes. . . ." She also explores the potential molecular links among MCS, fibromyalgia and chronic fatigue syndrome and explains how cellular changes induced by chemical exposure cause or contribute to patient symptoms.

References

Ashford, N. S. and C. S. Miller. *Chemical Exposures: Low Levels and High Stakes.* New York: Van Nostrand Reinhnold, 1991.

Cullen, M. R. "The Worker with Multiple Chemical Sensitivities." *Occupational Medicine* 2 (1987): 655–662. Also referenced in Ziem, G. E. "Profile of Patients with Chemical Injury and Sensitivity, Part II." *International Journal of Toxicology* 18 (1999): 401–409.

Donnay, A. and G. Ziem. "Prevalence and Overlap of Chronic Fatigue Syndrome and Fibromyalgia Syndrome Among 100 New Patients with Multiple Chemical Sensitivity." Published simultaneously in *Journal of Chronic Fatigue Syndrome* 5, no. 3/4 (1999): 71–80 (The Haworth Medical Press, an imprint of The Haworth Press, Inc.) and in *Chronic Fatigue Syndrome: Advances in Epidemiologic, Clinical and Basic Science Research,* ed. Roberto Patarca-Montero. The Haworth Medical Press, an imprint of The Haworth Press, Inc., 1999.

Miller, C. S. "Chemical Sensitivity: History and Phenomenology." White Paper: *Toxicology and Industrial Health* 10, no. 4/5 (1994): 253–276.

National Institute of Environmental Health Sciences: Environmental Health Perspectives Supplements. *Chemical Sensitivity.* National Institute of Environmental Health Sciences 105, Supplement 2, March 1997.

U.S. Department of Health and Human Services. *Multiple Chemical Sensitivity: A Scientific Overview.* U.S. Department of Health and Human Services: Public Health Service and Agency for Toxic Substances and Disease Registry, 1995.

Ziem, G. E. "Multiple Chemical Sensitivity: Treatment and Follow-Up with Avoidance and Control of Chemical Exposures." *Toxicology and Industrial Health* 8, no. 4 (1992).

———. "Profile of Patients with Chemical Injury and Sensitivity." *Environmental Health Perspectives* 105, Supplement 7 (March 1997): 417–436.

———. "Profile of Patients with Chemical Injury and Sensitivity, Part II." *International Journal of Toxicology* 18 (1999): 401–409.

A Closer Look at Healing Herbs
"I bet my prostate and won."

In the early 1990s, James A. Duke, Ph.D., bet his prostate in front of dozens of federal officials from the Food and Drug Administration (FDA) and the National Institutes of Health (NIH). "I wanted to publicly challenge the first FDA-approved pharmaceutical (Proscar, finasteride) developed for benign prostatic hypertrophy (BPH)," says Duke, a world authority on herbal medicine and the author of several bestselling books on the subject, including *The Green Pharmacy* and his latest *CRC Handbook of Medicinal Plants.*

BPH—an enlargement of the prostate gland—is a condition affecting nearly half of all men over fifty, causing urinary problems and other symptoms. "I told the FDA and NIH officials that a mixture of saw palmetto, pumpkin seeds and licorice would be cheaper, have fewer side effects, and be at least as effective at reducing the symptoms of enlarged prostate as the *new* drug then on the market," says Duke. "I was willing to offer up my own prostate gland. Some of us would be better off without the gland anyhow, especially at my age."

That was around a decade ago. "After that meeting, I got several calls from a number of the older officials at the meeting who wanted to know how much saw palmetto to take," says Duke. "I've converted my physician as well." Duke's challenge to the FDA helped to fulfill what he describes as one of his life's ambitions. "I want the FDA to make the drug companies test their new synthetic drugs not only against an inactive substance (a placebo) but also against most competitive herbal alternatives—and there are many competitive alternatives."

As evidence for his herbal advocacy, Duke cites a recent article by Lasser, et al., in the *Journal of the American Medical Association* (*JAMA*) which suggests that the leading cause of death in the United States may be adverse drug reactions. "Still, the media frenzy feeds on the erroneous anti-herb hype," fumes Duke, "and continues to frighten American citizens away from the safer herbs to the number-one killer in America: adverse drug reactions to pharmaceuticals. They warn of the dangers of ephedra, garlic, kava, St. John's wort and other herbs, which in total kill fewer than fifty Americans a year, to the best of my knowledge, while the more expensive pharmaceuticals kill more than 100,000 Americans a year and tend to lead towards infections that kill 90,000 Americans a year." To support this last contention, Duke cites a second recent *JAMA* article by Stephenson, et al., describing a Centers for Disease Control campaign to target infections in hospitals.

Duke is now seventy-three years old, with a healthy, normal prostate gland. "The FDA-approved drugs for BPH contain synthetic or semi-synthetic sterols, very similar to the natural phytochemical found in plants, notably saw palmetto," he says. "There are at least six well-designed clinical studies that have been done in

Germany showing that saw palmetto is as effective at reducing the symptoms of swollen prostate as the FDA-approved drugs, with fewer side effects and at about one-tenth of the cost. As an added bonus, saw palmetto also helps control male pattern baldness. For the past twenty years, I have taken only dietary sitosterol, using saw palmetto, pumpkin seeds, Brazil nuts and beans. I also eat tomatoes for lycopene to prevent prostate cancer. So far, I'm doing just fine."

WHAT IS A PHYTOCHEMICAL?

"A phytochemical is a chemical produced in or by a plant," says botanist Jim Duke. "Every plant probably contains more than a thousand, probably closer to a million different phytochemicals. Most are biologically active and when you give your body an herb, you are giving it a menu of biologically active compounds from which it can select those that it needs. Sounds pretty flakey, but through proven homeostasis (the process of maintaining physiological equilibrium), your body does take the compounds it needs and excludes those it does not need, up to a degree."

A Dream Job for an Herbalist

James Duke is an ethnobotanist, studying how native people use local plants for food and medicine in different cultures around the world. He spent the bulk of his thirty-year career working for the U.S. Department of Agriculture (USDA) as an expert in medicinal plants, with time out for travel and study in China, Costa Rica, Peru, the Amazon and a lengthy stay in Panama. In *The Green Pharmacy,* he writes, "I've personally seen medicinal herbs successfully treat conditions that high-tech pharmaceuticals could scarcely touch."

In 1977 he was appointed chief of the U.S. Department of Agriculture (USDA) Medicinal Plant Laboratory—a "dream job for a medicinal herbalist," he says. By the time he assumed this leadership, the laboratory was collecting and screening 10 percent of the world's known plant species, seeking anti-tumor activities. This work, in cooperation with the National Cancer Institute, contributed to the NIH and pharmaceutical firms developing several chemotherapy drugs, including Taxol from the yew tree, which is used to fight advanced breast and ovarian cancer; etoposide, from the mayapple, used for testicular and lung cancer; and camptothecin, made from extracts of a Chinese tree, for prostate and other cancers.

What Duke describes as his "love affair" with plants began at the age of five, when an elderly neighbor showed him how to find edible wild plants in the forest. After doing graduate work in botany and taxonomy and beginning work with the USDA, he took two years off to do environmental feasibility studies in Panama for a research institute that was contracted by the old Atomic Energy Commission. "I studied the relationship between the native people and the land," he says. "I learned about everything that they consumed from the land and how they used their environment not only for food, but also for housing and medicine. I saw that their children were as happy and healthy as my own and decided that they must be doing something right."

Becoming even more intrigued by the potential of medicinal plants, Duke began to build a computerized database of the information he was gathering from folk medicine and scientific sources. The database, now very large, is still available on the Internet (*www.ars-grin.gov/duke/*) even though Duke has retired. "It is the ghost of Jim Duke at the USDA," he laughs. "And it still gets sixty thousand visits a year." The site offers cross-referenced and easily retrievable information about the chemistry and uses of medicinal plants.

Duke has not let retirement slow him down. He still writes, gives about two hundred lectures a year on herbal medicine and tends his own half-acre "teaching" garden in which he grows more than three hundred of the most important medicinal plants. "Lots of allopathic physicians come to photograph my garden, even though they bad-mouth herbs in public," he says. "One documentary maker had male pattern baldness, for which he was taking a manufactured drug. After a tour of my garden, he told me—off camera—that he was going to switch to saw palmetto." Duke also teaches a regular herbal healing class, using his garden to teach students what blooms and can be used at different times of the year.

"Our genes have spent millions of years living in the same environment as these plants and herbs," he says. "If you name almost any pharmaceutical, I can come up with an herb that does the same job and is more familiar to your genes." (Please see below for information on the medical benefits of plants.) "For example, we have recently learned that deficiencies in choline, which is in all plants, can contribute to increased homocysteine, which has been linked to Parkinson's, Alzheimer's and heart problems," he says.

Jim Duke's teaching, research and writing are all aimed at his life's mission. "I am on a crusade for more comparative trials of the herbal alternatives to synthetic pharmaceuticals," he says. In *The Green Pharmacy,* he explains why. "Our challenge is to think green—not the mercenary, monetary green of the pharmaceutical firms but the cleansing, empowering green of chlorophyll, the green that feeds, fuels, oxygenates and medicates our planet."

A NOTE ON SAFETY

While James Duke, Ph.D., is an advocate of herbal medicine, he is also quick to emphasize that you should exercise caution in using herbs. Always consult a professional before using herbs. His safety recommendations in *The Green Pharmacy* include:

1. Make sure you know what the herb is, particularly if you find it in the wild.
2. Open the lines of communication; make sure that both your conventional doctor and your herbalist know what you are taking to prevent possible harmful interactions.
3. Make sure that your diagnosis is correct.
4. Watch out for side effects such as dizziness, nausea or headache. Listen to your body.
5. Be alert for allergic reactions; if you have difficulty breathing within thirty minutes of taking an herb, call 911 immediately.
6. Beware of interactions. If you suspect that the herb is interacting with a drug or food, consult your physician or pharmacist. Some examples of potentially dangerous interactions:
   - Coumadin (warfarin) is an anti-coagulant drug (prevents blood clotting). There is potential for excessive bleeding when it is combined with other drugs or herbs that have similar properties, including aspirin, gingko, garlic and ginger.
   - Echinacea, an immune booster, may cause complications in people taking conventional medicines for autoimmune diseases, including lupus and multiple sclerosis, although Duke points out that there are no studies to support this conclusion.

Herbal Medicine: What's the Evidence?

In his fascinating history of Western herbal medicine, Kenneth R. Pelletier, Ph.D., M.D. (hc), notes that "about one-third of all Americans, or some sixty million people, use herbal medicinal products each year, spending over $3.2 billion." The danger, he points out, is that "Without official standards of quality, herbal preparations may not always be pure, and may not be accurately labeled." He cites as examples studies showing that two out of three products claiming to contain feverfew, an herb used to treat migraines, actually contained no feverfew at all. And a study of echinacea, used for colds and flu, found that more than half of the echinacea sold in the United States from 1908 through 1991 was actually *Parthenium integrifolium,* and not echinacea.

Herbs by the evidence: selected clinical studies showing mixed results

Note: for the many herbs not mentioned here, including hawthorne for cardiovascular disease and milk thistle for the liver, please refer to the excellent and readable information in The Green Pharmacy, *by James Duke, as well as the books by Kenneth Pelletier, Edzard Ernst, Wayne Jonas and others listed in the bibliography in Appendix II.*

- **Black cohosh** has been found effective for menopausal and perimenopausal symptoms. (Please see chapter 10 for detailed research data.)
- **Echinacea** is primarily used to prevent and treat common colds, flu, upper respiratory tract infections and to enhance immune system functions. In a review of twenty-six controlled clinical studies, researchers concluded that the "most striking effects of echinacea were a reduction in susceptibility to infection and a decrease in the incidence of colds." In other studies, the herb was found effective in treating *Candida albicans* vaginal yeast infections and enhancing the immune function of patients with mononucleosis.

  Edzard Ernst, in his *Desktop Guide to Complementary and Alternative Medicine,* expresses less enthusiasm. He reports that the results of a Cochrane review of echinacea trials were inconclusive. "The authors conclude that, to date, there is insufficient evidence to recommend a specific echinacea product."
- **Feverfew** is currently popular as a remedy for preventing and treating migraine, due in part to the publication of a number of clinical studies in British medical journals, according to Pelletier. The studies show reduction in frequency, pain and nausea and vomiting of migraine. However, two studies, one using dried alcohol extract of feverfew leaves and the other using dried feverfew leaves did not substantiate these positive results. Despite these findings

however, Pelletier notes that feverfew has been proposed for adoption and "appears to have won acceptance" as a migraine prevention by the European Union.

In his *Desktop Guide,* Ernst cites a systematic review of double-blind randomized controlled trials in which three of four trials found that feverfew is beneficial for the prevention of migraine in terms of attack severity and symptoms such as pain, nausea and vomiting. One study found no significant benefit in the treatment of rheumatoid arthritis.

- **Garlic** has become popular for reducing cardiovascular risk factors, including lowering cholesterol, according to Pelletier. "By 1993, at least 1,088 scientific studies dealt with garlic's medicinal effects for both healthy people and ill people." In order to be effective, however, it should be taken as "carefully dried garlic powder" to preserve the activity of allicin, its principal active ingredient, and "the powder should be ingested in enteric-coated tablets to protect it from inactivation by stomach acid." Two meta-analyses of garlic research found that a dosage of about one-half to one clove a day (600 to 900 mg) was able to reduce total serum cholesterol.

  Sounding a cautionary note, Ernst cites recent randomized controlled trials that are more negative. Summarizing the results, however, he concludes that "garlic probably does lower total cholesterol but only to a minor degree." It might also have a "significant, albeit small antihypertensive (blood-pressure lowering) effect." In fact, the regular intake of garlic "might prevent or delay the development of arteriosclerosis" (clogged arteries) and might also have a protective effect on intestinal cancers."

- **Ginger** has been proven effective in the treatment of nausea in several clinical studies, according to both Pelletier and Ernst. One study compared ginger with Dramamine and a placebo using blindfolded subjects in a tilted rotating chair; and one involved 1,741 participants on a whale-watching cruise, in which ginger proved as effective as five other medications. (Please also see chapter 5 for the use of ginger to prevent nausea from chemotherapy treatment.)

- **Gingko** has been approved by Commission E in Germany (a research compendium that Pelletier calls the "definitive tract" on herbal medicine) for the "symptomatic treatment of dementia-related memory deficits, concentration problems, and depression; for intermittent claudication (pain on walking caused by compromised blood flow to the extremities); and for vertigo and tinnitus (ringing in the ears) of senile vascular origin. Daily doses of 120 to 240 mg have been shown to elicit a response."

  A meta-analysis (summary of the results of several studies) reviewed by Ernst suggested a "significant but modest increase of pain-free walking distance compared with placebo. Another systematic review, corroborated by three other studies—including a meta-analysis assessing patients with Alzheimer's disease—suggests that ginkgo is effective in the treatment of dementia." (Please see chapter 11 for more about ginkgo biloba and other herbs for the elderly.)

- **Ginseng** has become one of the top three herbs in the United States and this Asian root has been the subject of thousands of studies, according to Pelletier. He cites several that have been done using a proprietary extract of *Panax ginseng* manufactured in Europe, called Ginsana: It was shown to improve mental functioning, immunity and to prevent colds and flu. And a recent University of Illinois monograph supported the use of ginseng as a "mental and physical preventive and restorative agent in some cases of weakness, exhaustion, tiredness, loss of concentration, and during convalescence." However, in a 1997 study of thirty-one men, a standardized ginseng extract did not produce any improvement in work performance and recovery, nor a change in energy metabolism.

- **Saw palmetto** has had mixed clinical results, according to Pelletier. "Although a number of controlled clinical studies have verified the use of saw palmetto preparations as a safe and effective treatment for relieving the symptoms associated with BPH (benign prostatic hyperplasia), results overall have been somewhat variable. Claims that the herb reduces prostate enlargement, or helps prevent the onset of prostate cancer, are not well documented."

    Ernst, however, cites a systematic review of eighteen randomized controlled studies of saw palmetto for the treatment of benign prostatic hyperplasia. While he cautions that data from long-term clinical studies are not available, "there is good evidence for the effectiveness of saw palmetto for BPH. It seems to improve the symptoms and objective signs . . . to the same extent as finasteride (the commonly prescribed drug). The encouraging safety profile of saw palmetto renders it an attractive option for patients with this condition."

References

Baker, B. "Be Smart, Beware: Herbs and Botanicals Can Help—But Can Also Harm." *AARP Bulletin* 40, no. 5 (1999): 14–15, 17.

Blumenthal, M., ed. *The Complete German Commission E Monographs: Therapeutic Guide to Herbal Medicines*. Austin, TX: American Botanical Council, 1998. Published by Integrative Medicine Communications.

Breithaupt-Grogler, K., et al. "Protective Effects of Chronic Garlic Intake on Elastic Properties of Aorta in the Elderly." *Circulation* 6 (1997): 2469–2655.

De Weerdt, C. J., et al. "Herbal Medicines in Migraine Prevention: Randomized Double-Blind Placebo-Controlled Crossover Trial of a Feverfew Preparation." *Phytomedicine* 3, no. 3 (1996): 225–230.

Duke, J. A. *The Green Pharmacy*. Emmaus, PA: The Rodale Press, 1997.

Eastman, P. "Drugs That Fight . . ." *AARP Bulletin* 40, no. 3 (1999): 14–16.

Ernst, E. "Can Allium Vegetables Prevent Cancer?" *Phytomedicine* 4 (1997): 79–83.

Ernst, E., ed. *The Desktop Guide to Complementary and Alternative Medicine: An Evidence-Based Approach*. London: Harcourt Publishers Limited, 2001.

Ernst, E. and M. H. Pittler. "Ginkgo Biloba for Dementia: A Systematic Review of Double-Blind, Placebo-Controlled Trials." *Clinical Drug Investigation* 17 (1999): 301–308.

Heptinstall, S., et al. "Parthenolide Content and Bioactivity of Feverfew (*Tanacetum Parthenium*)." *Journal of Pharmacology* 44 (1992): 391–395.

Johnson, E. S., et al. "Efficacy of Feverfew as Prophylactic Treatment of Migraine." *British Medical Journal* 291 (1985): 569–573.

Lasser, K. E., et al. "Timing of New Black Box Warnings and Withdrawals for Prescription Medications." *Journal of the American Medical Association* 282, no. 17 (May 2002): 2215–2220.

Melchart, D., et al. "Immunomodulation with Echinacea: A Systematic Review of Controlled Clinical Trials." *Phytomedicine* 1 (1994): 245–254.

Mowrey, D. B., et al. "Motion Sickness, Ginger and Psychophysics." *Lancet* 1 (1982): 655–657.

Murphy, J. J., S. Heptinstall, and J. R. A. Mitchell. "Randomised Double-Blind Placebo-Controlled Trial of Feverfew in Migraine Prevention." *Lancet* 2, no. 8604 (1988): 189–192.

Palevitch, D., et al. "Feverfew (*Tanacetum Parthenium*) as a Prophylactic Treatment for Migraine: A Double-Blind Placebo-Controlled Study." *Phytotherapy Research* 11, no. 7 (1997): 508–511.

Pelletier, K. R. *The Best Alternative Medicine: What Works? What Does Not?* New York: Simon & Schuster, 2000.

Pittler, M. H. and E. Ernst. "The Efficacy of Ginkgo Biloba Extract for the Treatment of Intermittent Claudication: A Meta-Analysis of Randomized Clinical Trials." *American Journal of Medicine* 108 (2000): 276–281.

Schmid, R., et al. "Comparison of Seven Commonly Used Agents for Prophylaxis of Seasickness." *Journal of Travel Medicine* 1, no. 4 (1994): 203–206.

Silagy, C., et al. "A Meta-Analysis of the Effect of Garlic on Blood Pressure." *Journal of Hypertension* 12 (1994): 463–468.

Stephenson, J. "CDC Campaign Targets Antimicrobial Resistance in Hospitals." *Journal of the American Medical Association* 287, no. 19 (May 2002).

Stevinson, C., et al. "Garlic for Treating Hypercholesterolemia: A Meta-Analysis of Randomized Clinical Trials." *Annals of Internal Medicine* 133 (2000): 420–429.

Vogler, B. K., et al. "Feverfew as a Preventive Treatment for Migraine: A Systematic Review." *Cephalagia* 18 (1998): 704–708.

7

PAIN: LISTENING TO THE WISDOM OF THE BODY

"The pain was the catalyst that helped me rewrite the story of my life."

Barbara Kivowitz thought that she was having another urinary tract infection. "I had had those before, and this pain felt similar," she says. "I assumed that, as usual, antibiotics would take care of it." She called her primary care doctor, but because she was traveling when the symptoms started, she could not undergo the usual laboratory testing. Because the symptoms were so similar to her other urinary tract infections, however, her doctor started her on a course of antibiotics. But this time, the pain did not go away. In fact, it got worse. "During the next few days, it began to feel as if there were knives in my pelvis," says Barbara. "Over the course of the next several weeks, both my bladder and pelvis became so excruciatingly painful that I could no longer sit down. In fact, I spent the next seven months either standing up or lying down with a complex pillow arrangement. When I did manage to fall asleep, I could usually stay that way for a few hours. In the beginning, that was one of the only respites. The other was when I was standing at my computer, writing."

The pain began in 1999, when Barbara was in her mid-forties, and it remained the dominant force in her life for more than two years. Until then, she had lived a life free of any major health problems. Married for sixteen years and with no children, she and her husband enjoyed being physically active. "We especially loved hiking," she says. "All of our vacations together were focused on climbing mountains and eating good food." At the time that the pain started, Barbara had a successful, home-based corporate consulting business. "I provided organizational development and collaborative technology consulting to my clients," she says. "I helped them plan strategic change which included the use of technology." Her educational background includes languages and literature— her other love is writing—as well as advanced degrees in psychology and organizational development. "Luckily, I was well positioned both to understand and manage the medical system," she says.

During the next two years, these analytic and management skills were to become Barbara's lifeline.

When the antibiotics did not help, Barbara's doctor referred her to specialists, including a urogynecologist, an orthopedist and a neurologist. "The neurologist ordered a brain MRI and other neurological tests," says Barbara. "Everything came back negative." Laboratory tests as well as pelvic exams and ultrasounds also yielded no diagnostically useful information. "My doctor seemed at a loss," says Barbara. "'I don't really know what's going on,' he told me. 'Sometimes these conditions go away as quickly as they come. Exercising sometimes helps.' I had always loved to exercise, so I gave it a try."

Barbara developed a home routine of stretching and using a treadmill or exercise bicycle. "I found that exercising provided some relief," she says. "I also tried hot baths, meditation, a very slow form of meditative walking, as well as yoga. They helped somewhat, but most of the day was filled with pain, periods of which I can only describe as hellish." (Please see Appendix I for a description of alternative practices.) In addition to exercising, the only other time that Barbara felt no pain was when she was standing at her raised computer table and writing. "So I wrote," she says. During the two years that followed, she kept a journal of her experiences and completed a professional book on knowledge management with a colleague. "One of the many life changes that came out of this pain was that I began to take my writing more seriously," says Barbara.

By this time, Barbara had stopped working. She could no longer drive or sit at meetings with clients. "Despite continued testing, my primary care doctor and the various specialists could still come up with no organic reason for the pain," says Barbara. "I was becoming desperate. It was beginning to dawn on me that I had to give up the fantasy that some wise, all-knowing person would appear who would help me figure out what to do. Instead, I realized that I had to be the one to take control of my pain: to pursue a diagnosis and find ways to manage it. And this also meant that I had to be the integrator—the one who would bring together allopathic and complementary medicine. It was in my hands."

Chronic Pain: Treating the Whole Person

Let us leave Barbara Kivowitz for the moment in order to talk about the problem of chronic pain. (Her story continues later in this chapter.) Our expert on this subject is Brian Berman, M.D., founder and director of the Complementary Medicine Program at the University of Maryland, the first university-based center of its kind in the United States focusing on research. Berman is professor of family medicine at the University of Maryland School of Medicine and has trained extensively in complementary therapies such as acupuncture and homeopathy. He is principal investigator of a National Institutes of Health (NIH) center grant for the study of complementary alternative medicine in the treatment of pain and is principal or co-investigator of a number of other large clinical trials in complementary medicine. In addition to publishing widely in the national and international literature on complementary medicine, Berman also helped establish and now directs the Complementary Medicine Field of the international Cochrane Collaboration, an organization dedicated to evaluating all medical practices.

Chronic pain is the nation's third-greatest health-care problem after heart disease and cancer. Barbara Kivowitz's experience is shared by millions of Americans, notes Berman. Surveys have shown that 30 percent of the population in developed countries (which amounts to some eighty million people in this country alone) report some form of chronic pain during their lifetimes— and half of these people are either partially or totally disabled for periods of a few days to several months. Chronic pain costs the United States approximately $65 billion in health care and lost productivity every year.

"We know that 70 percent of people who seek out alternative or complementary therapies do so for pain-related problems," says Berman. "They are looking for relief from their pain, but they also want to be listened to and understood by their doctors. They do not want to be seen as a collection of defective molecules. They want a relationship with their physicians that is humane as well as healing." The International Association for the Study of Pain defines pain as "an unpleasant sensory and emotional experience associated with actual or potential tissue damage, or described in terms of such damage. *It is always subjective in nature.*"

What does this mean, "Always subjective in nature?" "It means," says Berman, "that whether or not we can find the physical cause of your pain, if you are feeling it, *it is real.* Our job as doctors is to find ways to stop it," he says. "We may try to stop it in the laboratory, by looking for ways to repair damaged nerve cells that are sending you pain messages." For example, see "The Science of Pain" in this chapter. We may use some combination of drugs that decrease the intensity of pain messages that originate in the brain. We may also try to understand not only the physical experience of your pain, but also the mental, emotional and perhaps even the spiritual meaning of the pain." Remember (from chapter 2) that this book is based on the premise that people are more than just a collection of molecules that can be chemically adjusted to solve health problems. This is particularly true when we are in pain.

Not all pain is bad, points out Berman: "Sometimes, pain can be an early warning sign of a potentially serious illness or a tumor," he says. "Also, *acute* pain (coming from an actual or potential injury) keeps us safe: jerking our hand away from a hot stove or boiling water will prevent a burn, for example. People without adequate pain warning sensations can seriously injure themselves without realizing it."

But chronic pain—which persists after an injury has healed and becomes itself a major focus of disability or dysfunction—is a multidimensional problem, says Berman. "This kind of pain can evoke an overlay of fear, depression (because we can see no end in sight), hopelessness, despair and isolation, coupled with the feeling of being out of control, a victim of our bodies. Pain needs a holistic, multidimensional solution, one that focuses not only on the physical cause, but also on each person's emotions, spirit and life coping skills."

Consider one patient who came to see Berman at the Complementary Medicine Center nine years ago. Mrs. Davis (not her real name), a financial analyst in her mid-forties, had osteoarthritis in her neck that was causing chronic, unrelenting pain so severe that she could barely turn her head. She had tried drugs as well as physical therapy, with little success. Examination revealed that a compressed disk in her neck was inflamed and pressing on a nerve. Other doctors had advised her that surgery was the solution, but she was reluctant to undergo an operation.

"I have found that acupuncture of the ear is often helpful for musculoskeletal problems," says Berman. (In Chinese medicine, every part of the body is represented by a point on the ear.) "I decided to begin with ear acupuncture every week to reduce the inflammation of the disk, followed by acupuncture along the 'meridians' (energy pathways) in the body that relate to the area that was inflamed." (Please see chapters 2 and 6, as well as Appendix I, for more about acupuncture.) Over the next couple of months, Mrs. Davis reported that her pain was reduced to the point that she felt she did not need surgery. Berman stretched out her sessions to every other week.

"As we worked together, Mrs. Davis and I got to know each other a little better," says Berman. "She began to talk about the 'pressure cooker' atmosphere of the world of finance, as well as family issues that were causing stress in her life. I suggested that she try meditation and relaxation exercises." (Please see "A Closer Look at Meditation.") Mrs. Davis agreed to work with a staff member in the pain clinic to learn some techniques that she could use on her own, at home. "Often, meditation and relaxation exercises help reduce some of our perceptions of pain which, as noted above, is always *subjective* in nature," says Berman. "We have found that meditation helps to modulate pain signals sent to the brain by sending other signals back to the site of the pain that, in effect, 'turn down the volume.'"

From Victim of Pain to Being in Control

Within a few months, Mrs. Davis was able to manage her pain so that it no longer interfered with her life. When she had flare-ups, Berman sent her for physical therapy exercises in mobility and strengthening that she could do at home. She learned other ways to help herself as well: improving her diet, for example, reducing caffeine and sodas, white flour and sugar, and adding more soy, fish and complex carbohydrates. (Please see "The Joy of Soy" in this chapter for recent research on diet and pain.) She also began taking supplements such as calcium/magnesium and glucosamine/chondroitin sulfate, both of which have been found to reduce the symptoms of osteoarthritis.

Nine years later, Mrs. Davis has still not had surgery and feels no need to do so. Her pain occurs sporadically, since the osteoarthritis is still present, but she has learned how to manage and reduce the discomfort through a program that combines acupuncture, meditation, dietary changes and exercises, she is now less a victim and more in control of the pain. *She has begun to own her health.* Every story in this book, including Barbara Kivowitz's story in this chapter, describes the healing benefits of feeling in control of your health care. In chapter 1, health psychologist Ester Shapiro, Ph.D., cites research findings that "self-efficacy"—which is the same thing as patients feeling that they own their health—is related to better health and recovery from illness.

The pain treatment model used in the University of Maryland Complementary Medicine clinic is called the "biopsychosocial" approach. First described in 1984 by British surgeon Gordon Waddell, this method treats the physical symptoms of pain while also taking into account patients' beliefs, psychological stress and attitudes toward their bodies. "We must never forget," says Berman, "that those painful vertebrae are connected to a human being with a life history, certain ways of coping, personal values, a family, a job, relationships and financial pressures."

Describing his approach to pain patients, Berman says that he uses his combined medical training and knowledge of complementary and alternative modalities. "I recently saw one man with chronic headaches, pain on the inside of his legs and problems and discomfort with his digestion," says Berman. "If I were to consider his problems only from the perspective of Western medicine, I might refer him to a neurologist, a vascular specialist and a gastrointestinal expert to rule out peptic ulcer disease or cancer, for example."

From the perspective of Chinese medicine, explains Berman, all of these problems stem from one cause: stagnation of the liver energy. "By using acupuncture and herbs to clear the blockage of this energy and restore the flow of qi or life force, all of these symptoms were alleviated," he says. But he also points out that creating a healing relationship with each patient is just as important as the particular treatment that is used. "Through such a relationship, a doctor can understand each patient's life and personality and treat the whole person, rather than just the symptoms," says Berman. "Using integrative medicine gives us additional diagnostic and treatment paradigms, and this is particularly useful when no reason for the symptoms seems clear from the Western perspective. With integrative medicine, we as doctors have more medical tools in our toolbox with which to help our patients."

REDUCING CHRONIC PAIN:
THE BEST TOOLS FROM BOTH WORLDS OF MEDICINE.

Recommendations from the University of Maryland Complementary Medicine Program:

Conventional tools for pain control:

Nonsteroidal anti-inflammatories, including aspirin, ibuprofen, indomethacine, naproxene. The side effects can include high blood pressure, intestinal bleeding and liver and kidney damage.

Analgesics, including the anti-inflammatories mentioned above, plus acetaminophen, and narcotics, such as morphine, which are by prescription only. Side effects of narcotics include drowsiness, confusion and constipation.

Neuropathic pain medications, which target pain that seems to have no obvious cause, or that remains after the original injury has healed. Neuropathic pain is thought to come from the central nervous system. (See, for example, "The Science of Pain," in this chapter.)

Transcutaneous nerve stimulation (TENS) uses a small, battery-powered stimulator to apply a gentle, painless electrical current to a certain area of the skin. The electrical current may block pain signals or cause the body to release endorphins (one of the body's natural painkillers). This technique must be done by a professional. TENS may help some people and some types of pain more than others.

Physical therapy for help with posture, movement and exercise; and occupational therapy to help you learn ways to do work and activities more easily.

Biofeedback uses a machine to help you be aware of—and eventually control—muscle tension, pulse, blood pressure and skin temperature.

Heat and/or cold therapy, under the advice of a health-care professional.

Complementary methods of pain management

Regular exercise is an important part of pain management, but you should consult with your doctor to make sure that the exercise is appropriate for your pain and your physical condition. Exercise releases endorphins (natural painkillers), strengthens muscles and bones, keeps joints more flexible, reduces stress, increases energy, improves sleep and helps with weight control. Choose activities you enjoy, start slowly and try to build up to thirty minutes of moderate exercise on most, preferably all, days of the week.

Traditional Chinese Medicine (TCM) includes several methods that studies have found effective in pain reduction. These include:

- Acupuncture (which uses thin needles) and acupressure (manual pressure) to stimulate some of the more than four hundred "acupoints" on the body's surface. (Please see "A Closer Look at Acupuncture" in chapter 6 for more about TCM.) Stimulation of certain points in particular has been associated with pain reduction.

- Traditional Chinese herbs. The use of herbs comes from three thousand years of observation and practice. There are more than twelve thousand known plants in China that can be used as medicine, but practitioners generally use about three hundred. Always consult with your doctor and a qualified TCM practitioner before using any herbs.

- Movement therapies. These include qigong exercises and tai chi (see chapter 6). These slow, meditative movements are thought to increase the flow of qi (life force) in the body, improve energy and balance and provide a feeling of general well-being. They teach you to associate movement with relaxation and health.

(continued)

Bioelectric magnetic therapies include the use of acupuncture and magnets. These therapies are primarily complementary and may be helpful for symptom management. Acupuncture is the one therapy in this category that has positive results in pain management documented by research studies. For some of the other therapies, research is scant but the interest in funded research is increasing.

Pulsed electromagnetic fields (EMFs) vary in terms of frequency (measured in Hz or oscillations per second) and strength (measured in gauss or tesla). Preliminary studies have examined the effects of both high strength, high frequency stimulation, and low strength, low frequency stimulation on pain. EMFs were found to be effective in reducing the pain of osteoarthritis.

Fasting or elimination diets. Fasting has been shown to influence arthritis pain. Several studies also have shown that humans with rheumatoid arthritis have temporary improvement in their joint inflammation when they fast for seven to ten days. Fasting is not a practical long-term therapy and unsupervised fasting is dangerous. Yet, these observations lend additional support to the idea that diet affects joint inflammation.

Dietary changes. For some people, avoiding nightshade vegetables such as tomatoes and eggplant, as well as dairy and wheat, has been helpful.

Pain-reducing herbs and supplements include boswellia, green tea, Duhuo for arthritis, Yuan Hu-So, Devil's claw, certain types of willow bark and SAM-e (pronounced "Sammy"). SAM-e is the commonly used name for S-Adenosyl-Methionine. SAM-e occurs in every living cell and takes part in several biological reactions in the human body. It is thought to be effective for depression and arthritis. In addition, B-vitamins, calcium/magnesium and glucosamine/chondroitin sulfate have been helpful for some people.

NOTE: Before using supplements or vitamins, or making dietary changes to treat pain, you should first consult your physicians to make sure that they are safe for you.

Manipulative therapies, including most kinds of massage (especially trigger point, Shiatsu and deep tissue), chiropractic, osteopathic medicine and craniosacral therapy.

Mind-body therapies, including the Alexander Technique, Feldenkreis, meditation, hypnosis, guided imagery, biofeedback, behavioral therapy (please see story about Crohn's disease in this chapter for an explanation of biofeedback and behavioral therapy), and Trager Movement Education—which uses gentle, rhythmic movements to facilitate the release of stress patterns, on the mental, emotional or physical levels. Its aim is to achieve integration between the body and mind process. (See "Four Ways to Feel Better" for more about massage, Trager and muscular therapy.)

Searching for Meaning—and a Life Preserver

We are now back to Barbara Kivowitz's story. Her continual pain was rapidly causing her life to become closely circumscribed: "I was basically confined to the house, spending all of my energy on finding ways to stop the pain," she says. "The pain would fluctuate wildly during the course of a day, so I could no longer make assumptions about my life. A friend would ask if she could come over to visit, and I would have to say, 'It depends. Call me right before you come and I'll let you know.' I had to recreate my world at every moment. I couldn't assume that this moment would be the same as either the last one or the one to come."

Even while allopathic testing was going on, Barbara began exploring alternative therapies, along with her primary doctor. "After all of the tests and exams had ruled out any dangerous or acutely life-threatening conditions, I decided to try homeopathy while continuing to search for allopathic remedies," says Barbara. "I was also interested in acupuncture, but was able to get an appointment with a recommended homeopathic doctor first. I was in such desperate pain that I wanted to proceed on all fronts at once.

"Homeopathy is a slow method," she says. "Ideally, you should take a remedy for six weeks before deciding if it is working, and often remedies need to be adjusted. I went through four different trials, and although it did not really help physically, it did help me to deepen my understanding of the meaning of the pain. And this is an important part of dealing with any serious illness, including pain. The homeopathic process helped me look deep inside the past and present constructs of my life to hear the message that the pain was trying to convey. Often, this is a message that you might have ignored or overridden before." (Please see "A Closer Look at Homeopathy.")

It is also vital to have a good support system, says Barbara. "You need people who are excellent scientists, who take you seriously, and who believe that you will get better," she says. "Both the homeopath and my primary doctor would always return calls quickly, even over the weekend, and they, as well as my husband, kept telling me over and over again that things would get better. I felt like I was drowning, and their conviction gave me a life preserver to hang onto when I most needed it."

Barbara is careful to distinguish between "curing" and "healing," especially when one is dealing with pain. Even if you cannot control its intensity, you can control your own perceptions of the meaning of the pain in your life, she says. "I knew right from the beginning that the pain was appearing for a reason, and I needed to figure out that reason at this point in my life. I began to read everything I could find about illness as metaphor, to try to understand what my body was trying to tell me about my beliefs about myself, and about old wounds, both emotional and physical. Keeping a journal became one of my most important tools for self-understanding during that time, in addition to psychotherapy."

✓ TAKE ACTION ✓

When You Are in Pain[1]

NOTE: These are some of the methods that helped Barbara Kivowitz, *but you should always consult first with your doctor* before beginning any new practice, treatment or medication.

1. Keep a journal and a daily pain log, recording both the progression of the pain and what helps to reduce it.
2. Write your own case history and update it regularly, describing the onset of pain, tests and results, therapies you have tried and their effectiveness. Send a copy to any new doctor or practitioner *before* your appointment. This saves you the time of endlessly repeating your story and helps them get a fuller understanding of *you*.
3. Scour the world for information on your condition: Talk to everyone you know (perhaps someone plays golf with an expert!) and use the Internet to find support groups and experts wherever they are. Don't be afraid to "cold call" experts who might be helpful.
4. If you go to pain clinics, find doctors who are not only excellent scientists but who are also compassionate and who *take you seriously*. They should have a *belief* that you will get better. Don't accept any less from your caregivers.
5. Make as many appointments with different experts as you think you might need. Often these appointments take months to get, so it is better to have them and then cancel them later if you do not need them.

(continued)

---

[1] Useful organizations: American Chronic Pain Association, P.O. Box 850, Rocklin, CA 95677. Web site: *www.theacpa.org*. E-mail: ACPA@pacbell.net. American Pain Foundation, 111 South Calvert Street, Suite 2700, Baltimore, MD 21202. Web site: *www.painfoundation.org*.

6. Research every pain medication they want to put you on. Ask about side effects.
7. Practice whatever form of meditation you are comfortable with, including slow, meditative walking and/or Vipassana meditation (see "A Closer Look at Meditation.")
8. Daily practice of one or more of these: yoga, tai chi and qigong, all of which involve deep, cleansing breathing, and all of which have been useful for pain management. (See details in Appendix 1 and in the "Closer Look" sections of the text.)
9. Massage: There are many forms of massage that may be helpful, including Trager bodywork, craniosacral massage, tui na and qigong energy work, as well as Ayurvedic massage. (See details in Appendix I and in the "Closer Look" sections of the text.)
10. Barbara's practitioners advised her not to mix homeopathy with other energy-based work, such as acupuncture, to avoid "system overload." Other experts disagree, saying that as long as all practitioners involved know what you are doing, it is possible to combine treatments.
11. Try to get in touch with your spirituality: Often, finding a belief in a higher power, or some universal source of healing, can help make the unbearable more bearable.
12. Try to understand, through psychotherapy or by using your journal, any deeper message that the pain might have about your life, your relationship to your body or your relationships to those who are close to you. This might be a message that you have ignored or overlooked in the past.

The next step on Barbara's odyssey was an allopathic doctor specializing in urogynecology who performed invasive testing of her bladder and urinary tract. "The good news was that there was no finding," says Barbara. "So at least I knew that I didn't have a horrible bladder condition. But then I was left with a feeling of 'What do I do now?' This was the first of many points in my journey that I realized that it was up to me to make health-care decisions for myself." She also tried an antispasmodic medication, which was not helpful. "When you are desperate for relief, you don't care about the scientific method, you just want to feel better," says Barbara. "I was so desperate for this medication to work that my judgment was off. I convinced myself that the pain was better; but really, it was not."

Throughout her decision-making process, Barbara used her primary doctor as a kind of scientific sounding board. "He helped me weigh options analytically and also recommended further testing," she says. "Although he is not trained in complementary methods, he played a critical role in my care: He was compassionate, and he believed that I would recover. Often, he would call me from his car on his way home from work, and just talk to me while I was lying on the couch, crying. It was so important for me just to have that connection with a healing person."

She chose a pain clinic as her next step. "My fantasy was that at a pain clinic, there would be a team of people who would look at my case and pool their knowledge about the correct combination of conventional and complementary services," says Barbara. This is not what happened. "My first visit began with a half-hour interview with a white-coated doctor who took my history, asked questions and seemed interested," says Barbara. "At the end of that time, he said, 'I'll share this information with the doctor who will be in to see you shortly.' I was shocked. I hadn't been told that he was a resident in training. I thought I was seeing a senior physician."

After a time, the senior doctor finally did come in. "I had no time to build a relationship with her, because she did not hear my story from me," says Barbara. "Furthermore, she spent most of the visit teaching the resident how to assess me. She barely interacted with me at all. I was too desperate and in too much pain to walk out. But that is what I really wanted to do."

The pain specialist recommended a course of neuropathic medication (used for pain that is thought to originate in the central nervous system, rather than specific bones, muscles or organs). "While the medication did help reduce the pain—I was finally able to sit down—my two follow-up visits with her made me feel like the clock was ticking," says Barbara. "She would keep looking at her watch, and I wanted to grab the hem of her white robe to keep her in the room with me, to make her *relate* to me."

While she was taking the neuropathic pain medication, Barbara stopped the homeopathy and began seeing an acupuncturist, a chiropractor, a physical therapist who did craniosacral work and a biofeedback specialist. (Please see

Appendix I and the "Closer Look" sections for information about these modalities.) "But even with all of the specialists—both allopathic and alternative—the pain medication, yoga and meditation, I still could not control the pain enough to function normally," says Barbara. "Finding a solution to a serious illness is hard under the best of circumstances, but when you are feeling physically devastated, it is nearly impossible, especially when you try to deal with the insurance bureaucracy! I am so lucky that my husband was my unwavering caretaker. He would leave work early, do all the chores and sometimes just hold me when I needed it. Now, he became my research partner."

Desperate Times Call for Desperate Measures

Barbara and her husband turned to the Internet and also began talking to everyone they could think of. Barbara was determined not to give up, to keep looking for specialists—either allopathic or alternative—until she found those who could help her. "Desperate times call for desperate measures," says Barbara. "Through my sister-in-law, who is a pediatrician, we found one of the few biofeedback experts in the country who specialize in pelvic pain. We telephoned neurologists and pain experts all over the country to ask if they had ever seen anyone with my symptoms before, and if so, had they come upon a course of treatment that worked? We found a virtual community of neurologists in Europe who discussed my case. I realized that it would be efficient if I wrote up my own case history to e-mail or fax to all of the people we were talking to. I kept updating it. Everyone said it was the best case history they had ever seen."

Barbara learned a great deal from her Internet forays, saw pelvic pain specialists around the country, gynecologists and a neurologist who wanted to give her a spinal tap. (She refused.) Nothing was helping. Finally, the answer came from a basketball game. "My brother plays basketball on Sundays with a group of other doctors, and he asked them if they knew of any good pain specialists in my city," says Barbara. "We got one highly recommended name. It took three months to get an appointment. I learned, by the way, to make a lot of appointments prematurely, just in case you want to see that person in three or six months. I also learned how to work with secretaries to get notified of cancellations."

In this case, the three-month wait was worth it. "This doctor was absolutely the right person for me to see," says Barbara. "He is a brilliant scientist and researcher, as well as a healer. He spent an hour with me on the first appointment; he calls me back and responds to e-mails." This doctor recommended a *combination* of drugs to manage the pain and decrease the intensity of pain messages that originate in the brain. Combinations had been tried before, says Barbara, "but this doctor had more experience with the medication interactions than the previous doctors. The drug 'cocktail' he put together helped tremendously." At the same time, Barbara began seeing an energy healer, who does hands on healing. "He was the only one who could actually bring my pain down quickly." (See "A Closer Look at Energy Healing and Spirituality," as well as chapter 6, for more details about this practice.)

Barbara is still followed by her pain specialist, continues to practice meditation, yoga and other mind/body activities, and does an hour and a half of aerobic exercise every day. She has also changed her career focus: She is back to consulting, but on a more limited basis, and she is putting more energy into what she feels is her true vocation: writing. "The allopathic and complementary track were two of my three sources of healing," she says. "The third was my own emotional healing, nurtured by my psychotherapist and my journal. The pain was the catalyst that helped me to rewrite the story of my life. I began to understand that the pain was my body's way of helping me be more in alignment with who I was meant to be. I now know that I need to take my writing more seriously."

Barbara now says that she has her life back, and she looks it. Curly, shoulder-length light-gray hair frames a youthful face with a rosy complexion and dark eyes. Her body looks strong and muscular, and she is dressed for the outdoors—hiking-style boots, fleece jacket and jogging pants. "My pain is at a level that I can almost ignore," she says. "I have begun to reduce the medication 'cocktail' with my pain specialist. When I do have higher levels of pain, I now have tools that will bring it down, such as the energy person, whom I see twice a week."

She has even started hiking with her husband again. And, in addition to her writing and consulting work, she has started doing some *pro bono* work for non-profit organizations. "It's my way of giving something back," she says. She recently achieved one of her biggest milestones so far, a cross-country trip to see her family. This was the first time she had traveled in three years.

And one other important thing: She was given a dog. "I think everyone who is ill should have a little, empathic love-machine dog. Mine is magical. He keeps me company, gets me out of the house every day to walk and makes me laugh—all of which is good therapy."

 ## Pain Treatment: What's the Evidence?

Acupuncture

In 1997, the National Institutes of Health (NIH) released the findings of its Consensus Panel (reflecting the opinions of many experts) on acupuncture for pain. The panel found "clear or promising evidence" that acupuncture helps relieve adult postoperative pain, postoperative dental pain, myofascial pain and low back pain. (The *fascia* is fibrous tissue that envelopes muscles and organs and can become constricted, leading to pain. See also "A Closer Look at Muscular Therapy.")

The NIH Panel also found "some promising evidence" that acupuncture helps with menstrual cramps, "tennis elbow," fibromyalgia, osteoarthritis, carpal tunnel syndrome and headache.

When compared to standard biomedical therapies for all of these pain conditions, the NIH concluded that acupuncture has "low adverse effects" (fewer than fifty) reported in the nine to twelve million visits to acupuncturists in the United States each year. However, in a 1999 survey of the published literature, Edzard Ernst found reports of more than two thousand adverse effects, including drowsiness and fainting, increased pain, lung punctures (pneumothorax), infections (this latter category is reduced by the use of disposable needles), and forty-five fatalities. Still, these figures are relatively low considering the total number of acupuncture visits.

To be safe, however, be sure to seek trained, licensed acupuncture practitioners. (Information on Web sites and licensing organizations can be found in the appendices.)

Herbal Medicine

Of the 30,000 species of plants in China, 12,800 medicinal agents have been developed over 3,000 years of practice. Of these, some 300 are now generally used in clinical practice. (Also see "A Closer Look at Healing Herbs.")

- *Chronic colitis.* Researchers found that a gum resin preparation of Boswellia could be effective in reducing the pain of chronic colitis (a bowel disorder) with minimal side effects.

- *Low back pain.* Two independent, uncontrolled studies suggest that devil's claw (*Harpagophytum procumbens*) is effective in reducing low back pain. In a placebo-controlled, double-blind study, 118 patients received either devil's claw or a placebo for four weeks. The number of patients who were pain-free by the end of the study showed a significant difference in favor of devil's claw.

  In a double-blind, randomized parallel-group study, a capsicum plaster was compared with a placebo for three weeks in 154 patients with nonspecific back pain. On three separate pain measures, the capsicum group had marked decreases in pain, prompting the researchers to conclude that "the efficacy ratings by observers and patients were definitely in favor of capsicum. There were a few 'harmless' adverse effects, which resolved spontaneously."

- *Joint pain.* A systematic review of all randomized controlled trials on the effectiveness of herbal medicines in the treatment of osteoarthritis found "promising evidence" for some herbal preparations. The evidence also suggested that the use of herbal preparations reduced the use of nonsteroidal anti-inflammatory drugs. Weak evidence for "mild to moderate relief" of pain was found for willow bark, the common stinging nettle leaf (applied topically) and Articulin-F, an Ayurvedic herbal formulation. Moderately strong evidence was found for Phytodolor, a fixed herbal formulation, and capsaicin cream, which is derived from hot chili peppers. Two other treatments—extract of avocado and soya bean, and devil's claw—were found to significantly reduce pain symptoms as well.

Eighteen patients with joint pain used nettle stings from *Urtica doica*—the stinging nettle plant—to treat their joint pain. All patients but one were sure that nettles "had been very helpful" and several considered themselves cured. This exploratory study suggests nettle sting is a useful, safe and cheap therapy which needs further study. A randomized controlled trial is planned in collaboration with a rheumatology specialist.

Qigong and Tai Chi

The series of slow, ancient movements that make up qigong and tai chi practice may be helpful as part of a multicomponent mind/body therapy for pain conditions such as fibromyalgia, according to an ongoing study at the University of Maryland funded by NCCAM (The National Center for Complementary and Alternative Medicine).

Another study found that a combination of "back school," relaxation and qigong yielded promising preliminary results.

Other studies of qigong have found that while it may not be as effective for general pain or muscle spasms, patients with low back pain reported that tai chi helped to reduce their pain. Qigong was also found to increase energy levels.

Spinal Manipulation

In his evidence-based review of complementary treatments, Edzard Ernst reports that the "most authoritative" systematic reviews of chiropractic "cast considerable doubt on the assumption that its effectiveness has been demonstrated beyond reasonable doubt." The best that can be said for spinal manipulation, according to Ernst, are the conclusions of a Cochrane review in progress (chapter 1 explains the research of the Cochrane Collaboration), which suggest that "spinal manipulation as a treatment for acute or chronic back pain is supported by moderately conclusive evidence."

Although osteopathy (a method of spinal manipulation) has been evaluated less thoroughly than chiropractic, a recent randomized controlled trial, involving 178 patients with chronic or acute lower-back pain found "no significant difference" between osteopathic treatment and standard medical care in a twelve-week trial.

(See also "A Closer Look at Chiropractic and Craniosacral Therapy" and "A Closer Look at Osteopathy.")

Massage vs. Acupuncture

In a survey of chronic pain in spinal cord injury, patients reported acupuncture rated lowest for satisfaction in pain relief and massage rated highest). See also chapter 8 on Trauma.)

For more research data on massage and muscular therapy, please see "Four Ways to Feel Better.")

Aromatherapy

Increasingly, aromatherapy has been used as part of an integrated, multidisciplinary approach to pain management. "The medicinal use of plant oils has a long history in Ancient Egypt, China and India," according to Edzard Ernst. The oils can be applied directly to the skin, into baths or inhaled through steam or a diffuser.

This therapy is thought to enhance the parasympathetic response through the effects of touch and smell, encouraging relaxation at a deep level. Relaxation has been shown to alter perceptions of pain. Ernst also reports that "Laboratory studies suggest that molecules of the oil can affect organ function, although the clinical relevance of these findings is not clear." A systematic review of all randomized controlled trials of aromatherapy found that aromatherapy massage has a mild effect in the reduction of anxiety, although it is temporary. Even if one ignores the possibility that essential oils have pharmacologically active ingredients, aromatherapy might possibly play a role in the management of chronic pain through relaxation. Clinical trials are in the early stages, but evidence suggests that aromatherapy might be used as a complementary therapy for managing chronic pain. Although the use of aromatherapy is not restricted to nursing, at least one state board of nursing has recognized the therapeutic value of aromatherapy and voted to accept it as part of holistic nursing care.

References (pain treatment)

Acupuncture. NIH Consensus Statement Online 15, no. 5 (November 3–5, 1997): 1–34.

Andersson, G. B. J., et al. "A Comparison of Osteopathic Spinal Manipulation with Standard Care for Patients with Low Back Pain." *New England Journal of Medicine* 341 (1999): 1426–1431.

Berman, B. M. and B. B. Sing. "Chronic Lower Back Pain: An Outcome Analysis of a Mind/Body Intervention." *Complementary Therapies In Medicine* 5 (1997): 29–35.

Bhatti, T. I. et al. "T'ai Chi as a Treatment for Chronic Low Back Pain: A Randomized, Controlled Study" (abstract). *Alternative Therapies in Health and Medicine* 4 (1998): 90–91.

Bonfort, G. "Spinal Manipulation: Current State of Research and its Indications." *Neurological Clinics* 17, no. 1 (1999): 91–111.

Buckle, J. "Use of Aromatherapy as a Complementary Treatment for Chronic Pain." *Alternative Therapies in Health and Medicine* 5, no. 5 (1999): 42–51.

Chrubasik, S., et al. "Effectiveness of *Harpogophytum Procumbens* in Treatment of Acute Low Back Pain." *Phytomedicine* 3 (1996): 1–10.

Chrubasik, S., S. Pollak, and C. Conradt. "Clinical Trial of Willow Bark Extract." *MMW-Fortschritte Der Medizin* 144, no. 9 (2002): 10.

Cooke, B. and E. Ernst. "Aromatherapy: A Systematic Review." *British Journal of General Practice* 500 (2000): 493–496.

Gupta, I., et al. "Effects of Gum Resin of *Boswellia Serrata* in Patients with Chronic Colitis." *Planta Medica* 67, no. 5 (2001): 391–395.

Keitel, W., et al. "Capsicum Pain Plaster in Chronic Non-Specific Low Back Pain." *Arzneimittel-Forschung* 51, no. 11 (2001): 896–903.

Liu, C. "Reflections: Introduction to Qigong, Chinese Traditional Deep Breathing Exercises." *Health Values—Achieving High Level Wellness* 12, no. 1 (198): 47–50.

Long, L., K. Soeken, and E. Ernst. "Herbal Medicines for the Treatment of Osteoarthritis: A Systematic Review." *Rheumatology* 40 (2001): 779–793.

Nayak, S., et al. "The Use of Complementary and Alternative Therapies for Chronic Pain Following Spinal Cord Injury: A Pilot Survey." *Spinal Cord Medicine* 24, no. 1 (2001): 54–62.

Randall, C., et al. "Nettle Sting of *Urtica Dioica* for Joint Pain—An Exploratory Study of This Complementary Therapy." *Complementary Therapies in Medicine* 7, no. 3 (1999): 126–131.

Trock, D., et al. "A Double-Blind Trial of the Clinical Effects of Pulsed Electromagnetic Fields in Osteoarthritis." *Journal of Rheumatology* 20, no. 3 (1993): 456–460.

Wu, W. B. E., et al. "Effects of qigong on Late-Stage Complex Regional Pain Syndrome." *Alternative Therapies in Health and Medicine* 5 (1999): 45–54.

Promising Research: Can Food Reduce Your Pain?

Jill M. Tall, Ph.D., has a soy milkshake every day. "I mix a couple of scoops of soy protein isolate powder, a banana or strawberries, soymilk and ice in a blender," she says. "It's delicious and gives me about twenty-five grams of soy protein. I also take isoflavones (a component of soy) daily."

Why does she do this? "Well, seeing is believing," she says. "In the lab, we are seeing evidence that soy helps to reduce pain. In addition, the Food and Drug Administration recommends twenty-five grams of soy protein per day to reduce the risk of heart disease. So, what have I got to lose? I've even convinced my mom to try soy milkshakes to lower her cholesterol!"

Tall is a pharmacologist and is currently a postdoctoral fellow in the Department of Anesthesiology at the Johns Hopkins Medical Institutes. What she is seeing are laboratory animals whose pain is reduced when soy protein is added to their diets. Tall and Srinivasa N. Raja, M.D.—professor of anesthesiology and director of the Pain Division in the Department of Anesthesiology and Critical Care Medicine at the Johns Hopkins School of Medicine—recently presented these findings at a conference of the American Pain Society. Raja and Tall both point out that while these findings are promising, soy has not yet been tested as a pain reducer in human clinical trials.

The animal trials do, however, give rise to hypotheses: When you have an injury, one of the first things that happens is an inflammation of the area that causes pain and swelling, or "edema," says Tall. "Inflammation also occurs in other places in the body, such as the bronchial tubes, which causes asthma," she continues. "It has been hypothesized that the pain that cancer patients experience, particularly when the disease has metastasized, is caused by the actual tumors in addition to the local inflammation that results at the site of the tumor."

So when trying to reduce pain, an important step is to reduce the inflammation and swelling, according to Tall and Raja. And that is exactly what soy seems to do. In several animal studies, Tall and Raja compared animals that were otherwise identical. One group had a soy protein-based diet, the other group a diet based on milk protein (casein). "The initial findings from our laboratory indicated that if you gave soy to the animals before a nerve injury, the pain was much less severe as measured by objective pain response reactions than the milk protein group," Tall says. The preliminary studies showed no effect on pain if you gave the soy after the nerve injury (palliatively).

In follow-up studies, the researchers found that the addition of soy protein to the regular diet significantly reduced the pain and swelling caused by inflammation, according to Tall. "The soy-fed animals still displayed pain behaviors," she says. "But the pain was less severe and the animals tolerated it better."

The next step is to find out how this works and what the implications are for people suffering from chronic pain. "These findings could be important for cancer patients with tumor-related pain," says Raja. "And we anesthesologists also wonder if the addition of soy to the diet might reduce the need for traditional analgesics (pain medication)." Raja's areas of expertise include acute and chronic pain management, pain after amputation and "neuropathic" pain, which is perpetuated in the central nervous system even after the original injury has healed. (For more about neuropathic pain, please see "The Science of Pain" in this chapter, describing the research of Clifford Woolf, M.D., Ph.D.)

In their current research, Raja and Tall are trying to determine what components of soy are the most important in pain reduction, and, eventually, how much soy people should eat. "One possible mechanism might involve phytoestrogens (naturally occurring estrogen in plants), some of which have hormonal properties," says Raja. "We know that there are some gender differences in pain tolerance and we suspect that hormonal differences may account for that. There are also certain fatty acids in soy, called alpha-linolenic acids, that may have an anti-inflammatory effect." Another hypothesis, adds Tall, is that isoflavones, another component of soy, may play a role in pain reduction.

Neither Tall nor Raja set out to research the complementary treatment of pain. They describe themselves as evidence-based scientists who are primarily focused on conventional pain treatments. Raja, for example, has published several book chapters and more than a hundred articles on pain treatment; he is a senior editor for several journals, and in 2000 established a new section, called "Classic Papers Revisited," for the journal *Anesthesiology*.

For her part, Tall was investigating the effects of estrogen and testosterone on pain. "As a pharmacologist, my true passion is related to the study of drugs, any substance that alters ongoing processes in the body," she explains. "While I am becoming more open to alternative therapies, I am a strong proponent of well-designed studies that meet rigorous scientific standards." In her own research, Tall found that female animals, with obviously higher estrogen levels than male animals, had less pain. "I joined the soy research because I wanted to find out if the hormonal components of soy that resemble estrogen—phytoestrogens and isoflavones—had the same effect on pain."

A Fortuitous Accident that Led to a New Discovery

Raja discovered the pain-reducing qualities of soy by a fortuitous accident. Dr. Yoram Shir had come to Baltimore from Israel to continue his groundbreaking work in developing a model of neuropathic pain, but found that he could not duplicate the Israeli results in the Johns Hopkins laboratory. "We looked at every reason we could think of," recalls Raja. "We went through a whole series of controls, compared species of the laboratory animals, the nature of the injuries, the types of sutures that were used, and found nothing to account for our inability to replicate the Israeli pain studies."

Finally, the researchers looked at the animal food. "Laboratory rats in the United States are generally fed soy-based pellets, while the Israeli lab rat diet is milk-protein based, containing casein," says Raja. "So we immediately started importing the milk protein pellets from Israel, fed them to the control group, and found that they had persistent and more severe pain than the animals on a soy diet." Not only were the researchers able to replicate Shir's Israeli studies, but they had discovered the potential benefits of soy in pain reduction, quite by accident.

"We are now interested in finding out whether other dietary ingredients can reduce pain," says Raja. In collaboration with Dr. Muraleedharan G. Nair at the University of Michigan, Raja and his colleagues are investigating compounds found in tart cherries. "In earlier research, Dr. Nair has shown that tart cherry extract has an effect similar to nonsteroidal anti-inflammatories such as ibupro-fen," says Raja. "We have just completed a series of studies to determine whether this extract decreases inflammation and pain in animals. The results are promis-ing." The cherry extract, according to Raja, may interfere with an enzyme that produces inflammation. (But these results are still only true for animal studies, so don't rush out to buy cherries just yet.) Other researchers are looking at the role of sugars in reducing pain. In one study, newborns given a high sugar drink have less signs of pain. "The sugar may be stimulating or exciting the body's natural system that releases opiates, which reduce pain," says Raja.

THE JOY OF SOY

If you are inspired to include more soy in your diet, you are in good company. In addition to its potential for reducing pain and cholesterol, soy is recommended to help with menopause symptoms (see chapter 10), and in general as part of a healthy diet. In his book, *The Simple Soybean and Your Health,* Mark Messina, Ph.D., of Loma Linda University's Department of Nutrition cites research evidence that soy may reduce the risk of heart disease, osteoporosis, prostate and breast cancer and some of the complications of diabetes.

In addition to Dr. Jill Tall's soy milkshake recipe above, you can check the Web sites to follow for more tips on cooking with soy. Soy Protein Partners (*http://www. soybean.org/proteinpartners.html*) puts out an annual guide to finding and using soy products, including soymilk, soy yogurt, soy ice cream, soynut butter, soy "cheese," soy flour and traditional soy foods such as miso, edamame, tofu, tempeh and soy sauce. The publication also includes a weekly "twenty-five soy grams a day" meal planner.

Web sites with soy protein information:
www.unitedsoybean.org/
www.soyohio.org/health/index.htm
www.centralsoya.com/
www.protein.com/
www.soybean.on.ca/uses.htm

References (Soy)

Kanarek, R. B. and B. Homoleski. "Modulation of Morphine-Induced Aantinociception by Palatable Solutions in Male and Female Rats." *Pharmacology, Biochemistry and Behavior* 66, no. 3 (2000): 653–659 (sucrose study).

Messina, M., V. Messina, and K. Setchell. *The Simple Soybean and Your Health*. New York: Avery Publishing Group, 1994.

Seeram, N. P., et al. "Cyclooxygenase Inhibitory and Antioxidant Cyanidin Glycosides in Cherries and Berries." *Phytomedicine* 8, no. 5 (2001): 362–369.

Shir, Y., et al. "Neuropathic Pain Following Partial Nerve Injury in Rats Is Suppressed by Dietary Soy." *Neuroscience Letters* 240 (1998): 73–76.

Shir, Y., et al. "Pre- But Not Postoperative Consumption of Soy Suppresses Pain Behavior Following Partial Sciatic Ligation in Rats." In M. Devor, M. C. Rowbotham, and Z. Wiesenfeld-Hallin, eds., Proceedings of the 9th World Congress on Pain, 16. Seattle: IASP Press, 2000: 477–483.

Shir, Y., et al. "A Soy-Containing Diet Suppresses Chronic Neuropathic Sensory Disorders in Rats." *Anesthesia and Analgesia Current Researches* 92 (2001): 1029–1034.

Shir, Y., et al. "Consumption of Soy Diet Before Nerve Injury Preempts the Development of Neuropathic Pain in Rats." *Anesthesiology* 95, no. 5 (2001b): 1238–1244.

Tall, J. M. and S. N. Raja. "Complete Freund's Adjuvant Induced Edema and Thermal Hyperalgesia are Suppressed by Dietary Soy in Rats." *Journal of Pain* 3, Supplement 1 (2002): 45.

Wang, H., et al. "Antioxidant and Anti-inflammatory Activities of Anthocyanins and Their Aglycon, Cyanidin, From Tart Cherries." *Journal of Natural Products* 62 (1999): 294–296.

The Science of Pain

Clifford Woolf, M.D., Ph.D., is helping to change the conventional definition of pain, although his world is the world of biological science, not alternative or complementary medicine. While he acknowledges that such treatments as homeopathy and acupuncture may make people feel better, he does not believe that alternative methods are scientifically valid. "If they work at all," he says. "It is purely because of the patient's belief that they are effective, which is the same as the placebo effect. By contrast, my work is devoted to finding scientifically proven, statistically significant methods to block pain at the level of the cells."

Woolf holds the Richard Kitz Chair of Anesthesia Research at Boston's Massachusetts General Hospital (MGH) and directs the hospital's neuro-plasticity laboratory. "Unlike other sensations, such as warmth, the experience of pain has an emotional as well as a sensory component," he says. "Pain is a word we use to describe a multitude of symptoms, emotions and states of mind. It can describe a clear-cut symptom, like a broken leg, or the anguish at the loss of a loved one. However, for people with chronic pain, the experience becomes an overwhelming, primary drive—similar to the compulsions of extreme hunger or thirst—that takes over their lives, evoking powerful emotions, memories, fears and feelings of being out of control."

In any discussion of pain, stresses Woolf, it is important to distinguish *patho-logical*, chronic pain from *normal*, acute pain: "Pain that warns us when our bod-ies are in danger of being damaged, such as the pain we feel when we touch a burning ember or a sharp blade, is essential to survival. We must never interfere with that mechanism," he says.

Until very recently, points out Woolf, conventional medicine has diagnosed pain in association with what was thought to be its cause, whether disease, surgery or traumatic injury. "If the diagnosis was related to a disease, such as arthritis, shingles, diabetes or AIDS, for example, conventional pain treatments have always been aimed at modifying that condition," he explains. "In the last several years, however, a new perspective of pain has emerged."

This new perspective is that chronic pain can itself be seen as a disease that is caused by abnormal changes in the brain and spinal cord. The damaged nerve cells involved in chronic pain are the targets of Woolf's work. "When we can understand what the molecular damage is, and how it creates pain, we can design molecular ways to block it," he says. Woolf's laboratory is in the forefront of promising research that is identifying the biological, molecular mechanisms of chronic pain.

New technologies—including the use of "gene chips" that can rapidly analyze thousands of genes to identify abnormalities involved in chronic pain—are speeding up pain research more than ever before. In the past thirty years of pain research, Woolf says, scientists have found about sixty pain-related genes, searching one-by-one. But with gene chip technology, he and other pain researchers identified fifteen hundred pain-related genes in 2001 alone. Woolf and his colleagues, according to a report in *The New York Times*, were the first to demonstrate that the body's pain system is plastic and can therefore be molded by pain to cause *more* pain: "The whole central nervous system revs up and undergoes what Woolf calls 'central sensitization.'"[2]

Woolf explains further: "We are learning that in abnormal pain, some trigger—for example, trauma, chemical toxicity, nerve compression or autoimmune disease—may set off changes in the central nervous system that damage or change the function of neurons (nerve cells) and that this damage may be permanent: It doesn't go away even after the original damage heals. It is as if there is a 'wiring malfunction' in the way that nerve cells communicate with each other."

What does this mean for patients? The future is filled with hope, says Woolf. "Pain has been the 'junk heap' of medicine until recently," he comments. "Patients with chronic pain were difficult to diagnose; they were coping with lives that had been destroyed; and we had poor treatments to offer. But in the last ten years, our understanding has increased so rapidly that pain research is now leading the way to a deeper understanding of the central nervous system itself. We have, for example, already identified a molecule that gets 'switched on' in the sensation of extreme cold, and we are identifying other pain molecules as well. We are close to identifying which mechanisms in damaged neurons are most important for sending pain messages, and when we do, we can design ways to block that pain message."

---

[2] Melanie Thernstron, "Pain, the Disease," *The New York Times*, 16 Dec. 2001: 66.

Pain, Woolf says, is a biologic disease afflicting millions of people, but there is reason for optimism. "We are closing in on pain. Very soon, I believe, there will be effective treatments for pain because, for the first time in history, the tools are coming together to understand and treat it."

Crohn's Disease: "Instead of the Pain Happening to Me, I Learned to Make Something Happen to the Pain"

Erica Orloff had stomachaches growing up, but nothing like what she felt while she was trying to get pregnant with her first child. "I went to the hospital, doubled over in agony and screaming in pain," she recalls. "I had lost twenty-five pounds in one month and the pain in my stomach had been building steadily until I could no longer tolerate it." Tests found that she had a fever and an elevated white blood count; doctors initially assumed she had appendicitis. A sigmoidoscopy (examination of only the lower part of the large bowel) revealed nothing.

"To this day I feel I got a raw deal from those imperious male doctors," says Erica. "When appendicitis was ruled out and the partial intestinal scope was negative, they told me that my stomach was sensitive and that I should eat only white things: bread, rice and potatoes. One doctor also said to me, 'This is all in your head. You are so worried about losing weight that you lost more.' But this little voice inside me said, 'I don't think I can have this much pain, and a fever, and have it all be in my head.' Despite my doubts, I resolved to accept what he said."

The pain finally subsided on its own, and Erica became pregnant almost immediately. "During those nine months, I felt great," she says. "I assumed that the pregnancy had somehow put whatever this disease was into a kind of remission." But four days after giving birth, she was back in the hospital again. "The pain was as bad as ever," she remembers. "Only this time I began bleeding profusely every time I had a bowel movement. The blood just came pouring out of me."

She refused to go back to the doctor who had treated her before and found a new doctor. "He was wonderful," she says. "Very different. He would hop onto the table, look me in the eye and want to know about my life, about my new baby, was I happy? None of the other doctors had ever looked me in the eye before, and no one had been interested in my life."

The new doctor did something more; he decided to do a complete colonoscopy—examining the entire large bowel—which finally solved the mystery: He diagnosed Crohn's disease, a chronic digestive disorder that falls into the category of "inflammatory bowel disease" (IBD). There are two categories of IBD: Crohn's disease occurs in patches along the digestive tract, anywhere from the mouth to the anus; ulcerative colitis is restricted to the large intestine.

It is thought that Crohn's disease is caused by the body's immune system wrongly reacting to the lining of the digestive system as if it is "foreign" tissue and therefore dangerous. White blood cells rush to attack the "invader," creating holes or ulcerations in the lining of the intestine, giving it a "cobblestone" appearance. The holes cause pain and bleeding and, eventually, scar tissue, which can cause severe, sometimes fatal obstruction of the bowel.

"I learned that Crohn's disease plays hide and seek," says Erica. "It can skip part of the intestine, which is why the first doctor never saw it. He didn't look far enough inside my intestine." The new doctor prescribed medications that helped alleviate the pain and symptoms somewhat, but did not eliminate them. "I felt a profound sense of relief that I wasn't crazy, that I finally understood what was happening in my body," says Erica. "I almost didn't care that I still had some symptoms."

Erica is a professional writer and accustomed to research; during the next two years she learned everything she could about her disease and its treatment. With the new medication, her symptoms remained fairly mild, and she went back to a normal life, writing and raising her daughter. She also divorced and remarried. "I was very happy," she says. But about eight years ago—just two months after her second marriage—she started having full-blown episodes once again. (Crohn's disease can lie dormant for months or years, followed by intense periods of pain and symptoms that can last an equal amount of time.)

"One year I spent a whole winter in and out of hospitals and needed surgery to remove a blockage that had wrapped around my intestine," says Erica. "Then, a few weeks later, I collapsed on the living room floor, throwing up black blood.

Luckily, a friend was over and called an ambulance; otherwise I would have died." This second blockage began a four-month odyssey of hospitalizations for intense dehydration, bleeding and pain.

Trying to Cope: Forty-Four Pills a Day and Life on the Couch

"They gave me high doses of intravenous steroids and also tried organ transplant rejection drugs to try to stop my immune system from attacking my body," says Erica. "At that time, they also used chemotherapy for Crohn's, which I rejected because I wanted more children." To add to her woes, Erica was anemic from the loss of blood during bowel movements, and the disease was also attacking her joints, causing arthritis-like symptoms.

"By the time I got home, I was taking forty-four pills a day," says Erica. "These included arthritis medicine for the joints, high-dose steroids, anti-ulcer meds, anti-inflammatory pills, as well as pills for pain. I had to do this five times a day, around the clock."

The pain and diarrhea abated somewhat, but the side effects of the steroids were dramatic: "I gained forty pounds in two weeks," says Erica. "My face was so swollen that I could look down and see my cheeks. I couldn't even bear to look at myself in the mirror." The steroids also made her hyperactive. "I was up twenty-two out of twenty-four hours," she says. "We didn't have cable, and TV went off at two in the morning. So I tried to find a silver lining. Despite everything I've been through, I've always been an optimist. So I cleaned my kitchen floor and got all my Christmas presents wrapped and ready."

Then she developed "steroid myopathy," caused by the steroids "consuming" the muscles, which become atrophied and lose their tone. Her weakened legs, combined with the joint pain in both her ankles, meant that she could barely walk. "All I could do was crawl or hobble, like someone who had sprained both ankles," she says. "And I had a toddler to take care of!"

So Erica and her new husband devised a system. Every morning, she would slide down the stairs on her rear end, and then hobble to the couch. He would use the ironing board to block the staircase to prevent her daughter from climbing. Before he left for work, he would prepare sandwiches, snacks and juice to leave on the coffee table until he got home at the end of the day. "I spent four months, twenty-two hours a day, on that couch," says Erica. "It was a brutal lesson. I had to learn to separate my self-esteem from what I could do and what I looked like. Luckily, my daughter seemed to understand that Mommy couldn't chase her, so we watched a lot of TV, played quiet games and ate snacks."

Moving into Health

Desperate to help their daughter, Erica's parents, who live in Florida, turned to the Internet, where they found the Web site of the Crohn's and Colitis Foundation of America (*www.ccfa.org*) and learned about the work of Alvin Zfass, M.D., a specialist and professor at the Medical College of Virginia. "It took almost two months to get an appointment with him," says Erica. "So I lay on that couch until he could see me. But it was worth the wait. He saved my life in a lot of different ways."

At the first appointment, Zfass spent two hours with Erica and her family. "It was an amazing experience," she says. "He invited my husband and my parents to join us, and we crowded into his tiny office. He left no stone unturned, starting with my own mother's pregnancy, my birth and childhood, and through every detail of my health history. He wanted to know it all. He even asked my husband how he was doing—we had only been married six months—and my husband broke down. No doctor had ever asked him that before."

At the end of two hours, Zfass told Erica she was not to leave the hospital. "I was initially shocked and dismayed, but then quickly realized that this was a good thing," says Erica. "I was admitted to a special floor where a physical therapist, three different rheumatologists, X-ray technicians and other specialists came right to my bed. The whole idea was to get me weaned off steroids, and a team of nurses and nurse practitioners continually supervised and balanced my medication in order to do this. One night, I woke up at four in the morning, and Dr. Zfass was just sitting in a chair in my room, watching me. He said, 'You're going to be well, and you're going to go home.' I believed him."

Erica did go home after a couple of weeks and, with supervision, slowly cut down her use of steroids. "Dr. Zfass used some of the newer medicines to treat the symptoms—diarrhea, ulcers and pain. Slowly, my intestines and joints healed, and after about a year, I was off the steroids completely and had begun to lose the excess weight," says Erica. She, her husband and daughter moved to Florida to be closer to her parents, and life began to resume its normal rhythm. She began writing again, publishing several books; she had two more children, without incident. Her children are now twelve, seven and four. She also began to collect the menagerie that shares her home: a canary, two dogs, four fish, doves and finches (she raises them), a cockatoo and a rabbit. "My mother always told me when I had my own house I could have pets," says Erica. "So now I do."

She tries to stay off of steroids, taking medications only to treat her symptoms as they arise. "I believe that if a disease is based on exacerbation and remission, it is better to treat the symptoms and avoid decimating the immune system with steroids, if possible. So under the doctor's supervision, I would take prescription antidiarrhea, anticramping and antinausea medications as needed. And, if necessary, a short-term course of a new kind of steroid that does not make you blow up. But I would try to get off them as soon as possible, because they do interfere with sleeping." This system worked for a few years.

But in July 2001, severe symptoms began to return. "I started vomiting more than usual, even blacking out from it at times, having terrible diarrhea, and I lost twenty-two pounds," says Erica. "There were whole weeks when I couldn't leave the house, even for ten minutes to pick up my kids from school. I was run-down, bruising easily and unable to eat much of anything. My husband, who is a gourmet chef, began to make me fruit smoothies with soy powder, or strained potato soup blended with zucchini. These have become my staples, because I can digest them so easily. I treat my dehydration at home with electrolyte drinks, but when I notice bleeding, it's time to go to the hospital." Since this new episode began, she was in the hospital for dehydration and diarrhea three times. In between, she continued to use her "medication as needed" system.

New Strategies from "Integral Medicine"

Still coping with almost daily pain and diarrhea, Erica decided to explore some alternative treatments. "I figured I had nothing to lose," she says. "Western medicine was offering me its best, but I felt I needed some additional tools." Since the beginning of her illness nearly twelve years ago, Erica had been doing some soul-searching on her own to try to discover the meaning of what was happening to her.

"I had read the book, *Man's Search for Meaning*, by the late psychiatrist Viktor Frankl," she says. "It changed my life. He used his experiences in Auschwitz to find meaning in the midst of suffering. I was trying to do the same thing. Why should a young woman be suffering like this? I realized that if I waited for someone to give me an answer, I'd still be waiting. I had to make sense of my suffering, and this book helped me do that. I try to walk with grace, dignity and courage, and be good to those around me. I have four or five women friends who come forward to help me whenever I am sick. They bring food, drive my kids and help with the house. I offer them support as well. This is a gift of grace that we give to each other. I know that I am a writer, but now I feel more defined by this amorphous term of 'grace.' Erica also started using her treadmill regularly again. "I am stubborn and didn't want to give up exercising," she says. "I'm not going to let this disease beat me."

Recently, she heard about a class sponsored by Transformation Associates, Inc., of Delray Beach, Florida. "The class was called 'The Nervous Stomach.' I knew that it was primarily for people with irritable bowel syndrome (IBS), which is less serious than IBD and Crohn's, so I was initially skeptical. I also didn't want more wacky doctors telling me my disease was 'all in my head.'" But after consulting with Sarena Morello, a licensed mental health counselor and biofeedback expert who developed the program, Erica decided to give the class a try.

Sarena Morello began her medical career as a specialist in pain management, directing biofeedback programs for medical and rehabilitation centers. Biofeedback training uses instruments that measure body "language," including muscle tension and finger temperature. The instruments transmit this information to us, either on a screen or with sounds. "Research and clinical practice with biofeedback has shown that we can consciously use this information to self-regulate many of the functions of the autonomic nervous system, which includes the 'automatic' functions of your body, such as heart rate, blood pressure or finger temperature," says Sarena.

This information about what is going on inside our bodies is important if we want to reduce our stress, she explains. "In a stress response, the blood rushes to the heart from the extremities (hands and feet) and from the gastrointestinal (GI) tract. One of the effects is lowered temperature of our fingers. We use special thermometers that are placed on the finger to measure changes in the skin temperature." During relaxation, the normal blood flow returns to the gastrointestinal tract and the extremities. Through biofeedback, patients can learn to regulate this blood flow and can measure their success by seeing the rising temperature of their fingers. Increased blood flow in the GI tract helps with digestion and can help reduce some of the symptoms of digestive disorders, such as irritable bowel syndrome. (The same techniques are used to teach heart patients to regulate their cardiac rhythm, another part of the autonomic nervous system. See, for example, Charlotte Harrington's story in chapter 4.)

Sarena calls the program that she has developed "Integral Health Care." "In addition to the biofeedback training, we also teach a method of deep, diaphragmatic breathing—similar to the breathing methods of yoga—which calms and stills the mind, combined with health-promoting imagery and visualization (creating 'movies in the mind' that are positive and life-enhancing)," she says. "We use these methods to teach people how to reduce stress and enter a state of deep relaxation. In this state, there is a direct, positive effect that the brain can have on many physical problems, such as irregular bowel function and insomnia." Sarena has synthesized the program into a series of audio and videotapes, along with instruction booklets and finger temperature thermometers, for patients to use at home. She has recently completed a similar program for children aged seven to twelve, called "Peacemaking and Earthkeeping Skills for Children." Sarena produces these Integral Health Care multimedia learning kits through her own wellness consulting firm, Transformation Associates, Inc.

✦ ✦ ✦ ✦

Erica knew that Crohn's disease is not likely to be cured by biofeedback alone. "But I told Sarena that I wanted another tool to use when I was in pain, and she thought it might be helpful," says Erica. "The biofeedback training, combined with the breathing, positive imagery and visualization helped me to control my fear during pain episodes. When I am in pain, my hands and feet are freezing. Using the audiotape, I can usually raise the temperature of my extremities by several degrees. This increased blood flow also goes back to my GI tract and seems to calm down the intestinal area. Last week, I had pain that I managed to reduce from a level of 'ten,' the highest on my personal scale, to a level three or four. It seems to work every time."[3]

Now, says Erica, she has more of a feeling of control over her illness. "Instead of the pain happening to me, I can make something happen to the pain," she says. "I can control my fear and separate this pain from the years of horrible pain experiences in my past. I can stay calm, which relaxes my intestines and my whole body."

Shifting from the Power of a Diagnosis to Empowerment of Self

As a result of her own major physical challenges, Sarena has devoted her career to bringing the power of mind/body medicine into mainstream medical practice. A back injury in 1988 two weeks before her wedding forced her to be married in a wheelchair. Doctors told her she would never walk again without surgery. Sarena did not want surgery. In addition to her work in clinical pain management, she had also begun to study yoga, meditation and other forms of alternative healing. So she first tried a one-week, full-day intensive program of craniosacral therapy, along with deep relaxation through breathing and meditation, positive affirmations and visualizations to help her "reframe" her thoughts about her condition. As an example of a positive affirmation, she would repeat to herself such statements as, "I trust that I am healed in the way that is most perfect." She also tried to understand the core lesson of this injury for her life.

---

[3] Erica used a multimedia kit called Healing with Autogenics, available from Transformation Associates. (561-482-2345 or 877-482-5683 or online at *www.transformationmeditation.com.*)

"I did not want to fight this or drug it away. I wanted to be aware, and this awareness was, for me, a major part of my healing."

Sarena never had the surgery. Her back has healed, and she has completely normal function with no residual pain. "As a pain specialist, I realized that biofeedback was a perfect way to use the deep relaxation techniques of yoga and meditation alongside the conventional treatment of disease and injury," says Sarena, who spent twenty years developing and perfecting her training programs. "These programs, and the control they give people over their health, help to shift from the power of the 'diagnosis' to the empowerment of self," she says. "The diagnosis is important for the physician and for treatment, but then it can become a box that holds one down and can limit the potential for healing. I teach my patients to say 'I am a beautiful, healthy, whole person who is having some difficulty in one area of my body. This difficulty can be treated with medicine as well as my own natural healing ability.'" The method is particularly helpful for treating gastrointestinal problems, as well as anxiety and insomnia, points out Sarena. (Please see "A Second Brain in the Gut," below.)

A SECOND BRAIN IN THE GUT? EVIDENCE SAYS YES.

In addition to the brain and central nervous system we all know about, there is evidence that a second complex "brain" and nervous system also exist in the human gut. The gut brain, called the "enteric nervous system," has been described by Michael Gershon, M.D., professor of anatomy and cell biology at Columbia Presbyterian Medical Center in New York. In a 1996 interview with *The New York Times,* Gershon explained that nearly every substance that helps run and control the brain has turned up in the gut. These include serotonin, dopamine, glutamate, norephinephrine and nitric oxide, as well as two dozen small brain proteins, called neuropeptides, and major cells of the immune system.

This explains why so many emotional states affect the bowel and stomach. The reporter asks: "Ever wonder why people get 'butterflies' in the stomach before going on stage? Or why an impending job interview can cause an attack of intestinal cramps? And why antidepressants targeted for the brain cause nausea or abdominal upset in millions of people who take such drugs?"[4]

---

[4] Sandra Blakeslee, *The New York Times,* 23 Jan., 1996: 1.

Gershon is considered one of the founders of a new field of medicine called "neurogastroenterology," which forms one of the foundations of the "Nervous Stomach" program that Sarena Morello has developed and used with considerable success. She has also based her program on research generated by the International Foundation for Functional Gastrointestinal Disorders (*www.iffgd.org*), as well as the University of North Carolina Division of Digestive Diseases. "Since there is a 'mind' in the gut, then the idea of a mind/body program to treat intestinal problems makes a great deal of sense," she says.

"Biofeedback does not 'do' anything to the patient," says Sarena. "It is what the patient does inside her own mind and body when she receives information from the biofeedback instruments that makes the difference. To me, biofeedback training, combined with meditation, visualization and diaphragmatic breathing walk the fine line between Eastern and Western medicine. The biofeedback instruments tell you what is happening inside your body—what your muscle tension and finger temperature are, for example—and you use relaxation techniques to make changes. We have found that with training, patients can voluntarily self-regulate the operations of all autonomic nervous systems: cardiovascular (heart), gastrointestinal (gut), immune, respiratory (breathing) and circulatory (blood flow)."

Among the several relaxation techniques that Sarena uses in her program is a method called "autogenic training" (AT). Two German psychologists, Wolfgang Luthe and Johannes H. Schultz, developed autogenic training in 1932, according to Sarena. "The material we give to patients explains that autogenic training—like some forms of meditation—helps us develop an internal awareness, so that we can observe our thoughts and feelings without judging them or getting caught up in them. The technique involves the repetition of relaxing phrases to ourselves in order to relax our muscles, our visceral organs and our body tissue. The method trains people to use their own inner resources to help themselves." (Please also see "A Closer Look at Meditation.")

After several months on the program, Erica says she is making "good progress."

She uses the training tape (called "Healing with Autogenics") as a meditation guide twice a day, for at least twenty minutes each time. When she feels stress or pain, she practices the deep, yogic breathing to calm her mind and body. She takes the following supplements: lecithin, aloe vera, acidophilus, bifidus, vitamin C (in liquid form), Greens+ (in a smoothie drink), DHA and a multivitamin with energy boosters. "I avoid iron," she says. "It is too hard to digest. And when the complementary methods fail, I still have my Western medicine to fall back on to treat my symptoms, and I might also use a short-term dose of steroids."

Erica's attitude toward her illness continues to evolve. "I have become my own advocate," she says. "I treat doctors as people who work for me. The doctor I have now in Florida is wonderful. He gave me his cell phone number when I was at my sickest and told me to call him every day. He even suggested that I might want to look into Chinese medicine and herbs, in addition to the biofeedback and meditation/relaxation work I am doing."

But Erica still is puzzled about something: "Why do hospital rooms only have those televisions hanging from the ceiling? Why doesn't every patient have headphones and a library of these relaxation/meditation tapes with instructions on calming breathing techniques? When you're lying in a hospital bed in pain all day, why don't they give you tools that can help you take control of your pain?"

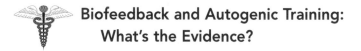

Biofeedback and Autogenic Training: What's the Evidence?

The "Integral Medicine" training programs for gastrointestinal problems and insomnia use two primary techniques: autogenic training (including relaxation, visualization and autosuggestion) and biofeedback. Research shows that both have been found to be effective in the treatment of certain conditions, including gastrointestinal disorders and insomnia.

Autogenic training: results are positive, but better research is needed

A systematic review of all controlled trials of autogenic training (AT) was conducted for some conditions: hypertension, asthma, intestinal diseases, glaucoma and eczema. This study, according to an analysis by Edzard Ernst, "reached positive conclusions," but it made no assessment of the quality of the research. Four out of five studies of AT for hypertension also yielded positive results, as did seven out of eight studies on the use of AT for anxiety. Ernst, who was a coauthor of both of these systematic reviews, cautions that despite the positive results, "the quality of studies was too poor to allow firm conclusions to be drawn."

Biofeedback works for headaches, diabetes, blood pressure, asthma and many other conditions, especially in combination with relaxation methods

The basic concept of biofeedback is that awareness of the processes in your body gives you the opportunity to change them. This is done through simple intention, not conscious effort (which may hinder the process.) Biofeedback is often used in combination with relaxation methods, such as autogenic training (see above), or meditation. Edzard Ernst reports that "Systematic reviews of clinical trials (including observational studies) of biofeedback in tension headaches, and migraines in adults and children found that the combination of biofeedback and relaxation is more effective than either therapy used alone." The technique can also be used directly clinically, for example, to teach people with diabetes to increase blood flow to their legs.

In his book, *The Best Alternative Medicine: What Works? What Does Not?* Dr. Kenneth R. Pelletier, Ph.D., M.D. (hc) former director of the Complementary and Alternative Medicine Program at Stanford University Medical School, cites several additional studies showing the effectiveness of biofeedback. In a 1992 review for the National Institutes of Health, biofeedback was found effective for 150 conditions. Another study found that patients with insulin-dependent diabetes were able to use biofeedback to improve blood sugar stability. In Japan, research found that patients using biofeedback learned to reduce stress-related increases in blood pressure. And a fifteen-month study of asthmatics found that biofeedback patients suffered fewer attacks and used less medicine.

For insomnia, "behavioral treatment" (such as autogenic training and biofeedback) works better than drugs

A two-year randomized controlled study published recently in the *Journal of the American Medical Association* concluded that "Behavioral and pharmacological approaches are effective for the short-term management of insomnia in late life; sleep improvements are better sustained over time with behavioral treatment." This study was designed to "evaluate the separate and combined effects of behavioral and pharmacological treatments for insomnia in older adults." The authors state, "Although such behavioral intervention is more time consuming than drug therapy, it is worth the investment because therapeutic gains are well maintained."

References

Achterberg, J., et al. "Mind-Body Interventions." In *Alternative Medicine: Expanding Medical Horizons—A Report to the National Institutes of Health on Alternative Medical Systems and Practices in the United States*. Prepared under the auspices of the Workshop on Alternative Medicine, Chantilly, VA and Washington DC: Government Printing Office (1992): 3–43.

Bogaards, M. C. D., et al. "Treatment of Recurrent Tension Headache: A Meta-Analytic Review." *Clinical Journal of Pain* 10 (1994): 174–190.

Ernst, E., ed. *The Desktop Guide to Complementary and Alternative Medicine: An Evidence-Based Approach*. London: Harcourt Publishers Limited, 2001.

Hermann, C., et al. "Behavioral and Prophylactic Pharmacological Intervention Studies of Pediatric Migraine: An Exploratory Meta-Analysis." *Pain* 60 (1995): 239–256.

Holroyd K. A., et al. "Pharmacological Versus Non-Pharmacological Prophylaxis of Recurrent Migraine Headache: A Meta-Analytic Review of Clinical Trials." *Pain* 42 (1990): 1–13.

Kanji, N., A. R. White, and E. Ernst. "Anti-Hypertensive Effects of Autogenic Training: A Systematic Review." *Perfusion* 12 (1999): 279–282.

Kanji, N. and E. Ernst. "Autogenic Training for Stress and Anxiety: A Systematic Review." *Complementary Therapies in Medicine* 8 (2000): 106–110.

McGrady, A., et al. "Biofeedback Assisted Relaxation in Insulin Dependent Diabetes: A Replication and Extension Study." *Annals of Behavioral Medicine* 18, no. 3 (1996): 185–189.

Morin, C. M., et al. "Behavioral and Pharmacological Therapies for Late-Life Insomnia: A Randomized Control Trial." *Journal of the American Medical Association* 281, no. 11 (1999): 991–999.

Nakao, M., et al. "Clinical Effects of Blood Pressure Biofeedback Treatment on Hypertension by Auto-Shaping." *Psychosomatic Medicine* 49 (1997): 493–507.

Pelletier, K. R. *The Best Alternative Medicine: What Works? What Does Not?* New York: Simon & Schuster, 2000.

Peper, E. and V. Tibbets. "Fifteen-Month Follow-Up with Asthmatics Utilizing EMG/Incentive Inspirometer Feedback." *Biofeedback and Self-Regulation* 17, no. 2 (1992): 143–51.

Rice, B. I., et al. "Effect of Thermal Biofeedback-Assisted Relaxation Training on Blood Circulation in the Lower Extremities of a Population with Diabetes." *Diabetes Care* 15 (1992): 853–858.

Stetter, F., et al. "Autogenes Training: Qualitative Meta-Analysis of Clinical Outcomes (*Kontrollierter Klinischer Studien und Beziehungen zur Naturheilkunde*)." *Forschende Komplementarmedizin* 5 (1998): 211–223.

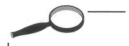

A Closer Look at Chiropractic and
Craniosacral Therapy:
Tapping into the Wellspring of the Body

Eurydice Hirsey first learned about alternative medicine when she was ten years old. She had just moved with her family to Madrid, Spain, from her native New York City. Her father was planning to write a play there. Shortly after the family's arrival in Spain, Eurydice came down with hepatitis from eating shellfish in a local restaurant. "I felt very weak and had yellow skin and eyes," she remembers. Her parents took her to a doctor in Madrid, who told them that she needed to be hospitalized for six months; otherwise she would die. "My parents were never big believers in conventional medicine," says Eurydice. "They were appalled at the thought of putting me in a hospital for six months, and the idea did not thrill me, either. So they began to research other cures. Somewhere, they found out about the 'grape cure' and together, we decided to try it."

The grape cure was simple: Eurydice was to eat nothing but grapes—big, Muscatel grapes—for seven days; five pounds of the grapes a day, chewing the skins and pits thoroughly, and drinking one to two gallons of warm water. Nothing else. "I felt so horribly weak that I was willing to do it," says Eurydice. "I followed the grape and water diet strictly for several days, and noticed that I was beginning to feel better. By the seventh day, I was totally healed, all the yellow was gone, and I felt once again full of energy. To this day I don't know why the grape diet worked—perhaps it cleanses the body, or perhaps there is some healing property in the skin or pits. But whatever the reason, this was the beginning of my evolution as a healer." (Note: there appears to be no research on grapes as a cure for hepatitis.)

Deciding to study medicine, Eurydice enrolled in pre-med at college, but discovered to her dismay that the entire orientation was to Western, conventional medicine. "By that time I was a vegetarian and never went to conventional doctors," she says. "I loved the idea of healing and working with people, and I felt that biology was magical, but I didn't believe in the strict paradigm of Western medicine. How could I devote my life to that?" She changed her major to geology and after graduation went to Israel to work on a kibbutz (an Israeli collective farm). She liked the hard, repetitive farm labor but soon after her arrival began having excruciating pain in her neck. (She found out later that she had herniated a disk.)

She kept on working for a few more weeks, but the pain became increasingly severe. She was twenty-one years old. "I had been accepted into a marine biology program at Hebrew University," she says. "But I knew that I needed medical care. I decided to go back home." Her parents were by then living in Boston and her father arranged for her to see a chiropractor. "I had no idea what chiropractic was," says Eurydice. "But I liked the man who treated me, and he was able to eliminate the pain in less than twelve visits!" By the following autumn, she had given up on going back to Israel and had become a student at a school for chiropractic in Davenport, Iowa. She graduated and began her practice in 1979.

Chiropractic: Realigning the Spine
to Help the Central Nervous System

The word chiropractic comes from the ancient Greek *cheiro* ("hand") and *praktikos* ("doing"). Chiropractors use their hands, as well as diagnostic tests and X-rays, to diagnose and treat disorders or misalignment of the spine. Distortions of the spine are thought to interrupt or damage messages that the brain sends through the central nervous system (the main branch of which is housed in the spine) to the rest of the body.

In her work as a chiropractor, Eurydice treats patients with problems that include headaches, back, neck, shoulder, arm and leg pain. "Chiropractic is based on the premise that pain and a sense of malaise or "dis-ease" (lack of ease) in the body come from a dysfunction in the spine, affecting both the central nervous system and the peripheral nervous system," says Eurydice. "The point of chiropractic is to get to the cause—where the nerves exit the spinal column, because distortions in these nerve messages can create problems throughout the body, affecting muscles, sensations, joints and organ systems."

The treatment involves orthopedic and neurological exams, as well as palpating (feeling) the muscles and joints to decide if there is a misalignment or mal-position in the joints, vertebrae or pelvis. Chiropractors then use their hands in a technique called an "adjustment" to realign the vertebrae of the spine and the large joints of the body. (They also use a variety of other alignment methods.)

The Craniosacral Rhythm: Going Deeper

After several years of practicing only chiropractic, Eurydice wanted to expand her practice by delving deeper into the relationship between body, mind and emotion. At about the same time, she had begun to climb mountains. "I enjoy not only the physical challenge of getting to the summit," she says, "but also looking out at the vast, expanse of space from the top of a mountain. I wanted to expand my knowledge as well, and learn more about our bodies and how we interact with the world."

Eurydice looks as if she could gracefully sprint up the side of a mountain. She is of medium height and very strong, built as efficiently as a mountain lion, with long, lean muscle. Her features are finely chiseled, and her face radiates a glow of vitality and a lightness, made more pronounced by the burnished glow of the tawny hair that she wears piled on top of her head.

In addition to mountain climbing, Eurydice had begun to learn Buddhist meditation from the master teacher Thich Nhat Hanh, periodically traveling overseas to study with him. "I wanted to explore how we can find a source of peace inside of us, and how we can use this peace to clearly see and understand our experiences from moment to moment—another way to expand the mind," says Eurydice. "My teacher was one of the people who brought this 'mindfulness' practice to the Western world." (See "A Closer Look at Meditation.")

A visit to Eurydice's office does much to describe who she is: On the walls are two of her own large pen and ink drawings filled with detail and bursting with color, inspired by ideas that range from quantum physics to biology. A stained glass "peace plate" from Israel reflects light from a window ledge. Eagle feathers and a parchment poem from a Navaho reservation adorn another wall, along with a row of color-filled sunbursts representing the "chakras" (energy centers in the body) from the Ayurvedic tradition. On a shelf is her special rock collection: crystals and minerals that she has collected on her travels and mountain-climbing expeditions.

Drawing on all of her interests and experiences, Eurydice added craniosacral therapy to her collection of skills. Developed by J. E. Upledger, an osteopathic physician, in the 1970s, craniosacral therapy is another way of looking at the central nervous system and its relationship to the spinal cord. The craniosacral "rhythm" within the body comes from the regular pulsing of the liquid—called cerebrospinal fluid—that bathes, nourishes and protects the spinal cord. It is through the regular pulses of the cerebrospinal fluid that the brain transmits nerve messages to keep the body alive and functioning.

"I begin to 'listen' to this rhythm—which is much slower than a heartbeat, pulsing only six to twelve cycles per minute—by placing my hands on the sacrum (base of the spine), other areas of the spine, and on the head, where I can feel the movement of the bones of the skull," says Eurydice. (The head is actually made of separate, movable "bony plates" that are connected at seams or "sutures.") "Through my hands, I feel the vitality, strength and symmetry of the craniosacral rhythm. I can also feel where there are restrictions to the flow of fluid throughout the body."

Blockages or restrictions in the craniosacral fluid can result from tension in the muscles or "fascia" (the tissue just under the skin that overlies muscle and some organs, like a kind of inner "sleeve"). These restrictions can be a response to physical or emotional trauma. "As I place my hands on the spine and head of my patient, I can often feel enormous resistance to the flow of cerebrospinal fluid, caused by blockages in the tissue," says Eurydice. "Any injury or trauma that alters or minimizes the flow of this fluid can have a negative effect on our well-being and health."

During a session of craniosacral therapy, you lie on your back, fully clothed, on a cushioned table. As Eurydice places her hands under your back on the connection between your head and neck, there is no sensation of "forcing" a movement. "I try to detect and focus on the deepest reservoir of the body, below the 'radar' of the conscious mind and even of the muscle," says Eurydice. "I often just follow the body's own impulse, gently helping it to undo the resistance in its own way, without pushing on the muscles or joints. This is how craniosacral work differs from chiropractic or even massage, where the practitioner might force or create a change in the body." It is the patient's own response to Eurydice's gentle touch that provides the release.

When the muscle resistance does finally relax, the sensation is one of deep release from a tension you might not have been aware of. "For some people this can be an enormous, sometimes volcanic release," said Eurydice. "They may cry, laugh or feel anger, often depending on whether the physical restriction in the body came from an emotional trauma."

◆ ◆ ◆ ◆

A woman in her fifties, whom we will call "Pamela," came to Eurydice for help with low back and pelvic pain that had become so severe that it was creating problems with walking. After several sessions it became clear to Eurydice that this particular pain was originating from tightness in Pamela's stomach and abdomen. "As I worked with Pamela, she began to talk about the horrible emotional abuse she had endured as a child," said Eurydice. "The safest way for her to deal with her anger and trauma was to hold it in check, and where she held it was in her stomach. Years of holding tension in her abdomen caused the muscles of her lower back and pelvis to remain chronically contracted, and the result was pain."

Slowly, over a period of months, Eurydice would place her hands gently on areas of tension in Pamela's body and "listen" for the pulsation of her craniosacral rhythm, deep in the spinal column. "I tried to guide her body to reduce its resistance to its own natural rhythm. Sometimes this would involve just waiting quietly. When Pamela's muscles relaxed, and the resistance melted away, I would often feel an actual motion, or a sensation of warmth under my hand. If the release was dramatic, she might cry or report that she was reliving feelings of anger."

Pamela still comes to see Eurydice, but less often now. She has begun to breathe deeply from her abdomen, the way children do naturally, and has regained movement in her pelvis and lower back. Her pain has been significantly reduced and she has started yoga classes. "Breathing from her abdomen has helped bring more oxygen into her system," says Eurydice. "She reports that she feels happier now, more energetic. The physical release is helping her heal emotionally and spiritually and she is continuing this work in psychotherapy."

When she is able to help patients like Pamela, Eurydice feels what she describes as a total joy. "To be the most complete person, you have to be a member of the world and do what you can to help others. I want people to be out of pain, to walk again, to be whole, and then to help make the world whole." she says. "The most important thing is love for ourselves and those around us. If you can heal yourself, you can heal the world." Not surprisingly, Eurydice's business cards, decorated with colorful drawings by Nicaraguan artists, bear the slogan, "Healing for Peace."

 ## Chiropractic and Craniosacral Therapy: What's the Evidence?

Chiropractic: the evidence is growing but mixed

Research on chiropractic is generally considered not adequate, but the evidence is growing, according to two summary reviews. "Historically, chiropractic has not had an adequate basis in scientific and academic research; it has not attained adequate research funding from government or the public sector," writes Kenneth R. Pelletier, Ph.D., M.D., (hc), author of *The Best Alternative Medicine: What Works? What Does Not?* former director of the Complementary and Alternative Medicine Program at Stanford University School of Medicine. "However, there are more than fifty RCTs (randomized controlled trials) in the chiropractic research literature, and the scientific basis for chiropractic is growing steadily."

Short-term help for acute low back pain

One of these studies is particularly noteworthy, according to Pelletier. In an evaluation of twenty-five controlled clinical trials of chiropractic, "there was a 17 percent greater likelihood of recovery from uncomplicated, acute low back pain within three weeks than without it."

Long-term benefits shown in at least one study

In a single long-term study of 741 patients, chiropractic was compared to hospital outpatient management for low back pain. "After three years, the chiropractic group had improved 29 percent more than the hospital group," summarizes Pelletier.

A second overall review of the literature is less encouraging:

The basic premise of chiropractic, which is that malalignment (subluxation) of the vertebrae causes disease, "has no scientific rationale," writes Edzard Ernst, M.D., Ph.D., FRCP (Edin), professor of complementary medicine and director of the Department of Complementary Medicine at the School of Postgraduate Medicine and Health Sciences, University of Exeter (UK). "However, numerous systematic reviews of (chiropractic) spinal manipulation have been published." One systematic review (by a chiropractor) suggests that "there is moderate evidence of short-term efficacy" in the treatment of acute low back pain when compared with placebo and commonly used therapies. For mixed chronic and acute back pain, and for sciatica, the evidence was inconclusive. Ernst also highlights two other recent trials which "did not demonstrate a convincing benefit of chiropractic over other forms of routine lower back pain treatments.

"The bottom line of this somewhat confusing situation," suggests Ernst, "is that the effectiveness of chiropractic treatment of back pain is uncertain."

And here is Pelletier's bottom line: "A small body of published clinical evidence now suggests that spinal manipulation may be helpful for fibromyalgia, high blood pressure, asthma, menstrual pain, infantile colic, otitis media, childhood enuresis (bedwetting), dizziness and vertigo, chronic pelvic pain, and other conditions."

Craniosacral therapy—not enough evidence

No controlled trials of craniosacral therapy seem to exist, according to Ernst, who points out that Upledger himself, who developed the technique, does not cite them in his own writing. "Even though small movements between cranial bones are possible, there is no good evidence to suggest that restrictions of these movements have any health related relevance," writes Ernst.

However, practitioners, patients and Upledger himself claim that the technique is beneficial for problems such as birth trauma, chronic pain, cerebral dysfunction, cerebral palsy, colic, depression, dyslexia, ear infections, headaches, learning disabilities, Méniere's disease, musculoskeletal problems, migraine, sinusitis and stroke. Young children are believed to respond particularly well.

Note: The Upledger Institute publishes a list of research studies that support the existence of a craniosacral system, as well as publications describing the uses of craniosacral work for a variety of conditions in adults and children.

References

Bronfort, G. "Spinal Manipulation: Current State of Research and its Indications." *Neurological Clinics* 17 (1999): 91–111.

Cherkin, D. C., et al. "A Comparison of Physical Therapy, Chiropractic Manipulation and Provision of an Educational Booklet for the Treatment of Patients with Low Back Pain." *New England Journal of Medicine* 339 (1998): 1021–1029.

Ernst, E., ed. *The Desktop Guide to Complementary and Alternative Medicine: An Evidence-Based Approach.* London: Harcourt Publishers Limited, 2001.

Green, C., et al. "A Systematic Review of Craniosacral Therapy: Biological Plausibility, Assessment Reliability and Clinical Effectiveness." *Complementary Therapies in Medicine* 7 (1999): 201–207.

Meade, T. W., et al. "Randomized Comparison of Chiropractic and Outpatient Management for Low Back Pain: Results from Extended Follow Up." *British Medical Journal* 300 (1995): 1431–37.

Pelletier, K. R. *The Best Alternative Medicine: What Works? What Does Not?* New York: Simon & Schuster, 2000.

Shekelle, P. G., et al. "Spinal Manipulation for Low Back Pain." *Annals of Internal Medicine* 117, no. 7 (1992): 590–598.

Skargren, E., et al. "Predictive Factors for 1-Year Outcome of Low-Back and Neck Pain in Patients Treated in Primary Care: Comparison Between the Treatment Strategies Chiropractic and Physiotherapy." *Pain* 77 (1998): 201–207.

Upledger, J. E. "Craniosacral Therapy." In D. W. Novey, ed., *The Complete Reference to Complementary and Alternative Medicine.* St. Louis: Mosby, 2000.

8

TRAUMA: WHEN LIFE CHANGES IN AN INSTANT
"All I wanted to do was hug my children, and I couldn't even do that."

One Sunday morning in February 1997, Jacqueline Miller was standing on a kitchen stool hanging curtains in her son's room. The last thing she remembers before she found herself covered in blood on the floor is beginning to get down off the stool. "We figured out later that I must have lost my balance," she says, sitting in a wheelchair in the living room of her home. "I had apparently hit my face—hard—on the corner of my son's desk." The impact had severely injured her spinal cord. Jackie is an attractive and youthful-looking woman in her early fifties, with shoulder-length brown hair and vibrant coloring. She offers a visitor a glass of water, wheeling herself into her kitchen. She pulls herself to a standing position by holding onto the counter to get a glass and fill it at the sink. (Her pots are low enough to reach from a sitting position.) She hands it to her visitor, her grip solid but somewhat stiff and awkward, lowers herself back into the wheelchair and steers it into the living room.

With effort, Jackie can now stand briefly on her own and walk slowly with a walker or two canes. Her balance has improved to the extent that she can throw a ball, catch it and even hit it with a bat. Although she still moves with deliberation and some difficulty, she does not look frail. Her arms and legs show strong muscles. She holds herself erect and her body seems to emanate physical strength, even when she is sitting in her wheelchair. She can use an elliptical walking machine at the gym and can swim with flippers. Last winter, she and her children got certified for scuba diving.

Five years ago, doctors told her that she would be permanently paralyzed below her waist, with minimal movement in her arms and hands. "They were wrong," says Jackie simply.

As Jackie thinks back to the day of her accident, she does not remember falling, only lying on the floor, her body numb and unable to move from the neck down. (She would later need 150 stitches for the lacerations on her face.) "I had no pain because I couldn't feel anything," she remembers. "I certainly couldn't move, all I could do was to call to my husband in a feeble, raspy voice." From downstairs, Jackie's husband, Bryan Roberts, heard a crash and then her weak call. "He thought I was kidding," she says. "Until he saw me."

An ambulance rushed Jackie to the hospital. "I didn't realize what was going on and felt no fear or panic," she recalls. "I assumed the numbness would go away, and I would be able to move. But we soon found out after a series of MRIs (magnetic resonance imaging) that I had a kind of 'super-whiplash' that had pinched or bruised the spinal cord in my neck, damaging or killing the nerve cells that transmit messages from the brain to the body. Luckily, though, I could still talk." When her boss came to see her in the hospital later that night, Jackie said, "I told you I didn't want to go to Iowa." Today, Jackie explains, "We were supposed to go there on a business trip the next day. I didn't want to go, but not *that* badly!"

Jackie's spinal cord injury had transformed her in an instant from an outdoor enthusiast, scientist and mother of two young boys to someone who could not walk, turn a page or feed herself. When the extent of the traumatic injury finally sank in, Jackie was in shock and disbelieving. "All I wanted to be able to do was hug my children," she says. "And I couldn't even do that." But she still held onto her characteristic resilience and determination; those who know Jackie say that those two qualities, along with her sense of humor, are helping her reclaim her life.

Refusing to accept the grim prognoses of her doctors and physical therapists (one of whom told her that the best recovery she could hope for was to be able to "shuffle ten feet down the aisle—with a walker—at my son's wedding."), Jackie took the best that conventional rehabilitative medicine had to offer and then struck out on her own in search of alternative and complementary thera-pies. "Conventional rehab just didn't go far enough," she says.

In a way, she was lucky. With a Ph.D. in molecular biology and a background that includes teaching at Harvard Medical School, developing high school sci-ence curricula and training teachers to use it, Jackie is naturally both curious and creative. And in her personal life she would seize every opportunity to share new experiences with her children. "I would drive the kids crazy on weekends," she says. "Always suggesting that we play baseball, go bike riding, ice skating, skiing or hiking." She had a woodworking shop in the basement where she made toys, puzzles and games. And one of the family's greatest joys was to go hiking near the house they were renovating in the mountains. It is this restless, seek-ing energy that still drives her to accept nothing less than full recovery.

"I Am Not a Spinal Cord—I Am a Person."

Within a week after her accident, Jackie began to make slight movements with her right arm, but still had no feeling from the chest down. "At the hospital, they just put me in a room and left me there," she says. "One of the neurosurgeons, whom I thought of as 'Kon Tiki Head,' would come into my room followed by an entourage of medical students and residents. He would tap my toes, shake his head and walk out. He never once smiled or looked directly at me. The only thing he said was, 'This is what you've got, and this is all you will ever have. You had better get used to it.' Finally, I said to him, 'You need a vacation.' He didn't react." As soon as Jackie was able to use her right hand to turn a page, she asked her husband to bring her *Crime and Punishment*. "I still don't know why I chose that book to read," she says. "Perhaps it was to see that things could be worse."

She also tried to keep up with her work. "I was in the midst of developing a new biology curriculum when the accident happened," she says. "I asked to have the notebook brought to me so I could do some editing. We supported the note-book in a cookbook holder; I could just about hold a big, chunky marker and use it to make marks on a page. Someone would then hold the phone to my ear so I could talk to people at work." After a few more days, she could wiggle her toes slightly (although she still could not feel them), and the decision was made to transfer her to a rehabilitation hospital. "But first, they sent a psychiatrist in to talk to me," she says. "They thought I needed help with the idea that I was going to be immobilized for life. But I couldn't believe it and didn't even want to entertain the idea."

Jackie describes the rehabilitation hospital as a "nightmare." The chief physiatrist (specialist in rehabilitative medicine) was "a nice person, but just didn't get it," says Jackie. "She treated the spinal cord injury patients as if we were barely conscious, because we couldn't move. The staff would leave helpless people in the halls for hours, and leave things out of our reach. They also weren't properly trained to transfer patients from bed to wheelchair. I was frantic to get to physical therapy (PT) every day, but they wouldn't take us if we weren't washed, dressed and catheterized (to collect urine through a tube), and since I couldn't do those things myself, I had to wait for someone to come in. When they didn't help me in time, I would miss PT. It was humiliating."

Jackie and several spinal cord injury patients finally got together to write a letter to the director, complaining in detail about their treatment. "My basic message was, 'I am not a spinal cord. I am a person,'" says Jackie. "Unfortunately nothing changed." By this time, Jackie's arms and hands were beginning to regain some function, so the exercises focused in that area. "They didn't work on my legs at all because they told me I'd be permanently in a wheelchair. They said I'd have to learn to get dressed in bed. I said, 'No way.'"

While she was still in the rehabilitation hospital, the occupational therapist and physical therapist visited her home in preparation for discharge planning. "They came back and told me to sell the house," says Jackie. "I was really mad. I said, 'Don't you think my kids have had enough trauma? Now you want to kick them out of their house?' So they agreed that I could move back there, if we put a bathroom on the first floor and I had a personal care attendant with me. They said the kitchen was fine the way it was, and my spirits soared. Then I realized that they thought I was never going to cook or walk again, so the kitchen was irrelevant. "

When Jackie moved back home, she decided she did not want a full-time personal care attendant. "I decided I didn't want a stranger in my house and could not accept that I would not be independent again," she says. For a time, a home health aide did come in two mornings a week to help her bathe and dress. "But very soon I was able to do everything with Bryan's help," says Jackie. "I began to even be able to catheterize and dress myself—we bought clothes that were easy to get in and out of."

"When I Realized I Might Never Hike Our Favorite Trail Again, I Knew I Couldn't Give Up."

Bryan and Jackie installed a wheelchair ramp to the house, enlarged the kitchen to accommodate a wheelchair, put in cabinets and added a first-floor bathroom. The occupational and physical therapists came three days a week to work with her. But her insurance company eventually ended coverage for walking rehabilitation. "They tried supporting my legs with braces, but they were too cumbersome for me to move," says Jackie. "My doctors told me there was no reason for the insurance to pay for further rehab because I was never going to walk anyway. That was like a death knell to me," says Jackie.

One weekend, the family went to their cottage in the mountains. "We had a favorite six-mile hiking trail up there," says Jackie. "That weekend, I was in my twelve-year-old son's room saying goodnight, and it hit me. I said to him, 'You know, I might never be able to take that hike with you again.' He started to cry. I knew then that I couldn't give up. I decided I would do anything to walk, even if the doctors and the insurance company thought it was impossible. I realized I had to move beyond what conventional medicine had to offer me."

Years earlier, when their children were babies, Jackie and Bryan had hired as a babysitter a woman who had just moved to the United States from China and who spoke no English. During the next fifteen years, Shu Xian Yang, M.D., would become another grandmother to Jackie's children and an important member of the Miller/Roberts family. In China, Dr. Yang had trained in both Western and Chinese medicine at Beijing Medical University. For twenty-five years she had practiced and taught oncology at a teaching hospital there, specializing in leukemia, lymphoma, aplastic anemia and hemophilia. "I always felt tired in China because I was working so hard, teaching medical students and taking care of patients," says Dr. Yang. "I had spent years working with high-dose radiation and chemotherapy, especially as part of bone marrow transplant procedures, and suspected that constant exposure to chemicals and radiation might be causing my symptoms. I have a family history of cancer, so I decided to come to the United States and try to find a job outside of medicine."

Now sixty-six, Dr. Yang not only speaks English, she has made a name for herself as an expert in shiatsu (acupressure) massage. Her work at a women's health center that later became part of the Brigham & Women's Hospital, won a "Best of Boston Award" from *Boston Magazine*; she was also featured in *Forbes* magazine. (In fact, several Western doctors still come to her home office for regular shiatsu treatments.) Although she is not licensed to practice Western medicine or acupuncture in this country, she uses her knowledge of Chinese medicine in her acupressure work, releasing the flow of qi to reduce pain and promote health. (Please see chapters 2 and 6 for more about traditional Chinese Medicine and the life force called qi.)

During the years that Dr. Yang babysat for Jackie and Bryan, she introduced the family to the principles of Chinese medicine as well as Chinese cooking and nutrition. As a result of this exposure, Jackie eventually became a board member of the New England School of Acupuncture. "Even though I am a conventionally trained scientist," says Jackie, "I am open to the healing possibilities of other methods of treatment. During the years before my accident, for example, Dr. Yang used her acupressure massage techniques to successfully treat my children for diarrhea, my mother-in-law for sciatica, my husband for his hypertension, and my own severe menstrual bleeding and cramps. I saw firsthand that these methods work." (Please see the "Closer Look" sections for more detailed explanations and research data on the efficacy of Chinese acupuncture, massage and herbal treatments.)

As we have seen in previous chapters, the practices of traditional Chinese Medicine—including acupressure, acupuncture, herbal treatments and massage—date back three thousand years. Medical students in China continue to learn these methods today, along with their Western training, according to Dr. Yang. "During the Cultural Revolution in China in the late 1960s, the farmers were very poor and couldn't afford medical care," she says. "We would take medical students into the country and teach them to pick special plants in the mountains and make herbal formulas. Along with the herbal medicine, we would also teach them how to use hands and needles to relieve pain and treat illnesses at a low cost. Some of my students are now doctors practicing conventional medicine in the United States," she adds proudly. "But they also know the Chinese ways."

Putting It All Together

"Bryan called Dr. Yang the day of the accident, and she came right to the hospital," says Jackie. Here, Dr. Yang takes up the story:

"When I saw Jackie, she was paralyzed from the neck down, no sensation," says Dr. Yang. "She was crying. She had two little boys. I felt so sorry for her. She said to me, 'I just want to see you.' I answered, 'I hope you can fight this and be well.' The whole family was in shock." Dr. Yang went to the hospital almost every day to massage Jackie's arms and legs. "From the Chinese medicine perspective, the meridians (invisible pathways) that carry the qi (life force or energy) were completely blocked by the injury," explains Dr. Yang. "The blood flow was blocked as well. Acupressure massage at the site of the injury and throughout the body helps to move the blood and qi, which helps with circulation and may help with the paralysis as well. This doesn't happen quickly, it takes time." At the same time, Jackie's doctors were also giving her high doses of cortisone to reduce the inflammation.

Using acupuncture points on the body, Dr. Yang worked to release some of the muscles that were in spasm. "Each day, the joints and muscles would get looser and have more range of motion," says Jackie. "While I was still in the hospital, I slowly began to get some control over these muscles and be able to move my arms and hands slightly." Dr. Yang continued to see Jackie several times a week while she was in the rehabilitation hospital, and continues to give her weekly massages at her home to this day. She will not accept any payment from the family. "I do this as a friend," she says.

After Jackie had been in the rehabilitation hospital for a month, she asked for acupuncture. "By that time I had been on the board of the New England School of Acupuncture for four years and was becoming convinced that qi is an energy or life force that exists and is related to our health," she says. "I dislike the arrogance of some Western medical doctors who disparage what they do not know." The rehabilitation doctor agreed that an acupuncturist could come to the hospital and treat Jackie, as long as it was not on or near the spinal cord.

"So every week, someone came to do acupuncture, and after each treatment, I could move a muscle I hadn't moved before, or extend my arm or hand a little further. He also gave me some herbs, and I am convinced without a doubt that the combination helped my recovery. I didn't really care why it worked, although as a scientist I am still curious; all I cared about at the time were the results. And they were convincing." (Please see the research section in this chapter for studies on acupuncture in the treatment of spinal cord injury and stroke.)

Through her experiences Jackie began to draw some conclusions about the differences between Chinese and conventional doctors. "Chinese doctors will spend ten minutes looking into your eyes and holding both of your wrists," she says. "Through their observation and the deep pulses they are feeling they can truly understand what is going on inside your body. Most of the conventional doctors who treated me rarely looked me in the eye and tended to see me as a collection of symptoms, rather than a whole person. Since then, I have only chosen doctors who are open-minded to the connection between mind, spirit and body, and who practice a more holistic form of medicine." For three years after her accident, Jackie also continued regular acupuncture treatments.

Spinal Cord Injury and Stroke: What's the Evidence?

In the United States, approximately 200,000 persons are now permanently confined to wheelchairs because of spinal cord injury. Each year, some 10,000 more people are injured, suffering paralysis and loss of sensation. Two-thirds of these people are under thirty years of age. The required specialized care costs approximately $5 billion each year in the United States (NIH report: National Institute of Neurological Disorders and Stroke, 1992).

Starting acupuncture treatments as soon as the injury occurs makes a difference

Studies have shown that both needle acupuncture and "laser" acupuncture (using beams of laser light) were beneficial in the treatment of both spinal cord injury and stroke, especially if the treatment is begun soon after the injury, even during the acute phase of spinal cord shock, to reduce the development of muscle spasms. These findings have been reported by neurology researcher and acupuncture specialist Margaret Naeser, Ph.D., Lic.Ac., Dipl.Ac., of the Department of Neurology, Boston University School of Medicine. Although Dr. Naeser is a licensed acupuncturist, she devotes most of her time now to research, writing and brain imaging for stroke patients.

Naeser highlights three studies performed in China before 1997, where acupuncture was successfully used to reduce the symptom severity in patients with spinal cord injury—although none had control groups. Overall, 340 out of 360 cases, or 94.4 percent, had an outcome level of beneficial progress, including reduction in muscle spasms, some increased level of sensation, and improved bladder and bowel function.

The authors recommend that acupuncture be initiated as soon as possible after spinal cord injury and that treatments continue for two to three or even five years. Electroacupuncture along the bladder meridian (paravertebral) area is especially recommended. Laser acupuncture can also be applied in a home treatment program to help reduce muscle spasms in the hands and feet. (Please see Appendix II for Web sites and other information about laser acupuncture.)

Exercise helps in rehabilitation of spinal cord injury

Thirteen volunteers with thoracic spinal cord injuries participated in a sixteen-week exercise rehabilitation program including mobility, strength, coordination, aerobic resistance and relaxation activities. Patients showed a significant and positive increase in several parameters measuring strength and "wheelchair skills."

Spinal cord injury patients rate massage best for chronic pain

This study surveyed seventy-seven people with spinal cord injury to find out which complementary and alternative medicine (CAM) treatments they used for chronic pain. The most common reason for choosing CAM treatments was dissatisfaction with conventional treatment. Acupuncture was the most frequently used modality, followed by massage, chiropractic manipulation and herbal medicine. Acupuncture was rated lowest for pain relief, and massage highest. The authors recommend more research and awareness of massage techniques.

The importance of nutrition, exercise and general health in recovery from SCI

Researchers from the Department of Rehabilitative Medicine of the University of Washington argue that neurologic recovery in spinal cord injury patients is facilitated by improving nutrition and general health, and by coordinating active exercise and functional training to enhance synapse growth in nerve cells, as well as motor learning (synapses are connections between nerve cells). This helps reverse muscle atrophy and control interfering muscle spasticity. They also advise monitoring for declining function both initially and later in life, diagnosing neurological decline promptly and accurately and using appropriate interventions.

References (spinal cord injury and stroke)

Duran, F. S., et al. "Effects of an Exercise Program on the Rehabilitation of Patients with Spinal Cord Injury." *Archives of Physical Medicine and Rehabilitation* 82, no. 10 (2001): 1349–54.

Gao, X. P. "Acupuncture for Traumatic Paraplegia." *International Journal of Chinese Medicine* 1, no. 2 (1984) :43–47.

Gao, X. P., et al. "Acupuncture Treatment of Complete Traumatic Paraplegia—Analysis of 261 Cases." *Journal of Traditional Chinese Medicine* 16, no. 2 (1996): 134–137.

Little, J. W., et al. "Neurologic Recovery and Neurologic Decline after Spinal Cord Injury." *Physical Medicine and Rehabilitation Clinics of North America* 111, no. 1 (2000): 73–89.

Nayak, S., et al. "The Use of Complementary and Alternative Therapies for Chronic Pain Following Spinal Cord Injury: A Pilot Survey." *Journal of Spinal Cord Medicine* 24 (Spring), no. 1 (2001): 54–62.

NIH Report: "Progress and Promise: A Status Report on the NINDS Implementation Plan for the Decade of the Brain." The National Advisory Neurological Disorders and Stroke Council, National Institute of Neurological Disorders and Stroke, National Institutes of Health, December 1992.

Wang, H. J. "A Survey of the Treatment of Traumatic Paraplegia by Traditional Chinese Medicine." *Journal of Chinese Medicine* 12, no. 4 (1992): 296–303.

The Next Phase: Getting the Legs Moving Again

The positive results from her massage and acupuncture treatments spurred Jackie to take on the battle of walking. "When they cut off my coverage for physical therapy because they thought I'd never walk again, my first reaction was despair," says Jackie. "Who would teach me to walk? My family? It was unthinkable that I would not walk." At first she tried to walk on her own, stiffly moving her legs while holding onto her walker and wearing the heavy leg braces that the rehabilitation hospital had sent home with her. "But I was doing everything wrong," she says. "I would go totally rigid, tightening the wrong muscles just to get my legs to work. I was desperate. To make matters even worse, my hairdresser's shop was too small for a wheelchair!"

Jackie then tried hiring people to come over and help her walk by supporting her. "This didn't work either, because these people were not trained," says Jackie. "Then I finally had an idea: Why not a professional trainer?" And this is when Susan Himmelman, another significant part of the recovery process, entered Jackie's life.

As a physical education teacher and coach turned personal trainer, Susan E. Himmelman, M.S., knows how to help people move. When Jackie contacted her, she was intrigued. "I had taught motor skills to thousands of children," says

Susan. "But I had never worked with someone who had been totally paralyzed from a spinal cord injury. It would be a challenge."

Susan started working with Jackie in September 1999. "When I met Jackie, she could not even stand for a second on her own. Her hands were curled up like claws. She had no balance and, because of all the time in a wheelchair, her hip, thigh and calf muscles had become so short from the constant sitting that she could not stand upright even with support. The range of motion in her ankles had decreased so much that she had difficulty getting her heels onto the floor when she tried to stand up."

Susan was undaunted. "I saw these first as mechanical problems that could be corrected by stretching, massage and strengthening," she says. "At the same time, we would work on re-educating healthy nerve cells in the brain and spinal cord to send the right messages to those muscles. I saw no reason why I could not teach her how to walk again. Perhaps I didn't know enough to get discouraged or quit."

For Jackie, Susan's optimism was a bright source of hope. "The first thing she did was to get rid of the braces because they were turning my legs into pendulums," says Jackie. "She said, 'You're not going to walk in a handicapped way. You're going to walk normally using normal muscle movements.' Every time I got discouraged, she would say, 'You can do this,' and she was usually right. One of my biggest goals was to get up to a room on the third floor that I was in the process of fixing up as an office before my accident. Susan put banisters on both sides of the staircase—she is also a carpenter—and taught me to use them. As soon as I could climb the stairs, we painted the room together."

As a first step, Susan began with massage and stretching to restore the range of motion to Jackie's ankles, knees and hips as well as to her hands. "Muscles have a protective 'spindle reflex' which prevents them from stretching more than they can," says Susan. "Jackie's muscles had been so tightened and shortened by the wheelchair that when I tried to assist her to stand upright as she held the walker, her legs would collapse, fold up like rulers. In the same way, whenever we tried to get her ankle to bend, the leg would go shooting straight out. These are both examples of spindle reflexes. So before we could work on movement, we had to stretch those muscles."

So each session began with massage. "Massage relaxes muscle tension, brings warmth and circulation to the area and makes joints less stiff by increasing their pliability," says Susan. "Within minutes, I could feel Jackie's muscles release. Then we could begin to work on gaining access to various muscle groups."

Susan decided that the best way to help Jackie learn to walk was to "reprogram" her spinal cord. "My own theory is to think of the spinal cord as a computer, separate from the brain," says Susan. "We move and keep our balance because instantaneous messages are constantly being sent back and forth between our muscles and the spinal cord. These are usually outside of our conscious mind. If we lose our balance, for example, our mind does not have time to tell us to lean in a certain direction; rather, an automatic correction is sent through the spinal cord to the muscles that need to be activated. But what happens if the muscle memory of how to do things is erased by a traumatic injury? As I thought about this, I kept going back to how a baby learns to walk and decided to try to replicate that. After all, babies are born without complex movement patterns."

So in the beginning, after massage, Susan had Jackie sit on the floor and practice supporting herself using her spinal muscles. Then Susan would sit in front of her and toss her a ball to catch. "Jackie had the strength to sit up on her own, but she needed to practice tapping into it, the same way a baby practices sitting up over and over again," says Susan. "Once she could do that, tossing a ball back and forth taught her to maintain her balance by adjusting changes to her center of gravity. She needed to re-educate her spinal cord to make constant, instant calculations and adjustments so she wouldn't fall over. Effortless movement happens when the spinal cord can send the correct nerve impulses to the correct muscles at the correct time."

When Jackie had her balance sitting, they moved to standing, and finally walking with support. At each step, Susan would figure out how to reprogram Jackie's muscles to perform normally, sometimes "tricking" the body by interfering with a movement pattern that did not work. For example, when Jackie had problems getting out of the wheelchair and standing upright because her knees kept coming together—the way they do when you sit in a wheelchair—Susan put a Styrofoam block between her knees to interrupt the nerve/muscle pattern, freeing Jackie to use her leg strength to stand up straight, ready for walking.

"I don't think of Jackie as a handicapped person," explains Susan. "I think of her as a person who needs to be taught motor skills. My job is to find the nerve pathway that the brain and spinal cord use to send messages to the muscles—and make sure that the correct messages get sent, either by blocking the wrong messages or by creating new ones. Then we enhance the 'motor memory' through constant repetition—the way a baby does—until the correct nerve pattern is established." In Susan's opinion, the leg braces were shortcuts, and not very effective ones. "It seems to me, if you're going to teach a motor skill, you need to use the proper biomechanics. And with heavy braces holding the legs rigid, the muscles will never learn on their own."

Susan's method is working. Lately, Jackie has begun to dispense with the two canes and walk holding onto Susan's hands. Her current distance is a quarter of a mile, but she expects that to increase (a far cry from the ten-foot "walker shuffle" that her doctors predicted would be her limit). Twice a week, Susan and Jackie go to the park, where Jackie stands on her own in front of her walker, a bench behind her, and plays catch with Susan. "Throwing a ball and batting helps Jackie deal with weight shifts," says Susan. "As soon as you reach out to throw or catch a ball, or swing a bat, your center of gravity shifts. This is teaching her to make those instant balance adjustments that she will need when she no longer needs the walker or canes—much more interesting than a boring balance drill! And having to swing a bat while watching the ball keeps her from looking down at her feet all the time."

It has been five years since that Sunday in February when Jackie's life changed forever. She is back at work now three days a week, typing with two fingers. She cooks, drives—with her walker or wheelchair in the car—and she is trying to play the piano again. "I hate relying on other people," says Jackie, "but I still need help with carrying heavy things, although I used to be very strong." She and her family are even planning to travel again, something she has always loved. "My stepdaughter is getting married in London next year, so I am practicing the skills I will need to walk down the aisle of the plane and use the bathroom."

Now Jackie has a new goal. Susan Himmelman was recently diagnosed with breast cancer and is undergoing treatment. "I am planning to walk in her honor during next year's Walk for Breast Cancer," says Jackie. "I expect to be up to a mile or two by then."

A HORIZON OF HOPE: SHEDDING LIGHT ON THE STEM CELL

Rudolf Jaenisch, M.D., is known throughout the scientific world as one of the founders of transgenic science. To Jacqueline Miller and Bryan Roberts, he is also a very good friend. Jaenisch was the first scientist to insert "foreign" (meaning from another species, such as human or bacterial) DNA into a laboratory mouse. These transgenic mice are now being used in laboratories throughout the world in the molecular study of human disease. Jaenisch's work is one of the foundations of therapeutic stem cell and cloning research into new treatments for cancer and neurological diseases.

While Jaenisch's international awards, symposia and groundbreaking publications are noteworthy, Jackie Miller values most the hours that he spent with her in the hospital after her accident. (Please see related story in this chapter.) "Rudolf would come to see me before I could move anything and just talk to me about the future of stem cell research," Jackie remembers. "The details didn't really matter to me at the time, but the message was one of hope as I lay unmoving and in despair. He was telling me about a world where one day people like me might be able to move again. Somehow, he knew that I needed something to hold onto, to give me the strength to fight back and not just give up."

Although Jaenisch cautions that there is not yet any concrete evidence that stem cells will be used in the near future to regenerate injured spinal cords, he does point to some hopeful clinical data in Parkinson's research. "When fetal brain cells are transplanted into patients with Parkinson's disease (a condition in which brain cells degenerate and die, causing loss of muscle control throughout the body), they seem to generate new, healthy brain cells and symptoms improve," he says. "The problem is, there is not enough of a supply of these cells."

(continued)

In Jaenisch's laboratory at MIT's Whitehead Institute, where he is also professor of biology, a dozen postdoctoral researchers and several students are working to find another way. "In the laboratory, we have taken skin cells from a sick animal, removed the nucleus (which contains all of the body's genetic "instructions") and transplanted it into an unfertilized egg cell from the same species in which the nucleus has already been removed," he explains. "This is how we create an embryonic stem cell, which is capable of growing into any type of cell the body needs. We bathe these stem cells with specific growth factor solutions, depending on whether we would like them to become brain cells, heart cells, liver or kidney cells, and when they multiply sufficiently, we inject them into the bloodstream of the diseased animal. There seems to be some evidence that this might work to cure disease, perhaps liver disease, anemia or diabetes (both types) for example, but much more research is needed."

Across the river from the Whitehead Institute, the multidisciplinary Tissue Engineering Team at Boston's Children's Hospital is using similar techniques to grow living tissue in the laboratory—but not just any tissue. The goal is to design individualized tissue and organs for particular patients, grown from embryonic stem cells created from their own cells to meet the specific medical needs of their bodies. The clinical applications are numerous, and include replacement heart valves, bladders and kidneys; cartilage for tracheas and esophagi and to replace joints eroded by arthritis; fat tissue to provide contours of the face or breast in plastic surgery; smooth muscle and bone to heal orthopedic deterioration or injury; cells of the inner ear to restore hearing; and brain and nerve cells to treat neurological problems such as stroke and spinal cord injury. A fully "engineered" trachea has already been successfully transplanted into large animal models, and human clinical trials are not too far away, according to surgeon and researcher Dario Fauza, M.D., F.R.C.S., a member of the Tissue Engineering Team.

For people like Jackie Miller with spinal cord injury, or for stroke patients, the hope is that this stem cell/cloning technique might be used one day to generate healthy nerve cells to replace those that have been damaged or destroyed, says Jaenisch. He has testified before Congress on the subject and recently spoke on a panel that included the actor Christopher Reeve, who was paralyzed in a riding accident. "Many people believe this is a possibility, but we do not have evidence yet," says Jaenisch. "We need to do more work."

(continued)

In March 2002, almost exactly five years after Jacqueline Miller fell and injured her spinal cord, she and Bryan were invited to a dinner at the Whitehead Institute honoring Jaenisch. The dining room was down a long hallway from the front door.

Jackie had decided to leave her wheelchair at home. She had walked, using her walker, from the car to the main lobby, where someone offered her a wheelchair to get down the hallway into the dining room. She demurred, saying, "I'll walk." And while all of the guests assembled at the dining tables, she grasped her walker and started down the hallway on foot. It took about ten minutes of hard concentration, but her feet and legs moved in even steps, her posture was upright, her head high and her balance firm. When she reached her seat at Jaenisch's table, everyone congratulated her. After the dinner, when someone asked why she had not used the wheelchair, she said, "I wanted to walk in Rudolf's honor."

✦ ✦ ✦ ✦

Coming Down on the Side of Hope and Possibility

Psychiatrist James S. Gordon, M.D., was running a mind/body workshop in a refugee camp for Kosovo Albanians in Macedonia. Two hundred refugees had assembled in a large open area hoping for some relief from the devastating emotional trauma of witnessing their loved ones killed and their homes destroyed in the war. About forty-five minutes into the session, when Gordon was talking about guided imagery and meditation as ways to cope with grief, one man raised his hand.

"Every time I close my eyes to try the meditation," the man said, "I see the same thing: twenty-one members of my family being massacred before my eyes. How can I get rid of this image?"

Remembering the incident, Gordon says, "I was floored. I did not have an answer. All I could say to him was, 'I appreciate your courage in talking about your pain and your willingness to try some of these mind/body techniques. I don't know how I can be helpful to you except to continue what we are doing.'" Gordon then led the group through several exercises that he had used in visits to more than a dozen refugee camps and ravaged villages in war-torn areas of the world, including Bosnia-Herzogovina, Kosovo and Mozambique. His mission: to help heal the psychological wounds that remain when the violence finally stops: to help terrified, traumatized children and the adults who suffer from the rage, grief, loss and despair that together have been called posttraumatic stress disorder. For all ages, the toll is both emotional and physical. The continuing stress caused by flashbacks and nightmares often leads to chronic illnesses, insomnia, rapid heartbeat and physical pain.

After speaking with the refugee from Kosovo, Gordon continued his program that day, including a period of dancing and shaking to various forms of music and drumming. "Moving their bodies to music often helps people unlock the sadness and lets them fully experience their grief," says Gordon. "Sometimes this can be freeing." At the end of the program, which also included guided meditation and visualization, breathing exercises and other relaxation and stress reduction techniques, the man came up to Gordon and asked if he could have his picture taken with him. "Of course," said Gordon, "but why?" The man smiled as he answered: "For two minutes during the dancing and shaking, I did not have the image of the massacre in my mind. Now I know that it is possible for me to go on living."

James Gordon started as a conventional physician, training in psychiatry at the Harvard Medical School. But an internship in a San Francisco youth health care center during the 1960s, as well as his own experience recovering from a back injury by using acupuncture and nutrition launched him on a more alternative path. Later, while working for the National Institute of Mental Health, he started the nation's first runaway teen program. Appointed by President Carter as part of a research team, he spent two months studying healing traditions in India and then became the first chair of the Advisory Council of the National Institutes of Health (NIH) Office of Alternative Medicine. From there, he was appointed by President Clinton to head the White House Advisory Commission on Complementary and Alternative Medicine.

Gordon now teaches at the Georgetown University School of Medicine and is founder and director of the Center for Mind-Body Medicine in Washington, D.C., whose board members include Dean Ornish, M.D., Jon Kabat-Zinn, Ph.D., and Joan Borysenko, Ph.D. He is the author of several books, including *Manifesto for a New Medicine: Your Guide to Healing Partnerships and the Wise Use of Alternative Therapies*. He describes himself as "a bridge between the modern medical establishment and the new medicine."

A Doorway to Compassion

"Psychological trauma is everywhere. We have all been traumatized, particularly after September 11," says Gordon. "For the past twenty-five years I have worked with people in other countries who have been politically tortured, who have lost family members, who have been raped and beaten, compounding their psychological trauma with physical injury. In our work, we teach health professionals in the areas of violence and conflict to provide mind/body and stress reduction services to people where they live." During the course of a dozen visits to Kosovo, for example, Gordon and his team have trained almost all of the mental health-care workers and many other physicians, along with rural teachers, in the use of mind/body medicine for reducing the effects of psychological trauma.

In Washington, Gordon's Center offers training for health professionals as well as patients in small group sessions. "In one of our patient groups, for example, we might have an elderly person who is depressed, a student suffering from gastrointestinal problems brought on by stress, and people of any age with cancer or heart disease," says Gordon. "They learn from and help each other."

Gordon has found that such skills as meditation, guided imagery, self-hypnosis, biofeedback, breath work, movement, journal writing, drawing and self-awareness training can contribute to emotional and physical health. "We have a great and largely untapped capacity to improve our own health," he says. "By teaching people the biology of stress and giving them simple techniques to affect their biology and physiology we can help them take control of their own health." In 1996, the Center launched an annual conference for doctors, patients and health professionals called Comprehensive Cancer Care:

Integrating Complementary and Alternative Therapies, co-sponsored by the National Center for Complementary and Alternative Medicine and the National Cancer Institute as well as private and nonprofit institutions. By the third year, more than a thousand people were attending the conference.

Since September 11, Gordon and his staff have been working in New York with firefighters, survivors from the buildings and bereaved family members. "We now know what the rest of the world experiences," he says. "The emotional and physical reactions to September 11 are not a disease. They are natural reactions to an overwhelming, threatening and disorganizing situation. I spoke with people who used to have a sense that there were rules, and if you followed them you would be okay. Now, the rules are gone, and we have learned how vulnerable we are, and we are deeply shaken."

Gordon draws parallels between national trauma and personal trauma. "The feelings of shock, vulnerability and a sudden change in the rules of life are similar when people are given a life-threatening diagnosis or have a serious injury," he says. "In both cases, however, there are potentials for positive experiences if we can enlarge our feelings to include compassion for ourselves and for others. After September 11, we no longer have a national sense of exemption from the horrors and misery that befall the rest of the world, and perhaps this can open the doorway to a healing compassion."

For people dealing with serious illness, the opportunity can also include a personal transformation, says Gordon. "If you have cancer or another life-threatening illness, or have to come back from a debilitating injury, heart attack or stroke, you can use this time to find people in your life who can be healing partners, and to discover who you are, what is important to you and what is the meaning of your life on this planet." (Please see box for Gordon's suggestions of ways to cope with serious physical challenges.)

✓ TAKE ACTION ✓

What you can do when the rules of life suddenly change: Guidance from experience and research

A frightening medical diagnosis or traumatic injury can make you feel suddenly vulnerable. James Gordon, M.D., has a few suggestions for ways to manage your stress and take control of your health.

1. Nothing anyone tells you about your condition is 100 percent true. Diagnoses are fallible and prognoses rely on statistics. You are unique, and the way you will react to disease and treatment is also unique.
2. Because of this, try to come down on the side of hope and what is possible.
3. Put together a healing team from the professionals you know, your friends and your family. Ask yourself, "Whom do I want around me? Who is in my life, and what do they have to offer me?"
4. Draw a picture of yourself and place these people in the picture. Drawing gets you out of your conscious, rational mind and allows you to access your intuition.
5. Understand that no matter what your situation, you always have the power to make a difference, even if only in your attitude. Try a variety of different approaches to managing anxiety, fear, frustration or despair. Choices might include meditation, guided imagery, self-hypnosis, biofeedback, breath work, movement (dancing or shaking to music or tribal drumming), playing a musical instrument, journal writing, drawing and self-awareness training. Sometimes it is a healing experience to find others who are suffering (perhaps more than you are) and to offer support and comfort to them.

Stress Reduction Techniques: What's the Evidence?

Studies show that people who believe they are healthier have lower stress and better physical outcomes. Research has also shown that relaxation training, guided imagery, and patients' perceptions of their quality of life can benefit the health outcomes and treatment reactions of cancer patients. And if you needed more evidence that stress is bad for you, an animal study found that stress stimulated tumor growth. (See "References" in this section.)

References

Bridge, L. R., et al. "Relaxation and Imagery in the Treatment of Breast Cancer." *British Medical Journal* 297 (198): 1169–72.

Buccheri, G. F., et al. "The Patient's Perception of His Own Quality of Life Might Have an Adjunctive Prognostic Significance in Lung Cancer." *Lung Cancer* 12, no. 1–2 (1995): 45–58.

Ganz, P. A., et al. "Quality of Life Assessment: An Independent Prognostic Variable for Survival in Lung Cancer." *Cancer* 67, no. 3 (1991): 131–135.

Gordon, J. S. *Manifesto for a New Medicine: Your Guide to Healing Partnerships and the Wise Use of Alternative Therapies.* Cambridge, MA: Perseus, 1996.

Gordon, J. S. and S. Curtin. *Comprehensive Cancer Care.* Cambridge, MA: Perseus, 2000.

Kobassa, S. C. "Commitment and Coping in Stress Resistance Among Lawyers." *Journal of Personality and Social Psychology* 37 (1982): 1–11.

Lyles, J. N., et al. "Efficacy of Relaxation Training and Guided Imagery in Reducing the Aversiveness of Cancer Chemotherapy." *Journal of Consulting and Clinical Psychology* 50, no. 4 (1982): 509–524.

Sapolsky, R. M., et al. "Vulnerability to Stress-Induced Tumor Growth Increases with Age in Rats: Role of Glucocorticoids." *Endocrinology* 117, no. 2 (1985): 662–666.

❖ ❖ ❖ ❖

Forgiveness for Health

Many years ago, someone hurt Frederic Luskin, Ph.D. "I just couldn't get over what this friend had done," says Luskin. "Every time I thought about it, I experienced the anger and resentment all over again, including the physical symptoms that these negative emotions release. This persisted long after I had lost contact with this person. After several years of this, I suddenly realized that the person who had hurt me was having a fine life, while I was still suffering over an incident that was long in the past. Why was I doing this to myself?"

Thus was born the Stanford University Forgiveness Project, one of the largest and most important studies of forgiveness ever conducted. Luskin, whose degree is in counseling and health psychology, developed a training program in forgiveness as part of his doctoral dissertation, and then conducted clinical research studies to see if it worked. After his initial research in 1996 showed that people could learn to forgive and that forgiveness was significantly correlated with improvements in health, Luskin and his colleagues at Stanford invited two groups of bereaved families from Northern Ireland to participate in the Forgiveness Project. "We felt that this was the ultimate test," he says. "There is perhaps no worse trauma than the loss of a child, a parent or another loved one to violence." His research corroborated the findings of previous studies of forgiveness, finding that people who were able to come to peace with their loss and grief had measurable health benefits.

In his book, *Forgive for Good*, Luskin describes the benefits that participants reported, which include fewer health problems, less stress, fewer physical symptoms of stress, and improvements in psychological and emotional well-being, even after devastating losses. Even *thinking* about forgiveness can make a difference, he writes: "People who imagine forgiving their offender note immediate improvement in their cardiovascular, muscular, and nervous systems."

The negative health effects of not forgiving are costly, writes Luskin: "Failure to forgive may be more important than hostility as a risk factor for heart disease. People who blame other people for their troubles have higher incidences of illnesses such as cardiovascular disease and cancers. People who imagine not forgiving someone show negative changes in blood pressure, muscle tension, and immune response."

Forgiveness, according to Luskin, does not mean condoning or forgetting what was done to you. "Forgiveness is the feeling of peace that merges as you take your hurt less personally, take responsibility for how you feel, and become a hero instead of a victim in the story you tell." In an interview, Luskin elaborates. "Forgiveness gives you access to more positive experiences," he says. "If you think of yourself as a victim, it will take your attention away from the beauty and love around you, and this is not good for your health. Each moment of appreciation, wonder and love helps to enhance your immune system and leads to improvements in your cardiovascular health."

Other health professionals support this view. Dean Ornish, M.D., for example, one of the first to prove that changes in lifestyle and nutrition can reverse cardiovascular disease, wrote a book called *Love and Survival*. In this book, he describes the powers of love and intimacy to improve physical health, pointing out that "emotional and spiritual" heart disease —caused by loneliness, isolation, alienation and depression—can be far more damaging to health than physical heart disease.

What happens when you cannot forgive? "One of the central mediating factors of the emotions relating to health is the sense of control and confidence in the present," says Luskin. "Every time you remind yourself of the experience that caused you pain, even if it happened years ago, your body responds by releasing stress hormones. One of the effects of these hormones—which activate our ancient 'fight-or-flight' response, is a change in the metabolism of fat in your body. The liver produces extra cholesterol, which is sent up to your heart to protect you from bleeding in case of attack. Your heart rate speeds up and blood is directed away from the brain and into the limbs, in case quick action is needed. Every time you activate this response system, there is a physical cost to your health."

People who completed the forgiveness training experienced "reduced anger, reduced depression, reduced symptoms of stress and greater hope and vitality," says Luskin. And according to questionnaires sent to participants months afterward, these benefits persisted. "People have the capacity to forgive, but they are not taught how," says Luskin. "In our culture, we are terrific at teaching anger, judgmental behavior and creating hostility. We are not as terrific at taking ourselves out of the center of the universe, not so terrific at hope, forgiveness or positive emotions."

These skills are particularly important as people age, says Luskin. "I see two types of older people in my training programs," he says. "One group realizes that life is short and they don't want to waste whatever time they have left in anger and negative emotions. These people are resilient and generally happy. Other people are more beaten down by life. They feel they have experienced too many insults, slights and disappointments and they are unhappy."

Luskin is now in the pilot stages of a project designed specifically for older people. "We have applied for a government grant to do an in-depth evaluation on the physical and emotional effects of forgiveness in older people," he says. "We're trying to answer the question, 'What helps people enjoy the life they have, despite the inevitable declines of aging?' It is almost easier to help people live longer than it is to help them enjoy, appreciate and feel gratitude for their lives." (Please see also chapter 11, "Aging Well.")

Luskin says he was surprised at the data that emerged from the Northern Ireland study. "We saw a 35 percent decrease in the physical symptoms of stress and a similar increase in people's feelings of physical vitality," he says. "You don't want to ever forget a tragic event in your life. But you do want to remember it through a different lens—not the lens that 'my life was ruined by the loss of my loved one,' because then the murderers will have killed two people instead of one. Rather, you want to remember through the lens of peace and appreciation of the present moment. Forgiveness does not change the past, but it can change the present. If you can do this for two minutes this week, perhaps you can do it for three minutes next week. After all, why should misery be more real than happiness?"

A Special Note About September 11

The terrorist attacks in the United States happened ten days before Luskin's manuscript was scheduled to go to the publisher. He added a postscript to readers before he sent it, describing his feelings of sadness and grief and examining the balance between forgiveness and vengeance. He writes that our first response must be to come to terms with what has happened, with an appreciation for "the collective outpouring of grief and support." Only then, he notes, can we begin to think about forgiveness. "With time, and once our safety has been ensured, each of us will be left with questions of forgiveness." In those early days after the attacks, Luskin urged that we "make peace wherever possible with family, friends and coworkers. In this time of great tragedy it is important for our health and happiness to heal the wounds of old. Working together and needing each other is crucial during this difficult time."

DR. LUSKIN'S NINE STEPS TO FORGIVENESS

In his book, *Forgive for Good,* Frederic Luskin, Ph.D., outlines a program to achieve peace and forgiveness. He explores each of these steps in detail and gives suggestions for how to achieve them.

1. Know exactly how you feel about what happened and be able to articulate what about the situation is not okay. Then, tell a couple of trusted people about your experience.
2. Make a commitment to yourself to do what you have to do to feel better. Forgiveness is for you and not for anyone else.
3. Forgiveness does not necessarily mean reconciliation with the person who upset you, or condoning their action. What you are after is peace. Forgiveness can be defined as the "peace and understanding that come from blaming that which has hurt you less, taking the life experience less personally, and changing your grievance story."
4. Get the right perspective on what is happening. Recognize that your primary distress is coming from the hurt feelings, thoughts and physical upset you are suffering now, not what offended you or hurt you two minutes—or ten years—ago.
5. At the moment you feel upset practice a simple stress management technique to soothe your body's "flight or fight" response.
6. Give up expecting things from other people, or your life, that they do not choose to give you. Recognize the "unenforceable rules" you have for your health or how you or other people must behave. Remind yourself that you can hope for health, love, friendship and prosperity and work hard to get them.
7. Put your energy into looking for another way to get your positive goals met than through the experience that has hurt you. Instead of mentally replaying your hurt seek out new ways to get what you want.
8. Remember that a life well lived is your best revenge. Instead of focusing on your wounded feelings, and thereby giving the person who caused you pain power over you, learn to look for the love, beauty and kindness around you.
9. Amend your grievance story to remind you of the heroic choice to forgive.[1]

---

[1] F. Luskin, *Forgive for Good* (New York: HarperCollins, 2002), 211.

Forgiveness: What's the Evidence?

In his book, *Forgive for Good,* Frederic Luskin, Ph.D., reviews scientific research—his own as well as others—demonstrating that forgiveness "helps people heal in physical, mental and emotional ways." Studies have shown, for example, that even thinking about something that makes you angry can suppress heart rate variability, which is a predictor of who will survive heart disease. Luskin also cites research showing that higher levels of hope help people deal successfully with pain and some forms of illness, as well as studies linking depression with greater risk of heart disease and stroke. On the positive side, learning to forgive might help prevent heart disease in middle-aged people, according to a study at the University of Wisconsin.

Luskin's own studies of people from Northern Ireland showed marked improvements in physical health among participants in the Forgiveness Project.

It seems safe to conclude that forgiveness, appreciation and love are better for your health than anger, resentment and harboring grudges.

References

Ferketich, A., et al. "Depression as an Antecedent to Heart Disease Among Women and Men in the NHANES I Study." *Archives of Internal Medicine* 160, no. 9 (2000).

Jonas, B. S. "Symptoms of Depression as a Prospective Risk Factor for Stroke." *Psychosomatic Medicine* 62, no. 4 (2000): 563–571.

Luskin, F. M. "A Review of the Effect of Spiritual and Religious Factors on Mortality and Morbidity with a Focus on Cardiovascular and Pulmonary Disease." *Journal of Cardiopulmonary Rehabilitation* 20, no. 1 (2000): 8–15.

Luskin, F. *Forgive for Good.* New York: HarperCollins, 2002.

Luskin, F. M. "The Effect of Forgiveness Training on Psychosocial Factors in College Age Adults." Unpublished Dissertation: Stanford University, 1999.

Ornish, D. *Love & Survival: 8 Pathways to Intimacy and Health.* New York: HarperCollins, 1998.

Sarinopoulos, S. "Forgiveness and Physical Health: A Doctoral Dissertation Summary." *World of Forgiveness* 3, no. 2 (2000): 16–18.

Van Oyen, C., et al. "Granting Forgiveness or Harboring Grudges: Implications for Emotions, Physiology and Health." *Psychological Science* 12 (2001): 117–123.

Tiller, W., et al. "Toward Cardiac Coherence: A New Non-Invasive Measure of Autonomic System Order." *Alternative Therapies in Health and Medicine* 2 (1996): 52–65.

Williams, R. and V. Williams. *Anger Kills: Seventeen Strategies for Controlling the Hostility that Can Harm Your Health*. New York: Random House, 1993.

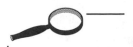

A Closer Look at Energy Healing, Spirituality and Therapeutic Touch

On one wall of Betty Solbjor's living room are two color photographs. They show different views of a woman of small stature whose entire body bulges with unusually large, powerful muscles. In both photos, she is wearing only a scanty bathing suit and posing to show off her muscles to best advantage. "This was during the body-building phase of my life," explains Betty with a smile. She had been a long-distance runner in her thirties, but had to give it up because of problems with her knees. "Bodybuilding kept me in shape, and I became quite serious about it for a time." Now fifty-one, Betty no longer has the bulging muscles, but with her bouncy haircut, ruddy complexion and vigorous body, she looks as if she just got off the ski slopes (her favorite sport now). The only reminders of her body-building days are the photos and a shelf full of trophies.

"I've always been healthy and attuned to my body," she says. So it came as quite a shock when she was diagnosed with thyroid cancer a few years ago. "I had been moving in a more contemplative direction and had been doing meditation and other spiritual practices," says Betty. She had heard about Reiki (a form of spiritual healing) and was about to start lessons when she had her annual physical. The doctor found a suspicious lump in Betty's neck and ordered an ultrasound and biopsy. The tests were inconclusive.

"They decided to take out that side of the thyroid as a precaution," says Betty. "The surgery was scheduled for mid-January, several weeks away." In the meantime, Betty had begun her Reiki lessons, and was becoming fascinated with the practice. "*Rei* means 'universal consciousness' and *ki* is like the Chinese qi, meaning life force,'" she explains. "So Reiki is the universally guided life force energy." Reiki practitioners learn to channel this universal life force, which is believed to exist in unlimited supply, into their own bodies, through the crown of the head. They then can transmit the energy through their hands to others, by gentle touch. Reiki sessions are done while fully clothed, lying on a table, and the sensation is a subtle feeling of relaxation and warmth throughout the body. One cancer patient described the feeling as "powerfully healing and peaceful. I really felt as if something wonderful were happening inside my body."

Reiki is one spiritual healing practice that can be done by the patient, without the intervention of a practitioner. In preparation for her surgery, for example, Betty Solbjor and her husband—to whom she had taught the technique—used their hands to direct Reiki energy into the lump in her neck. "We did it every day," says Betty. "By the time of the surgery several weeks later, we could see that the lump seemed to have gotten smaller by approximately 30 percent." The surgery found a Stage 1 malignancy, meaning the cancer was very small and had not spread outside the gland, and the rest of the thyroid was removed a week later, just to make sure. "My husband continued to do Reiki over my thyroid area every day, including in the preoperative holding area just before the surgery, and in the recovery room afterwards," says Betty. "I continued to do Reiki on myself every day after I was released from the hospital." She recovered with no complications. Three weeks after the surgery, she was back on the ski slopes. Five years later, she has had no further recurrence of the cancer.

"From the beginning, this type of healing called to me," says Betty, who is now a Reiki master, the most advanced level of practice. (During the regular work week, she manages administrative and computer systems for a small nonprofit organization.) Evenings and weekends, she sees clients and teaches aspiring Reiki practitioners in an upstairs room in her home. No remnants of her body-building life here. The room is filled with the calming scent of incense, the sounds of a small water fountain and the occasional tones of crystal bowls that she uses to help channel the energy. Several candles glow on a low table.

Betty tells the story of Reiki: Dr. Mikao Usui founded Reiki in the early-twentieth century in Japan. He began to use the technique to help his patients, with some success, and then trained sixteen other "masters" (which simply means "teacher"). At each level of training, the master gives an "attunement" to the student, which makes it possible to channel the Reiki energy. "Many people can lay their hands on others for healing touch," says Betty. "But they are not doing Reiki unless they have taken a class and received an attunement from a master teacher." The sixteen masters trained by Dr. Usui went on to train others. One of these masters trained Mrs. Hawayo Takata, who had been suffering from gallstones, asthma and appendicitis and was told she needed surgery. Instead, she received Reiki treatments every day. Her condition improved, and she did not have the surgery.

Mrs. Takata brought the technique to the United States, and trained twenty-two masters. Nearly all of the Reiki practitioners in this country, including Betty, can trace their training "lineage" back to Mrs. Takata, and through them, back to Dr. Usui.

Betty experiences the Reiki energy as tingling and warmth in her hands. "We call it 'heating pad hands,'" she says. Her clients come to her with both physical and emotional complaints. "Whatever the problem, the Reiki energy creates a womblike atmosphere in which people can truly relax and perhaps let go of the problem," says Betty. "One client was going through a difficult divorce, and burst into tears the moment I put my hands on her. With regular treatments, she became calmer, more even, better able to cope with her situation. Another had a badly swollen knee after a skiing accident. I spent a great deal of time with my hands on the knee, channeling Reiki energy, and could see the swelling begin to go down in the first treatment. The second time, the swelling, limp and pain were gone."

Betty stresses that while Reiki may complement conventional treatment, it should never replace it. "I insist that my clients with serious illnesses continue their medical treatments. Reiki does not interfere, and can often enhance treatment or help deal with the side effects of medication or chemotherapy." And for Betty, the wonder of Reiki is that the source of the energy seems never-ending. "As much as is needed flows abundantly from the universe," she says. "Often, I just have to think about the Reiki and I feel it flowing through my crown, down my arms, into my palms and directly where it is most needed in the client's body." And it is the energy, not the practitioner, that is the source of the healing, emphasizes Betty. "Sometimes people just need to relax enough to receive the energy. Then their bodies can heal themselves."

What Is Energy or Spiritual Healing?

Among the oldest-known therapies, dating back to the Bible, spiritual healing is defined as "The direct interaction between one individual (the healer) and a second (sick) individual with the intention of bringing about an improvement or cure of the illness." Almost every culture in the world has some form of spiritual healing, which may involve chanting or herbs in addition to touch and "focused intention" (using the mind to send healing energy). In addition to Reiki, other spiritual healing practices include Therapeutic Touch (TT), shamanism, laying on of hands, distant healing, faith healing, prayer, psychic healing and, from the tradition of Chinese medicine, qigong. Spiritual healers generally believe that they can channel "healing energy" from a universal source into the patient's body to stimulate the body's natural healing abilities.

"Religion and spirituality have been largely banished from modern science and medicine. In our zeal to free science from the constraints of religious dogma, we have neglected an important component of health and well-being, the spiritual factor," writes Kenneth R. Pelletier, Ph.D., M.D., (hc).[1]

In his book, Pelletier comments on the "irony" of considering spiritual healing as an "alternative" approach: "Throughout recorded history, community health care was typically delivered by religious figures, including medicine men, ministers, shamans, rabbis, priests, witch doctors and holy men. Such healers were often the tribal or community healers and the most educated members of the community. Even our modern health care delivery system traces its origins to the hospitals founded by the early Christian church."[2]

---

[1] K. R. Pelletier, *The Best of Alternative Medicine: What Works? What Does Not?* (New York: Simon & Schuster, 2000), 251.
[2] Ibid.

Energy Healing, Spirituality and Therapeutic Touch: What's the Evidence? The Faith Factor and Connections with Others May Be Good Medicine

Religious belief can speed healing, boost the immune system and even prolong life

Major work in this area is being done by Harold G. Koenig, M.D., founder and director of Duke University's Center for Religion/Spirituality and Health. "We began by looking at the relationship between religion and mental health," says Koenig, the author of several books on spirituality and health. "Then we began looking at the relationship between religious belief and physical health. Our research, as well as studies done by others, has shown that people who attend religious services and/or pray at home tend to have stronger immune systems (measured by lower levels of Interleukin-6, a stress hormone, in their blood) and lower blood pressure, and live longer than people without religious practices." By religion, Koenig means a belief in a higher power as well as a feeling of caring or responsibility toward other people.

Studies conducted at Duke and elsewhere have found that people who are more religious tend to recover more quickly from open heart surgery and from hip fractures, with less depression, than control groups of patients. "Studies of cancer patients have shown that those who are religious are more hopeful, less anxious and better able to cope with the stress of the disease and its treatment," says Koenig. "There is also data that religious people are less likely to develop and die from cancer." Religious belief can also have a negative effect on health: Patients who believe that their illness represents a punishment or abandonment by God were found to be at increased risk of death.

(In addition to the studies listed in the endnotes, other research on religious belief conducted at Duke and elsewhere can be found at the following Web site: (*www.garcia.geri.duke.edu/religion/index.html*)

Another opinion of spiritual healing

Here is a different view of spiritual healing: Edzard Ernst, M.D., Ph.D., F.R.C.P., writes that there is little *scientific* evidence of the efficacy of spiritual healing, although it seems to do no harm. He cites reviews of placebo-controlled randomized clinical trials involving almost three thousand patients. "Almost half of these studies yielded a positive result," reports Ernst. "However, due to methodological limitations of these trials, no firm conclusion could be drawn. . . . Whether spiritual healing is associated with specific therapeutic effects is unclear. Healing has few risks. There is insufficient evidence for or against this form of therapy."[3]

---

3 E. Ernst, ed., *The Desktop Guide to Complementary and Alternative Medicine: An Evidence-Based Approach* (London: Harcourt Publishers Limited, 2001), 273.

Kenneth Pelletier, Ph.D., M.D., (hc), presents a comprehensive survey of additional research studies that document which spiritual practices are most effective in his book, *The Best Alternative Medicine: What Works? What Does Not?* Faith and hope are associated with lower levels of stress hormones and fewer symptoms of distress among cancer patients, as well as less depression and speedier recovery in cardiac and other patients.[4]

Belief, hope and optimism are good for you

"For virtually any disease," writes Pelletier, "approximately one-third of patients will improve when given a placebo.[5] . . . In the absence of hope, people become depressed, and clear links have been established between depression and both physical and mental illness and mortality."[6] Studies have also found that optimism was linked with longer life and fewer illnesses (Peterson); and pessimism was linked with twice as many infectious illnesses and visits to doctors than people who were more hopeful.

Love and social support are also powerful sources of healing

Pelletier highlights several studies showing that social support is "a protective factor in preventing or alleviating many diseases."[7] In one classic study, a close-knit Italian community was found to have half the death rate from heart attack of neighboring communities, despite the fact that residents were overweight, sedentary and smoked. In other research, social isolation was implicated as a risk factor for recurrent heart attack and/or death. And two studies of cancer patients linked social isolation with greater incidence of disease and shorter survival time.

Additional Research

Distant healing

Daniel J. Benor, M.D., the author of *Healing Research,* Vols. I–IV, surveyed research on distant healing—which involves people praying or sending healing energy to groups of patients who are in another location, as well as therapeutic touch (TT), also called laying on of hands. He writes that, "An overall summary of healing research shows that of 155 controlled studies, 64 demonstrate effects at statistically significant levels."[8] Pain, reports Benor, seems to be the symptom most responsive to therapeutic touch, as well as anxiety, depression and relationship problems.

---

4 Also cited in Pelletier, *The Best of Alternative Medicine,* 257.
5 Ibid., 257.
6 Ibid., 258.
7 Ibid., 261.
8 W. B. Jonas and J. S. Levin, eds., *Essentials of Complementary and Alternative Medicine* (Baltimore: Lippincott, Williams & Wilkins, 1999), 369–382.

Benor describes one seminal study of distant healing by Randolph C. Byrd, M.D., in which a group of born-again Christians prayed for hospitalized heart patients in a coronary care unit. Healers were given only patients' first names, diagnoses and updates on their conditions and asked to pray daily for a rapid recovery and prevention of complications. No one prayed for a matched "control group" of patients in the same unit. The result, according to Benor's summary: Healing appeared to reduce the severity of cardiac pathology. The group that was prayed for had significantly fewer intubations/ventilations, required less antibiotics and diuretics, and had fewer cardiopulmonary arrests and cases of pneumonia than the control group. However, there were no differences in length of hospital stay.

A 2000 review of 23 randomized trials of distant healing involving 2,774 patients found that methodological difficulties made it difficult to draw definitive conclusions. "However, given that approximately 57 percent of patients showed a positive treatment effect," researchers noted, "the evidence thus far merits further study."

Therapeutic Touch (TT)

The laying on of hands has become a widespread practice in the nursing profession ever since Dolores Krieger, Ph.D., R.N., professor of nursing at New York University, and Dora Kunz, a clairvoyant and healer, developed it into the practice of therapeutic touch (TT). More than ninety nursing schools now teach the technique, and it is practiced by approximately forty thousand nurses in this country. Benor reports on studies that showed the potential effect of therapeutic touch on boosting immune function and pain reduction.

References

Astin, J. A., et al. "The Efficacy of 'Distant Healing': A Systematic Review of Randomized Trials." *Annals of Internal Medicine* 132, no. 11 (2000): 903–910.

Benor, D. J. "Spiritual Healing: Does it Work? Science Says, Yes!" In D. J. Benor, *Healing Research: Volume I; Spiritual Healing: Scientific Validation of a Healing Revolution.* Southfield, MI: Vision Publications, 2001.

Bruhn, J., et al. "Social Aspects of Coronary Heart Disease in Two Adjacent Ethnically Different Communities." *American Journal of Public Health* 56 (1966): 2493–2506.

Byrd, R. C. "Positive Therapeutic Effects of Intercessory Prayer in a Coronary Care Population." *Southern Medical Journal* 81, no. 7 (1988): 826–829.

Ernst, E., ed. *The Desktop Guide to Complementary and Alternative Medicine: An*

Evidence-Based Approach. London: Harcourt Publishers Limited, 2001.

Hodges, R. D. and A. M. Scofield. "Is Spiritual Healing a Valid and Effective Therapy?" *Journal of the Royal Society of Medicine* 88, no. 12 (December 1995): 722.

Helm, H., et al. "Effects of Private Religious Activity on Mortality of Elderly Disabled and Nondisabled Adults." *Journals of Gerontology Series A— Biological Sciences And Medical Sciences* 55A (2000): M400–M405.

Jonas, W. B. and J. S. Levin, eds. *Essentials of Complementary and Alternative Medicine.* Baltimore: Lippincott, Williams & Wilkins, 1999.

Koenig, H. G. and H. J. Cohen, eds. *The Link Between Religion and Health: Psychoneuroimmunology and the Faith Factor.* Oxford: Oxford University Press, 2002.

Maunsell, E., et al. "Social Support and Survival Among Women with Breast Cancer." *Cancer* 76 (1995): 631–637.

Ornstein R. and D. Sobel. *The Healing Brain: Breakthrough Discoveries About How the Brain Keeps Us Healthy.* New York: Simon & Schuster, 1987.

Pelletier, K. R. *The Best Alternative Medicine: What Works? What Does Not?* New York: Simon & Schuster, 2000.

Pergament, K. I., et al. "Religious Struggle as a Predictor of Mortality among Medically Ill Elderly Patients: A Two-Year Longitudinal Study." *Archives of Internal Medicine* 161 (2001): 1881–1885.

Peterson, C. "Explanatory Style as a Risk Factor for Illness." *Cognitive Therapy and Research* 12 (1988): 1191–1194.

Redner, R., B. Briner, and L. Snellman. "Effects of a Bioenergy Healing Technique on Chronic Pain." *Subtle Energies* 2, no. 3 (1991): 43–63.

Steffen, P. R., et al. "Religious Coping, Ethnicity and Ambulatory Blood Pressure." *Psychosomatic Medicine* 63 (2001): 523–530.

9

TAKING CARE OF OUR CHILDREN
"In one week, he was a changed child;
finally, we could all get some sleep."

Failure to Thrive: A Mystery Solved

From the time he was nine months until he was twenty-two months old, Emmett Mercer hardly slept in his crib. During that time, his parents took turns sitting up with him almost every night, holding him vertically on their chests. His chronic vomiting made it dangerous for him to sleep in any other position. "If he vomited while he was lying down, he could aspirate (breathe) the fluid into his lungs and choke," says Maureen O'Hare Mercer, mother of Emmett and two older children, Emileigh and Rett. "It was horrific. My ankles were swollen on the nights I was not able to lie down. I could barely function during the day, and my husband and I were exhausted all the time." Maureen and Walter, a real estate finance executive, have been married for twenty-five years. Before Emmett's illness, Maureen was the ultimate school and community volunteer. She also founded SenseAble Interiors/Facades, an interior and exterior design firm specializing in historic finishes and color restoration.

Emmett had begun having chronic vomiting and diarrhea almost as soon as he stopped breastfeeding and began eating baby food. "We were already going to a highly recommended pediatric practice, and they referred us to their top gastroenterology group," says Maureen. "The specialist tested him for Celiac's disease, fat absorption problems, multiple viruses, food allergies and cancer of the stomach and esophagus. Everything was negative. The doctor told us the problem was probably an 'echo' virus, a repeated exposure to viruses brought home by the older kids." Without a diagnosis, the doctor tried to reassure Maureen. "He told me that Emmett was not going to die, at least not from cancer, that his fat absorption rate was normal, and that I needed to calm down. He also said we'd probably have to wait until Emmett's stomach matured or he outgrew it. The only treatment he offered were antacids, which helped somewhat. I felt he was treating the symptoms but not the underlying problem."

In the meantime, Emmett was not growing properly (called "failure to thrive") because he was vomiting almost every day and was having diarrhea every couple of days. "It is devastating to be a parent and have a failure-to-thrive baby," says Maureen. "You can't fix it. He's neither on the way out nor on the way up. You can't have a normal life. It affects everyone in the family."

Maureen and Walter were trying to deal not only with Emmett's illness, but also with the needs of their other children. "When you have one child whom no one wants to babysit for because they don't want to get covered in vomit, one in nursery school, another one trying to learn to read, and the teachers calling to find out why they are 'out-of-sorts' in the classroom, you need a thoughtful, sensitive doctor," says Maureen. "This doctor was increasingly not sympathetic. I would talk to him on the phone, sleep-deprived and frantically worried, with Emmett throwing up on my shoulder, and he would say, 'Don't overreact. We just have to ride this last wave out.' But it was *never* the 'last wave.' I felt unheard."

Maureen and Walter decided to take Emmett to another doctor. "Five frustrating months was way too long to be trusting a doctor without even a possible potential diagnosis," says Maureen. They went to Children's Hospital in Boston. "What an awakening," says Maureen. "The first thing they did was to put Emmett on an elimination diet with a food journal, something no one had tried before. We stopped all food groups and reintroduced one at a time."

At the same time, the Mercers began to explore complementary medicine. "I had heard of homeopathy and wondered if it would be helpful to Emmett," says Maureen. (Please see "A Closer Look at Homeopathy.") A psychologist referred them to Ted Chapman, M.D., a conventionally trained physician as well as a respected homeopathy practitioner. "We waited months to see him," says

Maureen. "By the time we did, Emmett's diet was so limited; it consisted only of organic pear juice, goldfish crackers and chicken rice soup, but he was still vomiting." (Because the symptoms were continuing, they were still in the "food elimination" phase at this point.)

Chapman initially spent several hours with the Mercers and Emmett. "Dr. Chapman looked at Emmett's test results and did a detailed physical exam, even looking at his tongue, skin and hair follicles," says Maureen. "He asked us hundreds of questions. He was loving, nurturing and patient. He was as committed to communicating with Emmett as with us. He reviewed every facet of our physical and mental well-being, in conjunction with the medical problem. He wanted to know about our family life, stress, problems with other kids, the husband who travels on business. Can you imagine that not one other doctor had wanted to know these things?"

As a result of his homeopathic analysis, Chapman tried several remedies. One, called *Calcarea carbonica,* which is made of potentized oyster shells, seemed to bring Emmett the most relief, remembers Maureen. "Dr. Chapman explained to us that Emmett's response was related to the remedy's effect on his entire system and was reflected in an improvement in the efficiency of his digestive tract."

Maureen and Walter became the "integrators" of Emmett's medical care, learning and drawing from the worlds of allopathic medicine and homeopathy. "We made sure to share everything we were learning with both the Children's Hospital team and Dr. Chapman," says Maureen. By now, the Children's Hospital team had performed a food analysis of the pear juice, crackers and soup, focusing on Emmett's digestive tract. "They came up with sorbitol and fructose, both of which are fruit sugars. Sorbitol is highly concentrated in pear juice," says Maureen. "They finally determined that Emmett had been born without the enzymes to digest the sugars that are found in fruit, particularly sorbitol and fructose."

The Mercers put Emmett back on a normal diet, but eliminated all fruit and fruit by-products, carefully reading labels before they gave him anything. "In one week, he was a changed child," says Maureen. "He was eating and digesting normally. No more vomiting and diarrhea. Finally, we could all get some sleep."

Family Health Care Using the Best of Both Worlds

Their experience with Emmett prompted the Mercers to incorporate other alternative methods into their family medical care. Their large Victorian house is now filled with books on homeopathy and traditional Chinese medicine. (Please see chapters 2 and 6 for descriptions of Chinese acupuncture and herbal treatments.) "For the past ten years we have used the best family medicine from both worlds," says Maureen. This health strategy has helped the family cope not only with serious problems such as Emmett's, but also with the everyday problems of childhood illnesses for all three children. For example, Emmett's long bout with digestive problems has somewhat compromised his immune system, according to Maureen. "He has less stamina than other kids, and is more prone to colds and bronchitis," she says. "When he was nine, he had viral meningitis and mononucleosis. We found that combining alternative and complementary treatments with his conventional health care has helped him overcome illnesses fairly quickly."

Maureen also found that a Japanese style of acupuncture that includes magnet therapy is often helpful when the children feel rundown. "I learned to put the magnets on at home and it seems to help when they think they are coming down with something. Sometimes we can ward it off," she says. "Another preventive treatment is a constitutional remedy that Dr. Chapman has developed specifically for Emmett's personal characteristics. He takes this a few times year." Maureen also keeps a homeopathic remedy kit at home. "There are remedies for all kinds of acute ailments including colds, coughs, flu, stomach problems and ear infections. I have learned so much about using them through reading and consulting with Dr. Chapman, who is now our primary-care family practitioner," she says. "We have all benefited." (Please see "A Closer Look at Homeopathy" for explanations of homeopathic treatment as well as research evidence.)

Maureen used an additional complementary therapy for her daughter. "When Emileigh was in kindergarten, she fell and hit her head on a rock," says Maureen. "There was no concussion, but she needed stitches. We put ice on it and didn't think much more about it. But she soon began having headaches and reading problems, so we had her vision tested and found out that she needed glasses." Emileigh wore the glasses until second grade, but then Maureen decided once more to look beyond conventional medical treatment.

"The glasses did not seem to be alleviating all of her headaches and reading complaints, so I took her to a craniosacral practitioner," says Maureen. (Please see "A Closer Look at Chiropractic and Craniosacral Therapy" and "A Closer Look at Osteopathy.") "Cradling her head, the practitioner gently made tiny adjustments in the connections, called 'sutures,' that join the bones of the skull, particularly in the area that affects vision. We think that the fall knocked something out of alignment. After two sessions, her headaches were gone, and at her next vision checkup she no longer needed glasses." Emileigh, now a high school freshman, has not worn glasses since.

Today, Emmett Mercer is a happy, curious eleven-year-old with a great sense of humor. He is doing well in school, enjoys acting, singing and soccer (Maureen has been the coach for two successful seasons). "He understands very well the connection between fruit products and his digestion, and has learned to read labels and ask questions before he eats anything that might contain fruit by-products," says Maureen. Looking back on their experiences, she comments, "This diagnosis took fourteen months and showed us both the strengths and weaknesses of allopathic medicine. We feel that Emmett would not be who he is today without the interventions of conventional medical science together with homeopathy, acupuncture and other complementary treatments."

Breathing Easier: An Integrative Approach to Asthma

A four-year-old girl imagines a tightly closed rosebud opening its petals to become a beautiful flower. A twelve-year-old boy sees a complex arrangement of pipes with valves turned to the "on" position. A teenager visualizes a narrow stream that becomes a cascading mountain waterfall. As they close their eyes and think of these images, the children feel their airways open and they can breathe more freely. All three have asthma, a chronic inflammation of the lungs that restricts breathing, and all of them have learned "guided imagery" techniques that help open their airways, often without the use of asthma drugs.

Asthma is the leading cause of chronic illness in children and teens. National data indicate that the number of children with asthma in the Unites States has more than doubled in the past 15 years. In 1980, 2.3 million American children had asthma. In 1995, the most recent year for which data are available, the number of affected children has risen to 5.5 million. Asthma has reached epidemic proportions in preschool children (160 percent increase) and has increased 75 percent in school-aged children. The number of deaths related to asthma in children has nearly tripled over the last 15 years. Although the death rate has increased in all racial and ethnic groups, blacks experience a much higher death rate from asthma than any other group. In 1995, the death rate for African-American children was more than four times the rate in white American children.[1]

"Research has shown us that the mind can actually influence the body," says John D. Mark, M.D., assistant professor of clinical pediatrics at the University of Arizona. "We can teach children and adults to use visualization in their minds to open airways, reducing both mucous and inflammation in the lungs. The mind can actually change the immunological response to disease." (Please see Research boxes for studies on guided imagery and other complementary therapies for children.)

John Mark is board-certified in both pediatrics and pediatric pulmonology (childhood lung problems, including asthma, cystic fibrosis and chronic pneumonia). He became interested in complementary and alternative approaches for children when he was directing several pediatric outreach clinics that he had founded in conjunction with Stanford University and the University of California, San Francisco. "Patients and practitioners kept asking me about alternative therapies, not only for childhood lung diseases, but for other pediatric illnesses as well," he says. "I wanted to learn more about integrative medicine—combining conventional medicine with complementary and alternative treatment—so I applied to the University of Arizona Program in Integrative Medicine." Mark became one of the first two pediatricians in the United States

---

[1] Data is from "Asthma and the Environment: A Strategy to Protect Children," President's Task Force on Environmental Health Risks and Safety Risks to Children, 1999.

to be awarded a fellowship in integrative medicine from the National Institutes of Health. He spent two years in the Arizona program, seeing patients in the clinic as well as conducting research to investigate complementary and alternative treatments for children. After his fellowship, Mark joined the University of Arizona as assistant professor of clinical pediatrics, specializing in pediatric pulmonary integrative medicine.

"The primary conventional treatment for asthma is the use of steroids through an inhaler," says Mark. "My goal with children is to use the conventional treatment initially, for immediate relief and to establish control of their asthma, but then to try to taper off and even discontinue these medicines as soon as possible. We do this by finding out which alternative approaches both the child and the family can accept. This is what integrative medicine is all about."

Mark describes one five-year-old who was coughing almost all night long and whenever she tried to exercise. She also had frequent colds and bronchitis. "She was irritable and tired during the day because of her sleep interruptions, and she was often too sick to participate in family activities," says Mark. "The parents, however, did not want to accept the diagnosis of asthma, primarily because they did not like the idea of their child inhaling steroids." Mark worked with the family to help them see the need for medication, at least to give her some relief at night, and to control the chronic inflammation. "They were able to accept this after they understood it would not be permanent," he says. "They also saw that it helped her sleep."

After just a few weeks on the medication, this child was able to control her asthma symptoms on her own, through a combination of alternative techniques, including changes in her diet, guided imagery and the addition of dietary supplements. "Even very young children can learn guided imagery," says Mark. "Young kids are great at relaxing—they daydream naturally, and their imaginations are so active! Children between six and twelve have some of the most creative visualizations of any age group."

What Is Guided Imagery and Self-Hypnosis? What's the Evidence?

Advocates of guided imagery contend that the imagination is a potent healer. "Images and other senses are thought to be a way for the brain to communicate with organs of the body," says John Mark, M.D. "In fact, imagery has been called the 'language' that the mind uses to communicate with the body." (For more on guided imagery and visualization, please see also the story on Crohn's disease in chapter 7.)

Studies have shown that imagery, also referred to as self-hypnosis, is most successful when used in conjunction with such relaxation techniques as meditation and yoga, according to Mark. From this relaxed state patients can create images that include tumors shrinking, airways opening up, pain receding or a heart beating according to a normal rhythm. (In chapter 4, Charlotte Harrington describes how she uses imagery to restore regular heart rhythm.) These images can be powerful enough to actually induce physiological change. (Think of squeezing a tart lemon into your mouth. Do you begin to salivate?)

Do guided imagery, self-hypnosis and relaxation training help with asthma?

Several randomized controlled studies indicate that these techniques are beneficial for children and adults with asthma, according to Mark. However, he points out that these studies should be viewed with caution: With a few exceptions (see below) there has been little research in childhood asthma focusing on objective pulmonary (lung) function measurements and airway inflammation. Mark and his colleagues at the University of Arizona are currently involved in a study to measure airway function and inflammation in children who are using guided imagery to taper their inhaled steroids. (No results yet.)

—One study found that relaxation training in children not only helped their asthma, as measured by pulmonary function tests, medication use and symptoms, but also decreased airway inflammation.

—The use of storytelling, imagery and relaxation in a family asthma education program resulted in improvements in medication use, asthma scores and symptoms in preschool children.

—Young adults with asthma who practiced yoga reported fewer symptoms and medication use. (This study did not measure pulmonary function.)

—Another study found that treatment with a "hypnotic technique" resulted in improvements for adults with moderate asthma.

✓ TAKE ACTION ✓

"I can't go to school today!": Best things to do for asthma, allergies, viruses and ear infections

Homeopathy, while somewhat controversial (See "A Closer Look at Homeopathy.") has been a useful home-remedy method for many parents dealing with everyday problems that keep kids home from school. What else can parents do? Here are John Mark's integrative medicine suggestions for some common problems:

ASTHMA

Self-hypnosis and guided imagery (See "What Is Guided Imagery?" in this chapter for details).

Dietary changes. "Polyunsaturated fats, which are in almost every cookie, snack and cracker, can cause inflammatory precursors in the body, and remember that asthma is caused by inflammation in the lungs," says Mark. "I recommend staying away from processed foods and increasing consumption of fruits and vegetables."

Exercise. "I like to talk to kids about swimming, biking, roller skating, yoga or martial arts," says Mark. "Aerobic exercise helps with breathing and reducing the frequency and duration of colds. Martial arts and yoga are particularly beneficial for children with asthma because they teach control of the breath."[2]

Dietary supplements. With older children, between 10 and 15, Mark recommends dietary supplements, including a good multivitamin with vitamins C, A and E, as well as selenium. "There's been some research showing that B-complex and antioxidants help lung function," says Mark. "There is also evidence that fish oils, especially omega-3 fatty acids, are helpful. I encourage families to eat more salmon, sardines, mackerel and herring."

(continued)

---

[2] Some people's asthma may be made worse with exercise, says John Mark, especially if their asthma is not under control or they are exposed to adverse conditions such as cold, dry air, wind or particulates (like a dust storm or during an ozone warning). There is also a portion of the population with exercise-induced asthma (including famous Olympic athletes Nancy Hogshead and Jim Ryan).

However, says Mark, "Children and adults who have asthma that is stable and under control can often benefit from exercise. It helps them use their lungs to full capacity, helps them develop stamina and respiratory muscle strength, and often will help them decrease the amount of medication needed. Such activities as swimming and other sports that occur in a more 'humid' environment (since cold dry air can exacerbate asthma) are popular; however, studies show that any type of exercise is good for stable asthma. For folks with just exercise-induced asthma, one can pre-medicate with certain inhalers (albuterol, salmeterol, cromalyn sodium) and the symptoms can be 'blocked.' Also, slow warm-ups can also reduce the exercise symptoms."

Manual therapy. Osteopathy, massage therapy and other manual therapy techniques have been shown to improve symptoms of asthma and increase pulmonary function in both children and adults. (See "A Closer Look at Osteopathy.")

SINUS PROBLEMS AND ALLERGIES

The asthma remedies described above can also be helpful for allergy and sinus symptoms. In addition:

Environmental history and analysis can help determine if the symptoms may be coming from pets, dust mites (found in bedding, carpets and upholstery) or pollen.

Investigate possible food allergies. "Many children with chronic respiratory problems do better if they cut out milk, cheese, ice cream, butter and other dairy products," says Mark. "Other possible culprits are food dyes from processed foods. I suggest a trial of eliminating dairy to see if there is any improvement in symptoms and as many processed foods as possible for at least two weeks to see if there is any change in symptoms." Sometimes food cravings can be a clue to an allergy. One conventional allergist recommends eliminating any food that the child craves for two weeks to see if it makes a difference in symptoms.

Acupuncture (if children will tolerate it) helps alleviate asthma as well as allergy symptoms in some children.

EAR INFECTIONS

(See "A Closer Look at Homeopathy" for research relating to ear infections and homeopathic remedies.) The treatments described above for allergies and asthma can be helpful, as well as:

Osteopathy. This is a method of manual therapy involving massage, mobilization and gentle spinal manipulation. There is some research showing the benefits of osteopathy for relief of lower back pain. For ear infections, the theory is that a structure or function may not be working because it is blocked. "If a baby is stuck in the birth canal, for example, the function of their ear canals may be affected by structural changes from the delivery, making them more prone to ear infections," says Mark. "We are now conducting a study of children who are prone to ear infections who are being treated with gentle osteopathic craniofascial therapy, compared to children who receive conventional treatment. There are no results yet."

PAIN AND NAUSEA

Osteopathy may be helpful for headache pain and migraines, as well as other pain. "We have also used guided imagery to help children to cope with the pain and nausea of cancer treatment," says Mark.

(continued)

Music therapy. "There is evidence that the act of both choosing music and listening to the music you have chosen can reduce pain," says Mark. "In postoperative and intensive care units, music therapy has been found to reduce the need for pain medications and to promote faster recovery." (See *www.medicinehorizons.com.*)

Energy healing and therapeutic touch. (See also the "Closer Look" section on these topics.) "Energy healers believe that everyone has energy fields surrounding their bodies. Illness can result when these fields become unbalanced. Energy practitioners use their hands, either directly on the body as in therapeutic touch, or hovering above the body, to re-balance the energy," says Mark. "I have seen these methods used with children who are in the hospital, as well as outpatients, with some success. We are now conducting a study of premature infants in the intensive care unit to investigate therapeutic effects of healing touch during stressful procedures. We will evaluate the effects by measuring any changes in heart rate, breathing rate, oxygenation levels and stress hormones."

 Complementary Therapies for Asthma, Allergies and Upper-Respiratory Infections: What's the Evidence?

While these studies relate to asthma, they are also applicable to allergies and upper respiratory infections as well.

Herbs and supplements: what helps, what to stay away from

For a review of all the papers in the literature looking at herbal remedies and asthma, see Ernst for a good survey of what has been studied and where to go for more information. (See also "A Closer Look at Healing Herbs.") Individual studies look at ginkgo biloba, vitamin C and vitamin B_6. One study warns of the potential *dangers* of ephedra (also called Ma Huang), especially when used in combination with other drugs or chemicals.

Hands-on therapy works for children (and adults)

When parents, after instruction, spent twenty minutes a night giving massage therapy to their children, the children showed improved lung function, decreased medication and reduced asthma symptoms. Osteopathic manipulation in an emergency room improved lung function and breathing in adults. For a comprehensive review of the effects of chiropractic, massage, osteopathy and other manipulative therapies on asthma symptoms, see "Manual Therapy for Asthma," by M.A. Hondras, et al.

The mind/body connection

Yoga, acupuncture, and relaxation techniques, including guided imagery and self-hypnosis, were also found to be helpful for symptom relief. (Please see "A Closer Look at Yoga" and chapters 6 and 7 for information on acupuncture and guided imagery.)

References

Cohen, H. A., et al. "Blocking Effect of Vitamin C in Exercise-Induced Asthma." *Archives of Pediatric and Adolescent Medicine* 151 (1997): 367–370.

Collipp, P. J., et al. "Pyridoxine Treatment of Childhood Bronchial Asthma." *Annals of Allergy* 35 (1975): 93–97.

Ernst, A. H. "Herbal Medicine for Asthma: A Systematic Review." *Thorax* 55 (2000): 925–929.

Ewer, T. C., et al. "Improvement in Bronchial Hyper-Responsiveness in Patients with Moderate Asthma After Treatment with a Hypnotic Technique: A Randomized Controlled Trial." *British Medical Journal* 293 (1986): 1129–1132.

Field, T., et al. "Children with Asthma Have Improved Pulmonary Functions After Massage Therapy." *Journal of Pediatrics* 132 (1998): 854–858.

Fung, K. P., et al. "Attenuation of Exercise-Induced Asthma by Acupuncture." *Lancet* 2 (1986): 1419–1422.

Gaby, A. R. "Ginkgo Biloba Extract: A Review." *Alternative Medicine Review* 1 (1996): 236–242.

Haller, C. A., et al. "Adverse Cardiovascular and Central Nervous System Events Associated with Dietary Supplements Containing Ephedra Alkaloids." *New England Journal of Medicine* 343 (2000): 1833–1838.

Hondras, M. A., et al. "Manual Therapy for Asthma." *Cochrane Database of Systematic Reviews* 2 (2000): CD001002.

Jobst, K. A. "Acupuncture in Asthma and Pulmonary Disease: An Analysis of Efficacy and Safety." *Journal of Alternative and Complementary Medicine* 2 (199): 179–206.

Kohen, D. P., et al. "Applying Hypnosis in a Preschool Family Asthma Education Program: Uses of Storytelling, Imagery and Relaxation." *American Journal of Clinical Hypnosis* 39 (1997): 169–181.

Linde, K., K. Jobst, and J. Panton. "Acupuncture for Chronic Asthma." *Cochrane Database of Systematic Reviews* 2 (2000): CD00008.

Paul, F. A., et al. "Osteopathic Manipulative Treatment Applications for the Emergency Department Patient." *Journal of the American Osteopathic Association* 96 (1996): 403–409.

Vazquez, M. I., et al. "Psychological Treatment of Asthma: Effectiveness of a Self-Management Program with and Without Relaxation Training." *Journal of Asthma* 30 (1993): 171–183.

Vedanthan, P. K., et al. "Clinical Study of Yoga Techniques in University Students with Asthma: A Controlled Study." *Allergy and Asthma Proceedings* 19 (1998): 3–9.

Growing Up with Physical Problems

Benjamin Weisman was born with the spirit of an athlete and a body that can't play the game. He has a heart disorder, a long, lanky body and problems with his bones and muscles that give him less stamina, strength and speed than other kids. These problems are caused by Marfan syndrome, a genetic disorder of the connective tissue. Ben is my teenage son and he inherited the condition from me. Ben suggested that I include his story here because it might be helpful to other teens who are dealing with physical or emotional problems. I asked if he would want to use a pseudonym. "One of the important lessons I had to learn was to accept myself and not be afraid of what other people think," he said. "So I want to use my real name."

When he said this I realized that the message might be important not only for kids, but also for adults who might have trouble accepting physical disability. I was thinking of my late father, from whom I inherited the disorder. In the six years that he was married to my mother, he kept his illness a secret. It was not until after my father died that my mother finally learned of his diagnosis. Although my memories of my father are hazy, I know that his own denial of Marfan syndrome in himself left me with a legacy of shame and discomfort about my own body that took years to overcome.

Happily, Benjamin has vanquished that legacy of shame. He has charted his own path through the world of chronic illness, one filled with pride in his achievements, confidence in his ability to overcome challenges and a deep empathy for the suffering of others. I like to think that my father, had he lived, would have been proud of his grandson.

Parenting a Child with a Chronic Illness: Early Decision Making

When Ben was diagnosed with Marfan syndrome in infancy, Michael and I knew that he would have physical limitations that would require some decisions early in his life. First, we would try to introduce him to activities—such as playing in an orchestra—that would give him a way to relate to other kids. (We knew that he might well have cardiovascular and joint problems that would preclude competitive sports.) Second, we would deal with each symptom as it arose, so that he would understand the need to take care of himself without allowing the illness to define him. We hoped in the meantime to help him build enough positive self-esteem so that he could withstand the inevitable curiosity and teasing he would encounter. Third, Michael—a natural athlete—would work with Ben on developing baseball and basketball skills (contact sports like football and hockey were out of the question) so that he would feel comfortable participating at some level; Michael would also introduce him to the joys (and frustrations—especially in Boston) of being a professional sports fan.

Combining Complementary and Conventional Medicine

Fortunately, Ben has a relatively mild case of Marfan syndrome. (The gene has a "variable expression," which means that the symptoms vary from person to person, even within the same family.) He has had two major surgeries: one at the age of five to correct a protruding breast bone; and a spinal fusion at twelve that involved a bone graft and implanting steel rods to correct scoliosis (curvature of the spine). In his heart, he has a slight mitral valve prolapse, requiring daily beta-blockers and prophylactic antibiotics for all dental work and surgery, and he usually has chronic joint pain somewhere in his body. Despite this, he played for several years in Little League (those long arms were a boon at first base and for pitching) and still loves playing in pickup baseball and basketball games with his friends. He gave up being on the teams in high school—a difficult decision for him. However, he remains a rabid fan, with a command of statistics in every professional sport stretching back to the dawn of time.

He plays the double bass (the perfect instrument for his six-foot body and extra-long limbs) in youth orchestras, loves all kinds of music, from classical to rock to Broadway, and has become a talented actor, playwright and director. He is currently studying theater at Drew University. He has close, deep friendships and is truly happy in his life.

Most chronic illnesses requires long-term conventional medical care to monitor the condition and intervene when necessary and Marfan syndrome is no exception. This disorder may require physical therapy for musculoskeletal problems and medications to reduce stress on the heart. Surgery is often used to correct both curvature of the spine and to replace heart valves and tissues that have become so overstretched and thin that they are in danger of failure or rupture. (I had both back and heart surgery and my father, who did not have surgery, died of a ruptured aorta.) In addition to conventional medicine, complementary treatments can benefit people with Marfan syndrome, particularly the musculoskeletal problems, and Ben has taken advantage of several.

During his elementary school years, for example, it gradually became clear from X-ray monitoring that Ben was growing so quickly that he would need a back brace, physical therapy and possibly surgery to control the curvature of his spine. (The overly "stretchy" Marfan tendons and ligaments often do not hold the spine straight as the child grows.) He began wearing the brace at age seven, but by the time he was twelve, it became clear that he was growing so quickly (a foot in one year!) that the brace alone was not holding the spine in place. In an effort to avoid surgery, we tried weekly sessions of a form of Japanese acupuncture that is often used for scoliosis, as well as twice-weekly Pilates exercise workouts to build muscle strength and improve alignment. (Please see "A Closer Look at Pilates.") Despite the combined forces of conventional and alternative medicine, however, surgery became inevitable.

Ben had the spinal fusion in seventh grade. It required a week in the hospital and a month at home. After the operation, he spent a couple of days in the recovery room, quite uncomfortable, even with the conventional pain medication. His acupuncturist visited with her assistant and asked if we wanted to try a "hands on" type of healing. (Please see "A Closer Look at Energy Healing.") We agreed, and she instructed us to stand around his bed, put our hands somewhere on his body and envision healing energy flowing through our hands. (As you will see below, this was one of the few recovery room experiences that Ben actually remembers.) It seemed to relax him. Within a couple of days, he was walking and was home within a week, needing very little pain medication. He was back at school after a month and playing basketball in six months. His surgeon remarked that his recovery was unusually rapid. It is, of course, impossible to know if the "hands on" session, or even the weeks of Pilates and acupuncture before the surgery contributed to his recovery. But we feel they did not hurt.

During high school Ben began to have mild but annoying pain in his hips, shoulders, knees or ankles almost every day, stemming from muscle tightness, the lack of elasticity in his connective tissue and the slight asymmetry of his spine that still remained after the surgery. Weekly Alexander lessons taught him to move his body with less effort—whether he was playing sports, his double bass, dancing or performing as an actor—releasing muscles that did not need to be tense. (Please see "A Closer Look at the Alexander Technique.") As an added bonus, the Alexander teacher was also a professional voice teacher, and incorporated singing (and breathing) techniques into the sessions, both valuable for any aspiring stage performer. Regular craniosacral work also helped reduce his pain and encourage proper alignment. (See "A Closer Look at Chiropractic and Craniosacral Therapy.")

For Kids Only

This is where Ben talks about his health in his own words. He wanted to communicate directly with other kids:

One of the best things about being very young is that everyone is the same. Even if people look different, it doesn't matter, because you're too young to know that it's supposed to matter. So until second or third grade I didn't really feel different. Kids were curious about my body, but they weren't malicious, they just wanted to know why I was so long and skinny.

Then in second grade I had to wear a back brace for scoliosis. It covered my whole torso in thick molded plastic. That's when I realized there was something different about me. I was the only one. But my teacher made it into a status thing; she told everyone I was special. My family made me feel special, too. So after a while, even though the brace was painful and uncomfortable, I began to see it as part of me. I could still play sports, and I decided to have fun with it. I told kids to see how hard they could hit me in the stomach, and I didn't feel a thing. We also would play a game where we bounced balls off it. I was lucky because I had a lot of really good friends who liked me for who I was and for whom the brace didn't seem to matter.

In middle school things changed because people changed. In elementary school it was, "Let's find reasons to like everybody." In middle school, it was, "Let's find reasons to put people down and exclude them." And, guess what? I was a convenient target, not for the friends who had known me since kindergarten—some were protective and threatened to beat up anyone who teased me—but for the new kids I was meeting. For the first time in my life, I had the experience of being excluded because of the way I looked and my physical problems. There was one kid, for example, who made fun of me every time he could, saying things like, "Look at that thing sticking out of his shirt" (the brace), or "Don't touch him; he may break in half." He would even try to trip me or push me in the hallways. Once, a girl who was a year younger told him to leave me alone. That was nice, but I didn't like having to be protected by a younger kid!

Finally, I had had enough. I went to the guidance counselor, who called both of us into a meeting. When we were in the room, I pulled up my shirt and said, "This is my brace," and I explained to him why I had to wear it. Then I said, "Do you have a problem with that?" He never bothered me again.

In seventh grade, I had a spinal fusion, which kept me out of school for a month. But before the surgery they tried physical therapy—which consisted of boring exercises that I never wanted to do. My mother also took me for Pilates workouts, which were a lot more fun, and I could see how my muscles were growing. She also took me for acupuncture, which was very relaxing . . . after I got over the idea of needles. We were hoping that I wouldn't need the surgery, but I did.

I was pretty nervous when we arrived at the hospital on the day of the surgery, especially after they made me sign a paper saying all the terrible things that could happen to me, like dying or being paralyzed. After the surgery, I remember being in the recovery room—a scary place because of all the equipment and kids crying. In addition to being scared, I was also in a lot of pain. But I distinctly remember people, including my parents, standing around my bed and putting their hands on me. It made me feel safe and relaxed and free from the constraints of my body, as if my body were opening up. I also remember seeing my sister, and thinking that if they let her in, I was either dead or doing fine, and I was pretty sure I wasn't dead.

In six months I could play basketball again and felt like I was back to normal life. At that point, I made a conscious decision that I would never tell anyone else about my medical condition because I didn't like being treated differently. The brace and my crooked posture used to be the only real clues, and both were now gone. I had a straight back and no brace.

In ninth grade I switched to a small, private high school where no one knew me, a good time to put my plan into action. For a year and a half I told very few people (except the basketball coach) about my medical problems. But sophomore year was a turning point. Two major things happened to change how I felt. The first was an assignment to write a personal essay in the style of

George Orwell. I chose to write about having Marfan syndrome, thinking that no one but the English teacher would read it. But when she handed the essays back she surprised me by asking if I'd be willing to read mine out loud. At that moment, I made a decision. I felt like the fugitive who turns himself in after twenty years because he's tired of hiding. I was tired of dodging questions and pretending to be someone else and decided it was time to let people into the big secret of my life.

So I read my essay, right out loud to the class, most of whom had no idea. Then they knew, and you know something? Nothing changed. I walked out of that class the same person as when I walked in. No one treated me differently. No kid gloves, no teasing. All that was different was that my classmates knew a bit more about who I am. That taught me I didn't have to be afraid of who I was, just like when I talked to that kid in seventh grade.

The second big event was my decision to quit sports and take dance instead. I began to realize during my sophomore season on the team that basketball was not going to be my thing. I didn't have the endurance or the jump shot. And I had begun to read about kids with Marfan syndrome and similar heart conditions who had died playing sports. This was a painful decision, I loved playing basketball so much, and we had just won the championship, and my coach told me I was going to be a starter the next year.

But I knew I had two other things I loved. One was music, which has always been a constant in my life. I was lucky enough to perform in Symphony Hall and the Hatch Shell with the Greater Boston Youth Symphony Orchestras. And listening to music has always been a calming influence. I have CDs for every mood. When I am stressed I listen to Brahms' Tragic Overture. And my own frustrations could never hold a candle to the sense of frustration and despair in Beethoven's music, especially the second movement of his seventh symphony—Imagine how hard it must be for a musician to go deaf in the middle of his life. I also really love some rock groups, and I'm addicted to Broadway music (not a bad addiction at all!).

But my main passion is theater. I had started acting in freshman year and realized that I loved acting more than any sport. One of the reasons was that I could do it. And I could do it well. At an acting camp the summer after my sophomore year I created a performance art piece in which I acted out my transition from wanting to be a professional baseball or basketball player to wanting to be a professional actor. It was one of the most moving and revealing things I had ever done in front of an audience. Throughout the rest of high school, acting helped me become more open about who I was and more willing and able to share my emotions with other people, whether frustrations with my physical limitations or anything else.

In writing my college essay, I discovered another reason why acting is so much more valuable to me than sports could ever be. As an actor, I can step on the stage and all of a sudden I'm not Benjamin Weisman with physical problems any more. Acting allows me to take on another character and test out emotions in a "safe" setting—where they won't be reflected on me but rather on the character I am playing.

What I didn't expect was that by stepping out of myself, I would respect myself more. I saw that the characters I played had problems, too. In Brecht's *The Caucasian Chalk Circle*, my character, Azdak, has a drinking problem and likes to impress people with his stories. But he also likes to help poor people. In another play, *The Actor's Nightmare*, by Christopher Durang, my character, George, has a complete sense of helplessness. He is placed in a situation he can't control and desperately tries to figure out how to fit into his surroundings. Guess what? I have felt exactly the same way. With every play I act in, theatre teaches me that I am not so different after all. Everyone has problems and tries to cope as best they can. I can use my own experiences to help me interpret the characters I play and become a better actor. And I can use what they have discovered to help me in my "real" life.

Theater has also helped me accept and understand that it's important to get help when you need it. So I feel okay that yoga, the Alexander lessons and the craniosacral work help me feel better in my body. Doing these things has helped me feel freer to use my body onstage, to actually *become*, physically as well as emotionally, the characters I play.

I have had a lot more life experiences than most of the teenagers I know. Because of my problems with my body, I will never use drugs, smoke or drink too much, and my friends respect that. But I still like rock music, stupid movies, girls, yelling at Red Sox games until I can't even talk and hanging out with my friends. I finally realize that despite everything I've had to deal with because of my body and my genes, there's nothing about me that makes me less deserving of respect than anyone else.

A Closer Look at Homeopathy:
Like Cures Like

Twenty-five years ago, family practice physician Jennifer Jacobs, M.D., M.P.H., was looking for "a kinder, gentler way to treat people." She found what she was looking for in homeopathy, a medical system created two hundred years ago by German physician Dr. Samuel Hahnemann, who was himself on a similar quest. "Hahnemann was disillusioned by the harmful medical practices of his day, and set out to find a gentler approach," explains Kenneth R. Pelletier, Ph.D., M.D., (hc), in his comprehensive survey of complementary and alternative medicine.[1]

"Homeopathy is a wonderful way to treat children because it is gentle, nontoxic and effective," says Jacobs. The treatment is based on the principle that "like cures like." The theory is that tiny amounts of a substance that might cause disease symptoms in healthy people, when given in a highly diluted form to sick people, can stimulate their bodies' natural healing ability to fight the disease. Jacobs uses an onion to illustrate her point. "When we peel onions we get watery eyes, a runny nose and sometimes a hoarse cough, even though we are not sick," she points out. "If we take a homeopathic remedy called *Allium cepa,* which is made from the red onion, and give it in a highly diluted form to someone who has these cold symptoms, it helps to stimulate the body to fight the symptoms."

How does homeopathy work? The system is often explained through the concept of a "vital force," which has been called "the organizing, animating principle that maintains health in a living system. . . . A properly selected homeopathic remedy is believed to provoke the vital force, so that the body's own healing power can produce the cure."[2] The homeopathic vital force is similar to the Chinese qi or the Ayurvedic prana, both of which are considered to be the invisible "life force" or "energy" that flows in our bodies. When this energy flow is blocked or obstructed, disease results. (Please see chapters 2 and 6 for more about qi, vital force and prana.)

Jacobs grew so interested in homeopathy that she became not only a practitioner, but also earned a master's degree in public health, specializing in epidemiology and study design, to enable her to research its effectiveness. She now divides her time between seeing patients in her family practice clinic in Edmonds, Washington, and conducting research on homeopathy at the University of Washington in Seattle. In 1994, she published the first double-blind, placebo-controlled study of

---

[1] K. R. Pelletier, *The Best Alternative Medicine: What Works? What Does Not?* (New York: Simon & Schuster, 2000), 198–199.
[2] Ibid., 199–200.

homeopathy in a peer-reviewed U.S. journal (*Pediatrics*) demonstrating the effectiveness of homeopathy in childhood diarrhea. She has since published several follow-up studies on childhood illnesses, including diarrhea and ear infections, and coauthored the book *Healing with Homeopathy: The Doctor's Guide* with Wayne B. Jonas, M.D., former director of the National Institutes of Health National Center for Complementary and Alternative Medicine. (Dr. Jonas is featured in chapter 12.)

"Many parents do not want to keep giving their children antibiotics for ear infections," says Jacobs. "And in fact, an antibiotic crisis is underway in this country. Doctors are prescribing antibiotics for viral illnesses, colds and flu, when they are neither necessary nor appropriate. This is creating antibiotic-resistant bacteria, so that when we really do need these medicines—for such diseases as pneumonia, kidney infection or meningitis—they may not work."

Homeopathy is a possible solution to antibiotics, says Jacobs. "In twenty-five years of treating children with ear infections, I have prescribed antibiotics only once," she says. "With antibiotics, ear infections keep coming back, and they are harder and harder to get rid of. I often see children who are caught in this 'antibiotic treadmill'. I use homeopathic remedies to break the cycle, and they respond beautifully. The body's immune system is strengthened and there are fewer infections."

Jacobs's pilot study of ear infections, published in 2001, found that homeopathic remedies for ear infections produced significant decreases in overall symptoms, including pain and fever in the first twenty-four hours when compared to a placebo. "We did find enough positive evidence to apply to the NIH for a bigger study," says Jacobs. In his own review of other research studies, Pelletier cites evidence that supports the effectiveness of homeopathy for some conditions. "Homeopathy has always been considered particularly helpful for children," he writes. "It is reported to resolve, gently and effectively, such problems as teething pain, hyperactivity, emotional problems and even learning disabilities. . . . Many parents prefer homeopathy, since pharmaceutical drugs can have unpredictable and long-lasting, even toxic effects on children."[3]

Jacobs sees patients at the Evergreen Clinic, which she cofounded in the early 1980s with her husband, a physician who also specializes in family practice and homeopathy. When she first meets a new patient or family, she spends more than an hour in an initial interview and examination. "I take the health history, including details about current symptoms and past illnesses," she says. "I also ask about food cravings, sleep patterns, lifestyle, stress, the family

3. Ibid., 201.

situation and such personal details as whether they get cold or warm easily."

Jacobs then uses this information to perform a detailed analysis of the patient's health and to select which homeopathic remedies would be best. "There are thousands of homeopathic remedies," she says. "We have three thousand in our clinic alone, but we commonly use about one hundred. Each remedy is carefully selected to meet the particular constellation of symptoms of each patient." Jacobs stresses that homeopathy does not try to *suppress* symptoms in the way that antihistamines, for example, suppress cold or allergy symptoms. "These symptoms, whether they are sneezing, a runny nose or diarrhea, are the body's way of trying to heal itself," she explains. "The cold symptoms are a method for expelling bacteria and viruses out of the body. Through diarrhea, the body may be trying to quickly get rid of food-borne bacteria that are damaging the intestinal tract. Fever is a way for the body to kill disease-causing bacteria or viruses with high temperatures."

Jacobs explains that homeopathy does not mask or suppress the symptoms; it supports the body's natural ability to heal itself by *building up* the immune response, rather than trying to stop it. "We do this by trying to enhance the response that the body is already making, using the symptoms as a guide to the correct homeopathic remedy," she says. "Chronic diarrhea, for example, may be related to stress as well as physical or emotional upset in a person's life. We need to understand its cause in order to match the person with the best remedies." She says that homeopathy can be effective in the treatment of autoimmune diseases as well. "We have had good results with eczema, fibromyalgia, chronic fatigue and irritable bowel," she says. "We have even helped people with multiple sclerosis remain stable for five or six years, although we obviously can't reverse the course of the disease, especially if there has been damage to the tissues."

Doctors divide illness, particularly childhood illnesses, into two categories, acute and chronic. "With a homeopathic remedy kit at home and proper instruction about its use, parents can treat many acute illnesses themselves," says Jacobs. "These include colds, flu, earaches, diarrhea, teething, colic, chicken pox, croup, conjunctivitis." Chronic problems are more difficult to diagnose and treat at home, and for these—which include chronic skin problems, headaches, gastrointestinal problems, recurrent ear infections and behavior problems—parents should consult a homeopathic doctor. "We have, for example, used homeopathy to successfully treat children with sleep disorders and emotional problems," she says. "We are now in the beginning phases of a study on ADHD (attention deficit hyperactivity disorder). The study will include children who are currently taking Ritalin, as well as those who are not. We are looking for something that can be used to decrease or eliminate the need for Ritalin."

Homeopathy does not truly fall into the category of "complementary medicine," points out Jacobs, since it is best used as a stand-alone system. "The system was designed as an alternative to conventional medicine," she says. "Some conventional medical treatments may interfere with the homeopathic remedies. I usually ask my patients to give homeopathy six months to see if it works, and during that time not to add any new medicines or treatments to what they are already doing, so we can see clearly what the homeopathy is doing. If they are taking medicines that are optional, they may want to give them up during that time." She points out that diabetic patients who must take insulin or patients taking medication to lower their blood pressure should of course not stop taking these essential medications during homeopathic treatment.

Homeopathy: Research and Controversy: What's the Evidence?

Despite the research findings that point to its effectiveness for various medical problems, scientists and conventional medical professionals often criticize homeopathy. "The idea that microscopic amounts of medicine can cure disease goes against the principles of physics and modern medicine," says one researcher. Others argue that studies using principles of quantum physics and electromagnetic energy identified "measurable and unique electromagnetic signals emitted by homeopathic remedies. The signals produced specific dominant frequencies for each homeopathic substance tested."[4] This was found to be true even in remedies where no molecule of the original substance remained. (Several studies supporting this view are reviewed by Linda W. Freeman, Ph.D., in her 2001 article, "Homeopathy—a Scientific Enigma.") Supporters of homeopathy also point out that the principle of "like cures like" is the basis for the development of vaccines and allergy desensitization treatments. Kenneth R. Pelletier, Ph.D., M.D., (hc), takes some issue with this notion. "This analogy though, is not really accurate, since the substances used in immunization and desensitization are identical or similar to the disease-causing agents, whereas homeopathic remedies are usually substances different from those that cause disease."[5]

Despite the skepticism about homeopathy, clinical data, according to Wayne Jonas, M.D., "do not support the expected assumption that homeopathy operates entirely like a placebo. Basic research on homeopathy can help examine the

---

[4] L. W. Freeman, "Homeopathy—A Scientific Enigma," in *Best Practices in Complementary and Alternative Medicine: An Evidence-Based Approach with Nursing CE/CME* (Gaithersburg, MD: Aspen Publications, 2001).
[5] Pelletier, *The Best Alternative Medicine*, 199.

accumulating anomalous observations and experiments in this area."[6]

Even as the controversy continues, scientific evidence in support of homeopathy appears to be growing. Homeopathy has been reported as effective for digestive disorders, chronic fatigue, treatment for allergies, otitis media (acute or chronic ear infections), immune dysfunction, colic in babies, short-term, acute illnesses, such as influenza and chronic pain syndromes, such as migraine pain.

Two recent reviews of homeopathic research trials also showed the effectiveness of homeopathy. One, published in 1991 in the *British Medical Journal,* found that out of 107 controlled clinical trials of homeopathy, 81 showed that homeopathic medicines had some positive results and 24 showed "no positive effects." (Two were inconclusive). Conditions that benefited from homeopathy included vascular disease, respiratory infections, hay fever, faster return of bowel function following abdominal surgery, rheumatological disorders, pain or trauma, and mental or psychological problems. However, the authors caution that publication bias (because of the controversy surrounding homeopathy) and poor methodology may have complicated the results of the review.

A meta-analysis of homeopathic clinical trials published in the *Lancet* in 1997 by Klaus Linde, M.D., examined nearly ninety well-designed, randomized clinical trials. The combined results from all these studies also tended to support homeopathy compared to placebo. In addition to studies reporting homeopathy's effectiveness, there are also those that report its limitations. Pelletier, for example, points to studies that show that homeopathy is *unsuccessful* in treating plantar warts, osteoarthritis and in *preventing* illness. Both Pelletier and Linde stress the need for more well-designed studies of homeopathy.[7]

[6] W. B. Jonas and J. S. Levin, *Essentials of Complementary and Alternative Medicine* (Baltimore, MD: Lippincott, Williams & Wilkins, 1999), 7.
[7] Pelletier, *The Best Alternative Medicine,* 207–214.

References

Freeman, L. W. "Homeopathy—A Scientific Enigma," in *Best Practices in Complementary and Alternative Medicine: An Evidence-Based Approach with Nursing CE/CME*. Gaithersburg, MD: Aspen Publications, 2001.

Freeman, L. W. and G. F. Lawlis. *Mosby's Complementary and Alternative Medicine: A Research-Based Approach*. St. Louis, MO: Mosby, 2001.

Jacobs, J. J. and W. B. Jonas. *Healing with Homeopathy: The Doctor's Guide*. New York: Warner Books, 1998.

Jacobs, J. J., et al. "Treatment of Acute Childhood Diarrhea with Homeopathic Medicine: A Randomized Clinical Trial in Nicaragua." *Pediatrics* 93 (1994): 719–725.

Jacobs, J. J., et al. "Homeopathic Treatment of Acute Childhood Diarrhea: Results from a Clinical Trial in Nepal." *Journal of Alternative and Complementary Medicine* 6, no. 2 (2000): 131–139.

Jacobs, J. J., D. Springer, and D. Crothers. "Homeopathic Treatment of Acute Otitis Media in Children: A Preliminary Randomized Placebo-Controlled Trial." *Pediatric Infectious Disease Journal* 20, no. 2 (2001): 177–183.

Jonas, W. B. and J. S. Levin. *Essentials of Complementary and Alternative Medicine*. Baltimore: Lippincott, Williams & Wilkins, 1999.

Kleijnen, J., P. Knipschild, and G. Rieter. "Clinical Trials of Homeopathy." *British Medical Journal* 302 (1991): 316–323.

Linde, K., et al. "Are the Clinical Effects of Homeopathy Placebo Effects? A Meta-Analysis of Placebo-Controlled Trials." *Lancet* 350 (1997): 834–843.

Pelletier, K. R. *The Best Alternative Medicine: What Works? What Does Not?* New York: Simon & Schuster, 2000.

10

WOMEN AT MIDLIFE:
COMBINING ANCIENT WISDOM
WITH MODERN SCIENCE
"One day, I ripped the hormone patch off
and threw the entire box away."

In June 2000 Ellen Johnson (not her real name) was in her late forties and going through the early stages of menopause (called perimenopause). "I was experiencing suicidal thoughts, which at times were overwhelming," she says. "I would wake up at 3:00 A.M. almost every night unable to get back to sleep. I had hot flashes. Sex was painful because of thinning vaginal walls. I was depressed. My husband could barely recognize the woman I had become. I had two young children to take care of and I was trying to be a good psychotherapist for my patients, but I truly wanted to die."

Ellen's problems had started six months earlier. She had been having some mild perimenopausal symptoms, including hot flashes and insomnia, but was managing them with such herbal remedies as black cohosh, primrose oil, dong quai and soy products. In December 1999, however, she came down with viral meningitis and pneumonia. "I was in bed for six weeks with horrible head and neck pain and a gurgling in my lungs that sounded like soda popping," she remembers. With bedrest and conventional medical care, Ellen began to improve. By the end of January she was up and around, taking care of her children, then eight and four, and beginning to get back to work. By February, she felt fine.

"But one night, in the middle of March, I woke up at four in the morning, violently ill with diarrhea and vomiting and with a searing pain in my left side," she recalls. "I went to the ER, where they did a CAT scan and discovered a tumor in my kidney that had grown large enough to squeeze off the function of the ureter (the tube that brings urine from the kidney to the bladder). The doctor warned me that there was a 90 percent chance that the tumor was cancerous. I had to live with that knowledge until they removed it and did a biopsy." Three weeks later, the surgeon removed the entire kidney and part of the ureter. "The tumor was benign, thank goodness," says Ellen.

Although the tumor was out, the physical and emotional stress of her illness and surgery seemed to exacerbate Ellen's perimenopausal symptoms. "By the middle of May, I was a wreck: The insomnia, hot flashes and mood swings became severe, and I had lost twenty pounds, which was too much for me," she says. Over the summer she began taking conventional hormone replacement therapy, prescribed by the gynecologist at her HMO (health maintenance organization). "I used a patch that combined synthetic progesterone and estrogen," she says. "Within a week, I wasn't as depressed and was sleeping better, but then I began having intense menstrual periods with heavy bleeding every two weeks, almost like hemorrhaging. And my breasts were painfully engorged."

The doctor suggested a stronger dose of the synthetic hormones. "This only made matters worse," says Ellen. "Even though my mood swings and insomnia were better, I couldn't stand the heavy periods and painfully swollen breasts. One day, I just ripped the patch off and threw the entire box of them away." All of her symptoms soon returned, worse than ever.

"I remember going to meet a friend for lunch and sobbing into my salad," says Ellen. "I felt suicidal again and could barely continue to see my patients." The physical and emotional stress that Ellen was experiencing was unmatched in her life, including a demanding few years as vice-president of sales and marketing for a high technology company. ("I decided to get out of that world when my first child was born and needed open heart surgery," she says.)

She became a trained and licensed psychotherapist and has worked in conventional settings, along with psychiatrists, treating severe mental illness, substance abuse and post-traumatic stress disorders with cognitive behavioral therapy and psychopharmacology (psychiatric drugs). In recent years, however, she has switched her focus to a more Jungian-based psychotherapy in a private practice, seeing less severely ill patients and combining conventional treatment with what she calls a more "heart-centered" approach. "I work with people in difficult life transitions. I use dreams, repeating life patterns, meditation and imagery to help them get in touch with themselves and their psyches. It is less about drive, will and goals and more about understanding what is happening within the soul."

Accustomed as she was to managing difficult and challenging problems, Ellen knew she needed help with this one. During the lunch, her friend suggested that Ellen call Phuli Cohan, M.D., a specialist in women's health who was also trained in traditional Chinese medicine (TCM) and herbal medicine. "I called her office but they told me she had no appointments for a month," says Ellen. "I couldn't wait a month. I was on the edge, so I called the office again and left a desperate message on her answering machine, saying I needed help *right now*. Phuli called me right back and told me to come in the next day."

Menopause and Midlife: Caring for Body, Mind and Spirit

"Ellen was a mess," recalls Phuli. "I first saw her in the fall of 2000. She was forty-seven years old, and I believed she had been thrown into early menopause by the stress of her meningitis and the kidney surgery. She had also had children late in life, at thirty-seven. According to Chinese medicine, late pregnancies, as well as the normal aging process, deplete 'kidney energy,' which is thought to weaken the adrenal system, which the Chinese consider the most important organ system in menopause." (The adrenal glands, located on top of the kidneys, produce stress hormones, such as cortisol, as well as other hormones that are converted by the liver into sex hormones such as estrogen and testosterone.) As we have seen in previous chapters, TCM is based on the concept of energy—life force—that is called qi (pronounced "chi"). It is believed that qi travels along invisible pathways in the body, called "meridians," which have been well mapped over thousands of years of observation. (Please see Appendix I and chapters 2 and 6 for details about Chinese medicine and the concept of qi.)

"The Chinese notion of 'kidney energy' corresponds to what I learned in medical school about the adrenal glands, which are located on top of each kidney," says Phuli. Why are the adrenal glands and "kidney qi" so important in menopause? The explanation of this ancient belief, says Phuli, comes from conventional medicine: "As women age, the ovaries make fewer and fewer sex hormones (such as estrogen and progesterone). As the ovaries cease to function, sex hormones are still produced by the adrenal glands, as well as elsewhere in the body."

The role of the adrenal glands in sex hormone production is not well known, as Christiane Northrup points out in her book, *Women's Bodies, Women's Wisdom:*

"Though we've been taught to think of menopausal symptoms mostly as an estrogen deficiency state resulting from ovarian failure, this belief is based on incomplete information. First of all, estrogen is not the only hormone made by the ovaries. Androgens (male hormones), such as DHEA and testosterone, are also made by the ovaries, and so is progesterone. Total well-being at menopause and beyond depends at least as much on having adequate levels of these hormones as it does on estrogen."

These androgenic hormones, says Northrup, are produced by other sites in the body, including the adrenal glands, which increase their production of hormones as the ovaries decline. "Since androgens can act as weak estrogens and can also be precursors for the production of estrogens, it is clear that the healthy menopausal woman is naturally equipped to deal with hormonal changes in her ovaries. . . .

"In a healthy woman," continues Northrup, "the adrenal glands will be able to gradually take over hormonal production from the ovaries. Many women, however, approach menopause in a state of emotional and nutritional depletion that has affected optimal adrenal function. Under these conditions, a woman may require hormonal, nutritional, emotional and/or other support until her endocrine balance is restored."[1] (The endocrine system secretes hormones into the bloodstream to affect various processes throughout the body. It includes the thyroid, pituitary, pancreas and other glands.)

---

[1] C. Northrup, *Women's Bodies, Women's Wisdom* (New York: Bantam, 1998), 523–525.

From this perspective, Phuli explains how Ellen Johnson's weakened adrenals contributed to her menopause symptoms: "The adrenal glands also produce our 'fight-or-flight' stress- and disease-fighting hormones," says Phuli. "They give us our energy and vitality. But Ellen's adrenal glands were weakened from producing too much of these stress hormones and could not make up for the reduced estrogen production of her ovaries. Weak adrenal glands (conventional diagnosis) result in weakened kidney energy (Chinese diagnosis), but despite the differences in diagnoses, the result is the same: She was not producing adequate amounts of estrogen and other sex hormones and suffered from hot flashes, sleep disturbances and mood changes. She was also at risk for osteoporosis." (Please see "Building Healthy Bones" later in this chapter.)

Ellen, according to Phuli, was run down to begin with, both because of the normal aging process and by the toll on her body of childbirth late in life. "I believe the first signs of her weakened immune system due to adrenal deficiency were the viral meningitis and viral pneumonia, which occurred four years after the birth of her second child," she says. "Then, when they removed her kidney—possibly further weakening her adrenal gland—she was thrown into rather premature menopause."

Phuli points out that 20 percent of women go through menopause without symptoms. "I believe this is because they have strong and healthy adrenal glands. If we merely give women synthetic hormones, we are treating the 'leaf' (symptom) and not the 'root' (cause), as my first teacher of Chinese medicine would say. I believe it is far more effective to build up the adrenal function with a combination of herbs and acupuncture, as well as provide *natural*, low-dose hormone replacements if necessary."

For the past twenty years, Phuli has been treating women by combining her conventional medical training with training in Chinese and herbal medicine and homeopathy. After receiving her medical training from Brown University School of Medicine, she studied Chinese medicine, herbal medicine and homeopathy in New Zealand, Australia and India, where she worked alongside Ayurvedic physicians and homeopaths. She was certified in acupuncture at a program for physicians at the University of California and worked in private family medicine practice in that state. She also worked alongside *kahunas* (local healers) in Hawaii. She then became board-certified in emergency medicine and spent several years training and leading disaster teams as a "Med Flight" helicopter rescue physician. "I trained some of the first disaster medicine teams that eventually went to Ground Zero in New York," she says. (She has since become interested in exploring holistic approaches to the newly defined "World Trade Center Syndrome," now being described in survivors and rescue workers, which includes breathing problems, muscle pain, headache, cough and fatigue caused by exposure to asbestos and noxious gases. The "toxic injury" story in chapter 6 describes these illnesses in more detail.)

Phuli's interest in women's health came from her growing realization, both in medical school and in practice, that conventional medicine does not fully address many of the health problems specific to women. "Chinese medicine taught me to analyze pulses, the tongue, the eyes and to perform a detailed physical and psychological examination of a woman's symptoms, state of mind and subtle health conditions," says Phuli. "I then use biochemical methods, including twenty-four-hour hormone and metabolic analyses of urine and blood tests, to confirm what I see."

After examining Ellen from both the Western and Chinese perspectives, Phuli ordered blood tests and twenty-four-hour urine samples (requiring the patient to collect urine at various times over twenty-four hours). "I do twenty-four-hour tests because hormone levels fluctuate during the day, and I want to get the most accurate measurements," says Phuli. Ellen's single blood test showed a normal estrogen level, but the twenty-four-hour urine test told a different story: "Her adrenal hormone reserves were low; she had low thyroid function; and her DHEA level was very low," says Phuli. DHEA, produced by the adrenal glands, is the most abundant hormone in the body and is responsible for producing all of our sex hormones. The symptoms of DHEA deficiency include poor sleep (including REM sleep), depression, fatigue and poor memory. Both DHEA and thyroid deficiencies, according to Phuli, are common in women going through menopause. She is also interested in exploring the relationship between adrenal (kidney energy) weakness and such conditions as chronic fatigue, candidiasis (yeast infection), autoimmune diseases (in which the body attacks part of itself, such as multiple sclerosis and Crohn's disease—See chapter 6) and fibromyalgia (which is characterized by pain and fatigue, also described in chapter 6). "I routinely test my patients' adrenal hormone production when I am looking not only at menopause, but at these conditions as well," she says.

"All of the hormone-producing glands, including the pituitary, adrenals, ovaries and thyroid, are interrelated. When one is depleted, it 'borrows' from the next one," Phuli explains. "Ellen's thyroid was working overtime to fill the production gaps left by her weakened adrenals." To help Ellen, Phuli used a variety of conventional and complementary methods: "I used acupuncture to stimulate her immune function and to build up her weakened thyroid and kidney energy," she says. "I also gave her natural thyroid tablets, as well as natural estrogen and natural progesterone in skin creams, called 'transdermal' lotions. Unlike synthetic hormones, natural hormones closely mimic the molecular structure of the hormones in our bodies, without any 'foreign' additives or animal hormones. I also prescribed melatonin, a naturally occurring hormone, for temporary help with sleeping." Natural hormones are manufactured by specialized "compounding" pharmacies and can be tailor-made to fit the particular needs of any individual woman. Since they are applied in a cream, women can adjust the dosages as their symptoms change.

Phuli notes that she could also have used herbs to build up Ellen's thyroid and adrenal production, but that would have taken longer. "She was so miserable that I wanted her to have relief as soon as possible, and acupuncture and hormones work faster," she says. "Depending on the time of the cycle and a woman's particular condition, herbs, natural hormones and acupuncture can all be used to treat insomnia, fatigue, depression, hot flashes, low sex drive, hair loss, mood swings, vaginal dryness, urinary frequency and bone loss." Although Ellen had been taking herbs, they alone were not as effective when her symptoms became more severe.

Within weeks, Ellen was feeling better. "She had fewer headaches, the depression was lifting, and she was sleeping better," says Phuli. "The heavy periods began to taper off, and the breast soreness disappeared."

Two years later, Ellen, looking vibrant and youthful at forty-nine, reports on her condition: "There have been huge changes in my body, and they are reflected in the hormone measurements in periodic urine samples," she says. "I am only having very light periods every three months now, and Phuli taught me how to adjust the hormonal creams as my symptoms fluctuate. I feel as healthy and normal as I've ever felt. No insomnia, no mood swings. I'm back at work, exercising three times a week and using weight training to build bone density."

Phuli does not believe in long-term use of hormones, even natural ones. "You should be able to stabilize women by treating their underlying hormone deficiency with acupuncture, herbs and natural hormones, but eventually, you want women to go off the hormones as their bodies strengthen and are able to take over hormone production. I believe that even as women age, we should not have to suffer from the symptoms or signs of hormone deficiency. Ongoing health maintenance—diet, nutrition, lifestyle, supplements and hormonal replacements as needed, should be enough to sustain our health." Phuli is a member of the Anti-Aging Medical Society, which promotes this view. "There are now more than ten thousand physicians worldwide who are members and share this belief," she says.

Ellen says that her illness and recovery have taught her a great deal. "Phuli has inspired me to begin to learn about nutrition and health on my own," she says. "I still see my conventional doctor, through my health plan, but I continue to consult with Phuli every few months and to read." (Ellen's favorite books are those by Christiane Northrup on women's health and menopause, as well as *Nutritional Healing* by James F. Balch and Phyllis A. Balch. Please see Appendix II for other resources.) "This illness taught me to understand my body and my relationship to the world in a whole new way and has given new perspective and depth to my work as a psychotherapist."

✓ TAKE ACTION ✓

Best Ways to Cope with Menopause
Suggestions from Phuli Cohan, M.D.

There are many books and Web sites about combining conventional and complementary methods for relief of menopause symptoms. Some of the most useful are listed in Appendix II. Making decisions is even more difficult as the debate on the safety and efficacy of hormone replacement therapy (HRT) rages on, causing further confusion to woman and their doctors. Below is a summary of what are generally agreed to be some of the most helpful conventional and complementary methods, but you should consult with your doctors and practitioners and read as much as possible on the subject before embarking on any therapeutic program.

1. This is a time of great inner change. Consider your life and lifestyle. Are you happy in your life and work? What would you change?
2. Hot flashes: use 800 units a day of vitamin E and 1,500 to 3,000 mg of primrose oil.
3. Black cohosh works well for hot flashes if they are not too severe, but it may take three to six weeks for optimum benefit.
4. If hormones are needed, always use bioidentical natural forms. You can get these by prescription. There is no need for synthetic estrogen or progesterone. (See research note on hormone replacement.) Studies have shown that bioidentical hormones are at least as effective as synthetic hormones in reducing symptoms.
5. Don't use oral forms of estrogen. Use transdermal creams or patches. These are available by prescription. Transdermal creams or patches avoid excessive estrogen metabolism by the liver, are less toxic to use and easier to regulate. (Bioidentical transdermal hormone creams are available from specialized laboratories.)
6. Insomnia can be helped with progesterone and low doses of melatonin. (Note that doses of melatonin over .5–1 mg can worsen insomnia.)
7. Be assertive and diligent. Schedule a baseline bone density test at age fifty and do annual mammograms, particularly if you are on hormones.
8. If you do not feel good on hormones, stop, complain and change.
9. Always use DHEA with physician guidance. Most over-the-counter preparations are too high. Most women need only 10 to 20 mg per day and not for long-term use.
10. Don't use the same dose and the same supplements and hormones forever because your body changes. Take breaks and get update consultations each year about what you need.

The Life Cycle of a Woman: As a River Flows [2]

"A woman's health is like a riverbed," says Phuli Cohan, M.D. "The invisible life force called 'qi ' and the blood flow through a woman's body as water flows in a river. If the river is dry, or if boulders and twigs obstruct the flow of water, it will cause the water to stagnate in small pools. In a woman's body, when qi or blood flow is obstructed, patients complain of pain, such as breast pain or menstrual cramps; we might see fibroids or cysts in the breasts or ovaries. It is not necessary to have severe menstrual cramps or breast pain with your period. If you do, it's because you have obstructed flow of qi or blood. This is very treatable with herbs, acupuncture and/or natural hormones."

Traditional Chinese medicine explains a woman's health during the childbearing years as a function of the flow of qi through the liver meridian, according to Phuli. "This meridian goes around the pelvic organs and the rectum, wraps around the liver and gallbladder, goes through the breasts and thyroid gland and ends at the eye. From my observations, the liver meridian is women's health in a nutshell: For example, I don't think I have ever seen a woman with breast disease or breast cancer who also doesn't have some symptoms along this meridian, including pelvic disorders, hemorrhoids, gallbladder or liver disease, thyroid problems and migraines."

(Note: Blocked or "stuck" liver qi can also lead to the symptoms of premenstrual syndrome (PMS), according to Phuli. Please see the box for suggestions on how to deal with PMS.)

When puberty begins for a woman, the flow of blood and qi is downward, toward the ovaries and uterus, says Phuli. "This downward flow shifts in middle-age: Just as tides may shift the direction of a river's flow, a woman's qi and blood flow shift direction to flow upward, towards the heart." Phuli stresses that when most women reach their late forties, the kidney meridian and kidney energy become predominant: "At this time in a woman's life, we should enhance the function of the adrenal glands to produce enough hormones in order to avoid difficult menopause symptoms like those that Ellen was having."

---

2 Material in this section is drawn from interviews and from *Shifting Tides*, ©2002, an unpublished manuscript by Phuli Cohan, M.D. Used with permission of the author.

In her study of Chinese medicine, Phuli came across an ancient Chinese text that encapsulated this wisdom: "It is written that after 'seven times seven years,' [i.e., forty-nine], the sea of blood shall no longer flow downward to nourish the womb but alter its direction upward to nourish the heart." Rather than seeing menopause as a medical condition to be feared and treated, Phuli celebrates this change of life. "The shift in our tides brings us more in touch with our hearts and spirits," she says. "It is a time to draw our attention inward, to focus on our own growth, now that our children are grown, and to gain new insights about our life's purpose. We can use this time to nurture ourselves and to make a difference in our world."

AVOIDING PMS: PHULI'S RECOMMENDATIONS FOR NOURISHING THE BODY DURING THE MENSTRUAL CYCLE.

Many of the symptoms of PMS can be linked to "stuck liver qi," says Phuli Cohan, M.D. "The liver meridian is responsible for moving blood during the menstrual cycle. During the first half of the cycle, the body starts to store the fluid that is getting discarded from the lining of the uterus. If ovulation does not occur, the blood and fluid begins to move out of the body during the second half of the cycle. If the qi (energy) is blocked or disturbed, it can go upward, causing breast swelling, migraine, irritability, insomnia and neck tension. Or, the flow can be stuck in the lower channels, causing bloating, bowel problems and cramping. We can use herbs and acupuncture to open the channels and restore the flow of both qi and blood."
(Note: Always check with your doctor and practitioners before doing anything!)

During the first two weeks of the cycle:
This is the time to feed and nourish the blood and qi.
1. Foods that support the qi and blood: digestible, cooked orange and yellow vegetables, meat, such as lamb (unless you have a cholesterol problem) and other foods rich in blood, warm, cooked foods, root vegetables, "earthy" things.
2. Vitamins and minerals (only after you have been found to be deficient), including calcium and magnesium, iron, vitamin E (an antioxidant, which protects cells), vitamin B6 (from whole grains, nuts, legumes, brussels sprouts, cauliflower and potatoes), primrose oil/flax oil/borage oil (essential fatty acids). Black cohosh may also be helpful. The Chinese herb *rheumaniae* nourishes the blood and is an important component in most Chinese tonics for women. (See also the research section.)

During the second half of the cycle:

This is the time to support the liver function to help "move" the qi and blood to facilitate the menstrual flow. Avoid, if possible, anything that the liver must metabolize, or digest, such as excess caffeine or alcohol, rich foods or foods with preservatives, and almost any drug. Some people should avoid cold foods, such as salads, during this time.

1. *Herbs* (always in consultation with a professional) that cleanse and support the liver, such as dandelion root, burdock, milk thistle, bupleurum. The herb vitex (chaste tree) supports the progesterone function in the second half of the cycle.
2. *Acupuncture* along the liver meridian helps.
3. *Tai chi, yoga and qigong exercise* all help to free up the liver, as well as simple stretching and breathing exercises.

 ## Women at Midlife: What's the Evidence?

A note on hormone replacement: Because there is so much conflicting evidence about hormone replacement, it makes sense to follow Christiane Northrup's suggestion to have an individual hormone profile to determine where you are deficient. Then you can discuss the various options with your doctor. Northrup suggests that such a profile be done in the early to mid-forties, *before* the symptoms of menopause begin, so that you know which levels are right for you. "Then her ideal levels will be known beforehand, making it much easier to create a replacement regime that is tailor-made for her should she require it."[3] Northrup's book also contains comprehensive information, along with related evidence, of all the hormone options currently available. For example, she explains the meaning of bioidentical (also called natural) hormones. The bioidentical hormones are "derived from hormones found in soybeans and yams, but their molecular structure is modified in the laboratory to match those found in the human body exactly. . . . The amount of hormone is also standardized, so that its effects are measurable and predictable."[4]

---

[3] Northrup, *Women's Bodies, Women's Wisdom*, 540.
[4] Ibid., 539.

Imagine twenty-three menopausal women with hot flashes

A recent study appears to support the comments in this chapter about the importance of the kidney and adrenal system in menopause, at least from the perspective of TCM. Nine TCM practitioners independently examined twenty-three healthy menopausal women with hot flashes on the same day. The most frequent diagnosis made by the practitioners was kidney yin (energy) deficiency.

Well, at least they got some relief

In a study of acupuncture, eleven menopausal women with a variety of symptoms had five weekly sessions of acupuncture. According to questionnaires they filled out, acupuncture significantly improved hot flashes and other physical symptoms both during the treatment and up to three months after the last treatment. But it did not improve "psychosocial or sexual" symptoms and did not change the level of hormones in the body. (The women were not questioned after the three-month period.)

DHEA in a transdermal hormone cream

Christiane Northrup cites a study of postmenopausal women age sixty to seventy who used DHEA skin cream. "After a year of treatment, the women experienced a 10 percent decrease in body fat, a 10 percent increase in muscle mass, decreased blood-sugar levels, decreased insulin levels, and a decrease in cholesterol. Their vaginal tissue also showed a thickening similar to that seen with estrogen, but there was no increase in stimulation of the uterine lining. There was also an increase in bone density. Unfortunately, these women also experienced a 70 percent increase in the oiliness of their skin, which resulted in acne—an effect that could probably be reduced with somewhat lower doses."[5]

Synthetic vs. "natural" hormones?

One study tested the benefits of a "micronized" form of natural progesterone that is "readily absorbed and reaches peak concentrations" in one to four hours, when given with synthetic estrogen in postmenopausal women. This prospective, multicenter, randomized trial found that the micronized form of natural progesterone was a "clinically effective, well-tolerated, and cost comparable alternative to synthetic progesterone." The study found that "only patients receiving MP (the natural hormone) showed specific improvements in

---

[5] Ibid., 870.

the menstrual problems and cognitive domains" as reported in a questionnaire.

More about DHEA and herbs

Kenneth R. Pelletier, Ph.D., M.D., (hc), reports on several studies showing the benefits of DHEA for post-menopausal women in protection against cancer, osteoporosis and heart disease, and in conjunction with estrogen to treat hot flashes and other symptoms.[6] He also cites studies showing that herbs such as dong quai and black cohosh can help with menopausal symptoms, but should only be used under the supervision of a medical professional because of potential negative side effects.[7]

Beating premenstrual syndrome (PMS): Cut the fat, add herbs and supplements, and get moving

A study of the National Cancer Institute found that women with lower-fat diets (20 percent of calories) had significantly fewer PMS symptoms than women with higher-fat diets (40 percent of calories). Alpha-tocopheral and calcium carbonate supplements were both found to reduce PMS symptoms. In a 1985 study of 92 women, three grams daily of evening primrose oil for three to six months significantly reduced cyclical breast pain. In an even larger study of 165 women, ginkgo biloba significantly reduced "congestive" PMS symptoms, particularly breast complaints. And a 1994 study of 97 women with PMS symptoms at the University of Queensland in Australia found that regular exercise improved concentration, disposition and pain.[8]

A sobering view

Black cohosh, soy and relaxation techniques may have some benefit, but that's the only good news so far in complementary therapies for menopause symptoms according to Edzard Ernst in his review of randomized controlled trials. (Not all studies fall into this category, which use matched subjects randomly assigned to control groups and experimental groups.) "There is no compelling evidence for the efficacy of any complementary treatment for alleviating menopausal symptoms, particularly in comparison with hormone replacement therapy," he writes. "However, black cohosh looks encouraging in this respect and has a favorable safety profile. . . . Soy may have potential, particularly for reducing hot flushes, so efforts to increase consumption of soy products in the diet

---

[6] K. R. Pelletier, *The Best Alternative Medicine: What Works? What Does Not?* (New York: Simon & Schuster, 2000), 109.
[7] Ibid., 365.
[8] Ibid., 193.

may be worthwhile. Relaxation techniques also appear to have some benefits."[9] He also mentions kava as a "promising option." (Note that the FDA, however, is now requesting information about cases of liver failure being linked to excessive use of kava. See, for example, *www.fda.gov/medwatch/safety/2001/safety01.htm#kava*.)

Pelletier reports that Remifemin, a black cohosh extract manufactured in Germany, "is the most widely used natural alternative to hormone replacement therapy. More than 1.5 million women in Germany have used Remifemin since 1956 with remarkable effectiveness." He lists several studies conducted by the American Botanical Council that document the therapeutic effects of Remifemin in treating menopausal symptoms. However, he notes, "Although much of the research reported on black cohosh has not met the gold standard of RCTs (randomized controlled trials), the benefits of the herb are well-documented for treating premenstrual and menopausal conditions. Additional research with improved design will help to substantiate these findings."[10]

Other studies cited by Ernst showed only "transitory" improvement in symptoms with acupuncture and little or no benefit (when compared to placebo) of several herbs, including ginseng, red clover and evening primrose oil.[11]

RESEARCH IN THE PIPELINE:
STUDYING DIETARY SUPPLEMENTS FOR WOMEN

In 1999, the National Institutes of Health awarded a grant to the University of Illinois's Chicago College of Pharmacy to create one of the nation's first centers to research dietary supplements. The UIC Center for Botanical Dietary Supplement Research in Women's Health has begun to evaluate herbal supplements that are widely used by women in this country to treat menopausal symptoms, premenstrual syndrome and urinary tract problems. Studies will also focus on the risks and benefits of alternatives to estrogen replacement therapy.

---

[9] E. Ernst, ed., *The Desktop Guide to Complementary and Alternative Medicine: An Evidence Based Approach* (London: Harcourt Publishers Limited, 2001), 307.
[10] Pelletier, *The Best Alternative Medicine*, 158–159.
[11] Ernst, *The Desktop Guide to Complementary and Alternative Medicine*, 307.

The Center will be evaluating the following botanicals through basic research and clinical trials: black cohosh, red clover, chasteberry, hops, cranberry, black haw, dong quai, Asian ginseng, ginkgo, licorice and valerian. Clinical trials of black cohosh, red clover and chasteberry began in 2001. The studies will address the safety of these botanicals and their ability to reduce the frequency and intensity of hot flashes and other menopausal symptoms.[12]

References

Aganoff, J. A. and G. J. Boyle. "Aerobic Exercise, Mood States and Menstrual Cycle Symptoms." *Journal of Psychosomatic Research* 38, no. 3 (1994): 183–192.

Chen, F. P., et al. "Changes in the Lipoprotein Profile in Postmenopausal Women Receiving Hormone Replacement Therapy." *Journal of Reproductive Medicine* 43, no. 7 (July 1998): 568–574.

Dong, H., et al. "An Exploratory Pilot Study of Acupuncture on the Quality of Life and Reproductive Hormone Secretion in Menopausal Women." *Journal of Alternative and Complementary Medicine* 7, no. 6 (December 2001): 651–658.

Jones, D. Y. "Influence of Dietary Fat on Self-Reported Menstrual Symptoms." *Physiology and Behavior* 40, no. 4 (1987): 483–487.

London, R. S., et al. "Efficacy of Alpha-Tocopherol in the Treatment of the Premenstrual Syndrome." *Journal of Reproductive Medicine* 32, no. 6 (1987): 400–404.

Pye, J. K., et al. "Clinical Experience of Drug Treatments for Mastalgia." *Lancet* 2 (1985): 373–377.

Ryan, N., et al. "Quality of Life and Costs Associated with Micronized Progesterone and Medroxyprogesterone Acetate in Hormone Replacement Therapy for Nonhysterectomized, Postmenopausal Women." *Clinical Therapeutics* 23, no. 7 (July 200): 1099–1115.

Sahelian, R. "Landmark One-Year DHEA Study." *Health Counseling* 9, no. 2 (1997): 46–47.

Tamborini, A. T., et al. "Value of Standardized Gingko Biloba Extract (Egb761) in the

---

[12] For more information, the University of Illinois at Chicago/National Institutes of Health Center for Botanical Dietary Supplement Research in Women's Health can be reached at (312)-996-7253, or at *www.uic.edu/pharmacy/research/diet*.

Management of Congestive Symptoms of Premenstrual Syndrome." *Revue Francaise de Gynecologie et Obstetrique* 88, no. 7–9 (1993): 447–457.

Zoll, B., et al. "Diagnosis of Symptomatic Postmenopausal Women by Traditional Chinese Medicine Practitioners." *Menopause* 7, no. 2 (March–April 2000): 129–134.

Additional information on the adrenal glands and estrogen production can be found in J. Bullock, M. Wang, and J. Boyle, NMS (*National Medical Series) Physiology*, 2nd edition. Baltimore, MD: Lippincott, Williams & Wilkins, 1990. On the Internet, also see *www.helioshealth.com/menopause/estrogen*.

Building Healthy Bones[13]

Like a never-ending urban renewal project, the bones of the body are constantly being rebuilt. In the case of the human body, the renewal goes on at the rate of about 5 percent a year. "Every fifteen or twenty years, each person has a new, complete skeleton," says Michael Rosenblatt, M.D., former chief of the Bone and Mineral Metabolism Division of Boston's Beth Israel Deaconess Medical Center.

Each person, that is, except for postmenopausal women, whose reduced estrogen levels slow down the rebuilding process. The result is osteoporosis—thinner, more fragile bones that increase the risk of debilitating fractures of the spine, hip and wrist. "What a lot of people don't appreciate is that osteoporosis is a potentially lethal disease," says Rosenblatt, the George R. Minot Professor of Medicine at Harvard Medical School. "The risk of dying within twelve months of a hip fracture is 10 to 20 percent." Among those who survive, one half are unable to walk unassisted and 25 percent are confined to nursing homes for long-term care. (Osteoporosis also affects certain middle-aged and older men, for whom hip fractures are associated with more difficult recovery and higher mortality than for women.)

More than thirty million Americans, most of them women, suffer from osteoporosis, making this potentially debilitating disease more common than heart disease or diabetes. The lifetime risk of hip fracture for white women, in fact, is

---

[13] Some of the material in this section first appeared in an article by Roanne Weisman for *Pulse* magazine (published by Beth Israel Deaconess Medical Center, Spring, 2000). Used with permission.

as great as the risk of breast, ovarian and endometrial cancer combined, according to the National Institute of Arthritis and Musculoskeletal and Skin Diseases.

Two cells are responsible for the normal "bone renewal" process, Rosenblatt explains: one of these, called an osteoclast, carves its way through bone, leaving empty channels in its wake. This process is called bone *resorption*. "Osteoclasts are the only cells that can actually chew their way through bone," says Rosenblatt, "almost like little 'Pac Men.'"

Following close behind the osteoclasts are other cells, called osteoblasts, that rebuild bone in response to the body's needs, including changes in diet or exercise. "When things go right, the 'blasts' replace exactly the amount that the 'clasts' tear down, keeping the bones in a state of equilibrium," says Rosenblatt. But lowered estrogen levels during menopause result in resorption overtaking rebuilding. "Even a slight edge in resorption—as little as 2 percent per year—can result in a woman losing 40 percent of her bone mass over a period of twenty years," says Rosenblatt.

Osteoporosis is an insidious disease; other than bone density tests, there are no warning signs until a bone breaks, according to Rosenblatt and other osteoporosis experts. By the time the disease has progressed far enough for a woman to fracture her hip or spine, it is almost too late to rebuild her skeleton. Experts advise women to have bone-density tests and to make choices early—before and during menopause—about how to take care of their bones. Prevention strategies include a calcium-rich diet, along with vitamin D, and a regular routine of weight-bearing exercise.

✓ TAKE ACTION ✓

Best ways to prevent and reverse osteoporosis

Harold Rosen, M.D., is director of the Osteoporosis Prevention and Treatment Center at Beth Israel Deaconess Medical Center. "There is clearly an effect of diet and exercise on skeletal health, and not just for older people," says Rosen. "There are good data that *from childhood* on you can improve your bone density with weight-bearing exercise and adequate amounts of calcium and vitamin D. Developing high peak bone mass earlier in life is like putting "calcium in the bank" for use later on.

Some postmenopausal women, however, may also need estrogen and other hormone supplements, as well as drugs, to prevent bone resorption. (See the Research section.) Rosen's recommendations:

- **1,000 to 1,500 mg of calcium and 400 to 800 mg of vitamin D every day.** The benefits of these supplements have been well established. One study of more than three thousand healthy elderly women compared those who took the two supplements daily for eighteen months with those who took a placebo (the control group). The women taking calcium and vitamin D had greater increases in bone density and significantly fewer hip and other fractures than the placebo group.

  Based on studies showing that many menopausal women are also deficient in magnesium, Christiane Northrup, M.D., also recommends **300 to 800 mg of magnesium per day in the form of citrate or malate.**[14]

- **Thirty minutes of weight-bearing exercise five times a week.** "If you add an aerobic component, through brisk walking or jogging, you get added cardiovascular benefits," advises Rosen, noting that swimming, while aerobic, does not increase bone density. "There are data to suggest that the more you beat up on your skeleton, the more it will have to respond by thickening up," he says. That is why gymnasts have less bone loss than swimmers." "However," warns Rosen, "you must also be careful to avoid injury. Weight training is probably safer than tumbling on a mat." (See "A Closer Look at Pilates.")

- **Have a bone-density test at menopause when you need to decide about hormones or other drugs.** The test is to detect osteoporosis or osteopenia—a precursor condition leading to osteoporosis. After that test, Rosen notes, future bone density tests would depend on whether patients are taking hormones or good osteoporosis treatments and on "whether there is any reason to believe that she would not respond to the usual measures." Studies have shown that for postmenopausal women, calcium and exercise alone may not prevent bone

(continued)

---

[14] Northrup, *Women's Bodies, Women's Wisdom*, 553.

loss, says Rosen. "But when combined with estrogen, the result is better." Rosen also recommends that women at risk for osteoporosis consider Fosamax, Actonel or Evista, all of which are "anti-resorptive" (preventing bone loss).

- **Avoid foods and practices that hasten bone loss:** smoking, sugar, carbonated beverages. (See below, "Are You at Risk?"). While caffeine can accelerate bone loss, Rosen does not advise against it if you are taking enough calcium.

- **Eat a well-balanced diet.** "If you're starving, you won't build bone," says Rosen. In her book, Christiane Northrup provides a nutrient-rich, whole-foods diet, including vitamins K and C and zinc, in addition to vitamin D. She also warns that the phosphates contained in colas and root beer interfere with calcium absorption[15] and recommends many calcium-rich foods in addition to (or instead of) dairy products. These include green, leafy vegetables and green herbs, nuts, salmon, sardines, oysters, sea vegetables and legumes.[16]

- In addition to all of these suggestions, Glenn Rothfeld, M.D., (the integrative physician in chapter 6), points to the importance of **adequate sleep, stress reduction, as well as proper hormone balance** (not just estrogen). "Estrogen prevents bone loss, but does nothing to grow new bone," he says. "Progesterone, DHEA and testosterone all have the ability to promote bone growth, and all can be deficient, especially in the menopausal woman."

ARE YOU AT RISK FOR OSTEOPOROSIS?[17]

You might be if any of these risk factors apply to you:

— Smoking

— A history of excessive alcohol intake

— A mother with severe osteoporosis

— A sedentary lifestyle—lack of regular exercise

— A diet high in refined carbohydrates

— Deficiencies in calcium, boron, trace minerals and vitamin D

— Never having borne a child

— Depression and stress. These have also been shown to be a significant risk factor for osteoporosis, according to Christiane Northrup. This is most likely caused by the increased levels of cortisol (a stress hormone) usually associated with this condition.

---

[15] Ibid., 552
[16] Ibid., 716.
[17] Northrup, *Women's Bodies, Women's Wisdom,* 550; interview with Glenn Rothfeld, M.D.

Reversing Osteoporosis: What's the Evidence?

The most serious —and potentially life-threatening—dangers of osteoporosis are fractures, especially of the hip. Most research therefore focuses on ways to build and maintain strong bones (peak bone mass) and increase balance and strength to reduce the risk of falls and fractures. These goals can be achieved through diet, supplements, medication and weight-bearing exercise.

The National Institutes of Health, in a March 2000 conference on osteoporosis prevention, diagnosis and therapy, came up with the following recommendations, based on a review of scientific literature from 1995 to 1999 and nearly twenty-five hundred references:

—**Adequate calcium and vitamin D** intake is crucial to develop optimal peak bone mass and maintain it throughout life.

—**Regular exercise, especially resistance and high-impact activities in young adulthood,** contributes to development of high peak bone mass and may reduce risk of falls later in life.

There's more to bones than calcium

The effects of **calcium, vitamin D,** as well as estrogen, on osteoporosis prevention are well known. But research cited in Wayne B. Jonas's book tells us more: One study demonstrated that sixteen of nineteen women with osteoporosis were deficient in **magnesium**. As part of another study, postmenopausal women took magnesium supplements for one year. Twenty-two out of thirty-one women had increases in their bone density, and another five women remained stable. **Vitamin K** markedly reduced bone loss in postmenopausal women and **trace minerals, folic acid, vitamin B₆, vitamin D, boron, silicon and strontium** may also be important in osteoporosis prevention.

Strength training: Do as much as you can and your bones will get stronger

Even moderate physical activity has been associated with higher bone mineral density (stronger bones) in postmenopausal women, according to one study. A comment on that study was quick to point out that while moderate activity is beneficial, women should not be discouraged from performing vigorous exercise. "It is safe to conclude," wrote one researcher, "that an exercise prescription for the prevention of osteoporosis should include weight-bearing exercise, but the optimal intensity, frequency and duration of exercise remain to be established."[18] In other words: do what you can.

And in case you don't know where to begin . . .

In her book *Strong Women Stay Young,* Miriam E. Nelson of Tufts University presents a strength-training program that can be done at home, with weights. The program is based on her own research into the benefits of strength training.

NEW DEVELOPMENTS IN OSTEOPOROSIS: RESEARCH IN THE PIPELINE

Several conventional studies are testing promising treatments to reverse bone loss:

Viper venom to save bones. Osteoclast cells tear down bone by attaching to the surface of bones like tiny suction cups, with a tight seal surrounding a space, explains Michael Rosenblatt, M.D., of Beth Israel Deaconess Medical Center. (Please see text for a description of how osteoporosis causes bone loss.) "The osteoclast then secretes enzymes into the suction cup, literally 'digesting' the bone beneath it," he explains. A few years ago, researchers at Beth Israel Deaconess synthesized a molecule that can attach to the bone surface, forming a "competitive blockade" that prevents osteoclasts from sticking to bone cells and secreting their bone-digesting enzymes. This molecule was derived from a protein called echistatin, found in the venom of the saw-scaled viper. As of this writing, researchers are testing the effectiveness of this "blocking" treatment in clinical trials.

A different approach: a hormone that builds new bone. Another way to treat osteoporosis is to build new bone, rather than prevent bone resorption, as in the echistatin study. This method uses the actions of parathyroid hormone (PTH). Circulating normally throughout the body, PTH is responsible for keeping the correct amount of calcium in the bloodstream, ensuring that the heart beats, nerves fire and blood clots properly. When the calcium level in the body drops, the parathyroid gland releases PTH to go to the body's "calcium bank"—the bones—to cause the release of more calcium

(continued)

---

[18] W. M. Kohrt, "Osteoprotective Benefits of Exercise: More Pain, Less Gain?" *Journal of the American Geriatrics Society* 49, no. 11 (November 2001): 1411–1417.

into the bloodstream. "But when PTH is injected at low doses and intermittently, it has the exact opposite effect," says Joseph M. Alexander, Ph.D., who is working on the research. "It actually creates new bone; we do not yet understand the exact mechanism, however." A 2001 study of PTH involving more than 1600 post-menopausal women found that the hormone decreased the risk of fractures and increased bone density with minor side effects (occasional nausea and headache).

Researchers at Beth Israel Deaconess are now working to design smaller molecules that will mimic the function of PTH. An important caution: "While PTH is one of the only methods to build bone, rather than prevent bone loss, it has caused bone cancer in laboratory animals," says Harold Rosen, M.D. "While promising, this treatment should be viewed with caution, and clearly requires further research."

Osteoporosis: References

Chapuy, M. C. "Vitamin D₃ and Calcium to Prevent Hip Fractures in Elderly Women." *New England Journal of Medicine* 327, no. 23 (December 1992): 1637–1642.

Cohen, L. and R. Kitzes. "Infrared Spectroscopy and Magnesium Content of Bone Mineral in Osteoporotic Women." *Israel Journal of Medical Sciences* 17 (1981): 1123–1125.

Colbin, Annemarie. *Food and Our Bones.* New York: Penguin Putnam, 1998.

Friedlander, A. L., et al. "A Two-Year Program of Aerobics and Weight Training Enhances Bone Mineral Density of Young Women." *Journal of Bone and Mineral Research* 10, no. 4 (April 1995): 574–585.

Hagberg, J. M., et al. "Moderate Physical Activity Is Associated with Higher Bone Mineral Density in Postmenopausal Women." *Journal of the American Geriatrics Society* 49, no. 11 (November 2001): 1565–1567.

Johnston, C. C., et al. "Calcium Supplementation and Increases in Bone Mineral Density in Children." *New England Journal of Medicine* 327, no. 2 (July 1992): 82–87.

Jonas, W. B. and J. S. Levin, eds. *Essentials of Complementary and Alternative Medicine.* Baltimore: Lippincott, Williams & Wilkins, 1999, 465.

Kohrt, W. M. "Osteoprotective Benefits of Exercise: More Pain, Less Gain?" *Journal of the American Geriatrics Society* 49, no. 11 (November 2001): 1411–1417.

National Institutes of Health Consensus Panel on Osteoporosis Prevention, Diagnosis and Therapy. *Journal of the American Medical Association* 285 (2001): 7858–7895.

Neer, R. M., et al. "Effect of Parathyroid Hormone (1–34) on Fractures and Bone Mineral Density in Postmenopausal Women with Osteoporosis." *New England Journal of Medicine* 344, no. 19 (May 2001): 1434–1441.

Nelson, M. E. *Strong Women Stay Young.* New York: Bantam, 1998.

Northrup, C. *Women's Bodies, Women's Wisdom.* New York: Bantam, 1998. This huge and comprehensive book about all aspects of women's health contains a detailed program to prevent and reverse osteoporosis, evaluating the benefits of exercise, nutrition and herbal methods as well as such drugs as Fosamax (alendronate) and Miacalcin (calcitronin).

Riis, B., et al. "Does Calcium Supplementation Prevent Postmenopausal Bone Loss? A Double-Blind, Controlled Clinical Study." *New England Journal of Medicine* 316, no. 4 (January 1987): 173–177.

Sojka, J. E., and C. M. Weaver. "Magnesium Supplementation and Osteoporosis." *Nutritional Reviews* 53 (1995): 71–74.

Taeffe, D. R., et al. "Differential Effects of Swimming Versus Weight-Bearing Activity on Bone Mineral Status of Eumenorrheic Athletes." *Journal of Bone and Mineral Research* 10, no. 4 (April 1995): 586–593.

A Closer Look at
Osteopathy—Movement Is All

"Osteopaths focus on the structure of the body and how it functions," explains Rachel Brooks, M.D. "The goal is to restore the free, natural flow of movement at all levels, whether in the bones and joints, muscles and ligaments, the organs within their sheaths of connective tissue, or the flow of blood, lymph fluid or the cerebrospinal fluid that bathes and cushions the spinal cord and nerves throughout the body." Brooks lives in Portland, Oregon, is a graduate of the University of Michigan Medical School and is board-certified in physical medicine and rehabilitation. "Though an M.D. by training, I've devoted my whole professional life to osteopathy," she says. Just before entering medical school, Brooks met Rollin E. Becker, "a wonderful osteopathic physician who was my mentor until his death several years ago." Brooks has, in fact, edited several books about Becker and osteopathy.

Dr. Andrew Taylor Still, a physician who served in the Union Army, founded osteopathy in the late 1800s. "After his wife and children died in an epidemic of spinal meningitis, Still became disillusioned with the tools of allopathic medicine," says Brooks. "He developed osteopathy as a hands-on way to treat people that built on what he believed to be the body's own inherent capacity to heal." Some of the key principles of osteopathy are:

1. The body is a unit; the person is a unit of body, mind and spirit.
2. The body is capable of self-regulation, self-healing and health maintenance.
3. The structure and function of the whole body are related.

Dr. Still developed a method of using the hands to affect the structure of the body to encourage and restore the free and natural flow of movement on every level.

There are a number of manipulative approaches in osteopathy. Brooks practices a type called "cranial osteopathy," an extremely gentle practice that she uses to treat problems related to injury and illness. She can use the method to treat ear infections in children, pain throughout the body resulting from muscle strain or trauma, infections and menstrual problems.

Our bodies are never still, says Brooks. In addition to the beating of our hearts and the breath that flows in and out of our lungs, there is a constant pulse of movement throughout our organs and tissues. "Cranial osteopaths work from the principle that this constant, natural 'pulsing' within the body is how the body maintains itself in a state of health," she says, explaining that this pulsing has been linked to the slow, rhythmic movement of the cerebrospinal fluid originally described by osteopathic physician William Garner Sutherland in the 1930s. "By finding out where this rhythm is blocked, whether it is caused by injury or illness, and then helping the body to release that blockage, we can reduce pain and restore health," says Brooks. "For example, promoting a greater flow of lymph fluid, which helps to clear infection, allows the body to work more efficiently to recover from pneumonia and other infectious diseases."

Brooks explains how cranial osteopathy works, using childhood ear infections as an example. "Many people think of the adult head as a solid 'bowling ball' type of structure, but that is not the case," she says. "The bones of a newborn's skull are moveable and then become connected by seams called sutures as we grow. The skull solidifies but even in the adult it always retains a resilience in the suture connections. I could train you to place your hands on someone's head and feel the slight, rhythmic, rocking movement that is normally present." The ear, Brooks explains, is located in a chamber inside the "temporal bone" of the skull, on either side of the head. "If something, either a birth trauma or an injury, jams the temporal bone, limiting its natural rocking motion, the fluids that flow inside the ear cannot drain normally," she says. "And if fluid is relatively still and stagnant, it is more prone to infection."

Brooks explains that in every case she first examines the whole body to find out where the restrictions are, even if they are not located near the area of the symptoms. "Often, restrictions elsewhere in the body can have important effects on the area where the symptoms are," she explains. To treat the temporal bone, Brooks holds the head while the patient is lying on a table. Following the body's own rhythm she uses gentle, barely perceptible motions to encourage the free movement of the temporal bones. "I do not apply a significant force from the outside," she says. "I use my hands and my own intention to help the body find a state of balance and to support it while allowing the tissues to release. I have found colicky, irritable babies respond well to this treatment, as well as adults with head or neck injuries and pain."

Over the years since Still created the practice of osteopathy, it has entered into the field of mainstream medicine. Doctors of osteopathy (DO) are certified to practice all medical specialties, including surgery. However, they add a more holistic approach as well as their special training in osteopathic manipulation.

Osteopathy—What's the Evidence?

Research on osteopathy is not plentiful. But studies indicate that it is effective for musculoskeletal pain, especially for post-operative recovery and lower back pain, although one study found no significant difference between osteopathic treatment and standard medical care. In addition, Wayne Jonas, M.D., reports on several studies that show benefit for children with recurrent ear infections, developmental delays and attention-deficit disorders, although Jonas stresses the need for more research.[1]

---

[1] W. B. Jonas and J. S. Levin, *Essentials of Complementary and Alternative Medicine* (Baltimore, MD: Lippincott, Williams & Wilkins, 1999), 299.

In his review of the literature on osteopathy, Edzard Ernst, M.D., Ph.D., agrees that there is some evidence to suggest that osteopathy is helpful for low back pain, "particularly acute and subacute stages." For other indications, "the clinical trail evidence is sparse and not compelling."[2]

John Mark, M.D., at the University of Arizona Integrative Medicine Program, reports that research is currently underway to study children who are prone to ear infections who are being treated with gentle craniofascial massage and osteopathy, compared to children who receive conventional treatment. There are no results yet.

(See also "Breathing Easier" in chapter 9 for research on osteopathy in children and adults with asthma.)

References

Agresti, L. M. "Attention Deficit Disorder: The Hyperactive Child." *Osteopathic Annals* 14 (1989): 6–16.

Andersson, G. P., et al. "A Comparison of Osteopathic Spinal Manipulation with Standard Care for Patients with Low Back Pain." *New England Journal of Medicine* 341, no. 19 (November 1999): 1426–31.

Frymann, V., et al. "Effect of Osteopathic Medical Management on Neurologic Development in Children." *Journal of the American Osteopathic Association* 92 (1992): 729–744.

Gintis, B. "AAO Case Study: Recurrent Otitis Media." *Journal of the American Academy of Osteopathy* 6, no. 2 (Summer 1996): 16.

Jarski, R. W., et al. "The Effectiveness of Osteopathic Manipulative Treatment as Complementary Therapy Following Surgery: A Prospective, Match-Controlled Outcome Study." *Alternative Therapies in Health and Medicine* 6, no. 5 (September 2000): 77–81.

Lesho, E. P. "An Overview of Osteopathic Medicine." *Archives of Family Medicine* 8 (1999): 477–483.

---

[2] E. Ernst, ed., *The Desktop Guide to Complementary and Alternative Medicine: An Evidence-Based Approach* (London: Harcourt Publishers Limited, 2001), 65.

11

AGING WELL
"Don't fence me in."

Virginia ("Jinny") Chapin describes herself as an extrovert. "I like to connect with people. In Jungian terms, I like to imprint myself on my
environment."

Here is Jinny's environment: She lives alone with two golden cats in a sunny
apartment in Cambridge, Massachusetts, with a circular "tower" room; a walnut
farm table that seats ten; pots of herbs and plants thriving on window ledges; a
treadmill (for when she can't get out to exercise); a study lined with floor-to-
ceiling bookshelves displaying her passions for gourmet cooking, Jungian psychology, art, music and architectural history; and paintings, wall hangings,
prints, sculptures, maps and drawings from all over the world, gathered in her
travels. "I have met almost all the people whose art I have," she says. "I would
have loved to have known Rembrandt, but I can't afford him anyway."

Jinny spends her summers in a rental cottage in Maine, swimming regularly
in the frigid ocean. "It is very stimulating," she says. "I can spend about fifteen
minutes thrashing around and come out looking like a cooked lobster. I believe
seawater is therapeutic: The ocean is the mother of us all." (Please see chapter
3 for more about the health benefits of cold water.) During the summer, she also
works out three times a week at a nearby health club.

During the spring and fall, Jinny walks twenty-five minutes every week to her
community garden plot (She sold her car long ago and walks or takes public
transportation everywhere). On this early spring day, she has just planted her

peas, lugging forty pounds of topsoil in a grocery cart up the hill. When she first got the garden ten years ago, she spent eight hours "double-digging" down eighteen inches to aerate it. "I did it in two-hour shifts," she says. This spring, as usual, she will fertilize it with cow manure and topsoil as well as with minerals and fertilizer that she orders during the winter. When she needs help with transportation, a friend with a neighboring plot drives her. "She offered to be my chauffeur if I'd be her gardening guru," says Jinny. This year, she plans to grow her usual crops, including rhubarb, herbs, potatoes, tomatoes, eggplant, lettuces, beets, carrots, onions, arugula and tiny wild strawberries.

Did I mention that Jinny Chapin was born in 1915? No matter. It hardly seems relevant. "I guess I'm still a child at heart," she says. She's already planning her ninetieth birthday party: "It will be a dance party with a jazz combo," she says. "Stick around."

There is far more to Jinny's life than swimming and gardening. She has regular shiatsu massages and osteopathic treatments, practices yoga and has been working out at a Pilates exercise studio twice a week for the past seven years. "All of this keeps things moving and aligned," she says. (Please see "Closer Look" sections and Appendix I for descriptions of alternative practices.)

When she's not moving her body, she coordinates volunteers at the Harvard Institute for Learning in Retirement, where she also co-teaches a course in analytical psychology and is currently taking two courses: Cosmology, and Literature and Opera. She listens to the Metropolitan Opera every Saturday on the radio, and cooks herself a gourmet dinner most evenings. "Last night, I made golden beets with beet greens, a mélange of red peppers, okra, zucchini, onion and garlic, cooked in olive oil, served over gemelli pasta," she says. "I also like lamb and pork, but mostly fish."

Jinny has had only two major health problems in her long life: "Twenty years ago, when I was in my sixties, I had pneumonia, and it took me about a year to get my energy back," she says. "Then my knee began bothering me when I was eighty-three and I needed to use a cane. An arthroscopy didn't help, so I had the whole joint replaced. After a few months, I was better than ever!"

Today, at eighty-six, Jinny is a spry woman with short blond hair and clear blue eyes, wearing beige knit pants, a turtleneck sweater and sensible walking shoes. She moves gracefully through her apartment (no more cane), showing a visitor with pride how well her "new" knee works and sharing the story and artifacts of nearly nine decades of a well-lived life. Divorced twice and the mother of two, Jinny has been an amateur actress and a faculty wife, and has traveled extensively, living for a time in Costa Rica during World War II with her first husband and two small children. After her first divorce, she lived with her children in Washington, D.C., managed a bookstore and sold real estate. During and after her second marriage, she lived in Illinois and New York City, studied fine arts at NYU, became certified as a graphologist (handwriting expert) at the New School for Social Research and began what was to become a lifelong study of Jungian psychology at the C. G. Jung Foundation. She also became director of a committee providing service and information to United Nations delegations. "All of my life, I have refused to be tied down," she says. "Don't fence me in."

What Can We Learn from People Who Live to One Hundred?

Jinny Chapin is a mere youngster compared to more than a hundred people in New England who have passed their one-hundredth birthdays and who are participating in the New England Centenarian Study (NECS), a joint project of Boston Medical Center and the Harvard Medical School, founded and directed by geriatrics expert Thomas T. Perls, M.D., M.P.H. (The study was originally located at Beth Israel Deaconess Medical Center in Boston.) NECS is the first comprehensive investigation of the world's oldest people. Since 1994, Perls and associate director Margery Hutter Silver, Ed.D., have been analyzing the mental, physical, and emotional health of centenarians in New England. "Our goal is to use our discoveries about this group to expand our understanding of the aging process in the larger population," says Perls. Centenarians, in fact, are the fastest-growing age group in the United States, according to Perls.

The study has already resulted in significant findings. Perls and his colleagues have looked for clues to longevity in families with several centenarians, focusing especially on long-lived sibling pairs. They have analyzed data on everything from lifestyle and diet to the DNA found in blood samples. "The results seem to indicate a link between genetics and longevity," says Perls. "And once we discover which genes play a major role in aging, we can develop drugs that interfere with or potentiate the processes these genes regulate."

The centenarians in Perls's study not only have had long lives, they have also delayed or escaped many of the diseases commonly associated with aging, including cancer, Alzheimer's, stroke and heart disease. "We believe that there are a few genes that have powerful influences both on how fast we age and our susceptibility to the diseases of older people," says Perls. "This is the first time anyone has used humans to discover the genes associated with extreme old age. People with average genes have a life expectancy into the mid-80s. But there appear to be special genes that can get you past 100."

In their book, *Living to 100: Lessons in Living to Your Maximum Potential at Any Age*, Perls and Silver describe several centenarians who have reached extreme old age in good health, exploding the myth that aging has to be associated with disease and deterioration. "Contrary to the belief that 'the older you get, the sicker you are,' most of the people we studied weren't bed-bound, ill or demented," says Perls. "They were all independent until their early nineties, and only had illnesses at the very end of their lives. They got to one hundred because of extreme good health."

In presenting the findings of their research, Perls and Silver make it clear that even if you don't have the "extreme age" gene, it is possible to live a full, long, healthy life by following the examples of those who have done just that. "We look at aging as an opportunity rather than a curse," says Perls.

✓ TAKE ACTION ✓

Best ways to live a long, healthy life—Do what centenarians do

According to the New England Centenarian Study, directed by Thomas Perls, M.D., M.P.H., and Margery Hutton Silver, Ed.D., people who have passed their one-hundredth birthday may have the genes to help them, but they also have lifestyles that are remarkably similar. Some of their research findings:[1]

1. Healthy centenarians stay connected with others of all age groups and involved in their communities.
2. They keep physically active with regular, daily exercise. One woman in the study, 101 years old, had a habit of reading while riding a stationary bicycle. Other centenarians baked and cooked for family gatherings, went to the office and played golf.
3. They continue to use their brains throughout their lives. "Learning new skills all through life contributes to healthy brain function," says Perls.
4. They have learned how to handle stress and the many losses that happen on the way to one hundred. Perls describes the life of a Holocaust survivor as an example: "[She] never became trapped in anger or self-pity, nor did she expend undue energy on hatred toward the Nazis. All her resources were focused on engineering the survival of herself and her family."[2]

   "If people can emulate centenarians, either through stress reduction programs, alternative approaches like yoga, or a regular physical exercise program, we believe they stand a much better chance of coping with the mental and physical problems of old age," according to Perls.[3]
5. They use humor to cope with difficult times. The title of the section in Perls's book that describes the importance of humor for emotional and physical health is called "He who laughs lasts."
6. They find meaning in some kind of spiritual practice and seem to take a lively interest and joy in everything around them.

The centenarians in the NECS study have valuable lessons to teach, most of which are exemplified in the life of Jinny Chapin, who seems well on her way to becoming a centenarian herself. Like them, Jinny maintains a wide network

---

[1] T. T. Perls and M. H. Silver, *Living to 100: Lessons in Living to Your Maximum Potential at Any Age* (New York: Basic Books, 1999).
[2] Ibid., 63.
[3] Ibid., 70.

of social and family connections, stays physically active, has a varied diet, low alcohol consumption and does not smoke. She is a member of a group to help preserve Boston Harbor and has been a volunteer counselor to inmates at a county jail, using hand analysis (in which she has a private practice) as well as conventional counseling. She keeps in touch with her body through massage, yoga and Pilates exercise (See Appendix I and "Closer Look" sections) and keeps her brain alive as both a student and a teacher.

Perls and Silver explain in their book the importance of lifelong learning: It is possible for the brain to grow new "dendrites," branchlike extensions that reach out toward neighboring neurons (brain cells), enabling the exchange of electric and chemical messages in the brain. These new dendrites may replace or replicate existing connections or create new links to neurons. "Such cell growth takes place throughout life and compensates for cell loss," they write. "New dendritic formation may be stimulated by learning new skills or taking up new activities." In fact, report Perls and Silver, autopsy examinations of the brains of many centenarians who were part of the study has revealed no sign of "neuritic plaques" and "neurofibrillary tangles"—the telltale brain lesions that define Alzheimer's disease.[4]

Humor is another personality trait that Jinny Chapin shares with the centenarians in the NECS study. Perls and Silver use examples from their own research, as well as other studies, to point to the benefits of humor, which helps people "cope emotionally, think creatively and solve problems," as well as laughter, which increases the concentration of disease-fighting antibodies in the bloodstream. In addition, they write, "Laughing helps people relax and stay alert. During laughter, muscles throughout the body—in the head, neck, chest and pelvis—tense and relax, in the same way that they do during stress reduction techniques like yoga. This helps keep muscles limber when in use, and also allows them to rest more easily."[5]

The late Norman Cousins, former editor of *Saturday Review*, wrote about overcoming a crippling disease with humor and positive thinking. In his 1981 book *Anatomy of an Illness*, Cousins described how he used Marx Brothers films

---

[4] Ibid., 30.
[5] Ibid., 73.

and other sources of humor to cope with pain. "I made the joyous discovery that ten minutes of genuine belly laughter had an anesthetic effect and would give me at least two hours of pain-free sleep."[6] Later in the book, he describes how he became convinced that "creativity, the will to live, hope, faith, and love have biochemical significance and contribute strongly to healing and to well-being. The positive emotions are life-giving experiences."[7]

When asked for her own secrets of longevity, Jinny says, "I'm a bloody-minded optimist. You cannot foretell or foresee the future; you can learn from the past, but you cannot retrieve it. You can only live in the moment, because that's the only thing you have. I don't believe in guilt. I pay attention to my dreams because they are a part of my consciousness. One friend called me to say she dreamed she had lost her head. I said, 'Thank goodness! You've been in your head too long. It's time you got out of your head and into your heart.'"

A much older woman, a participant in the New England Centenarian Study, echoes Jinny's optimism and positive outlook. During a recent interview, this hundred-year-old woman showed her visitor a photograph and said, "I am particularly enjoying this photo my daughter just sent to me of a beautiful flowering plant in the desert, near where she lives." She handed over the photograph, her eyes lingering on the image of white flowers emerging from a bed of rock and sand. "Such beauty, pushing its way through the most difficult ground," she said with a smile. "What a miracle."

It's Not Just Your Genes, It's What You Do with Them: Reaching Our Biological Potential

Why are so many of us dying thirty or forty years before we are biologically programmed to do so? Kenneth R. Pelletier Ph.D., M.D., (hc), clinical professor of medicine at the University of Maryland and the University of Arizona Schools of Medicine, has been asking this question for more than twenty years. "There are well-documented cases of people living to the age of 120, without serious disease—the most recent example being Jeanne Calment of France, who died in 1997 after

---

[6] N. Cousins, *Anatomy of an Illness* (New York: Bantam, 1981), 39.
[7] Ibid., 86.

a brief illness at the age of 122," he says. "These people represent the upper limits of our life expectancy. We now know that it is biologically possible for the human species to have a healthy life for more than a century. What is preventing most people from fulfilling our biological potential for extreme longevity?"

Prior to his current medical school appointments, Pelletier investigated human health and longevity as director of the Complementary and Alternative Medicine Program of the Stanford University School of Medicine (funded by the National Institutes of Health). He is also an international health consultant for the World Health Organization, government and business. For many years, his research, clinical practice and publications have been the subjects of numerous national television programs. He has written ten major books on holistic, mind/body and alternative medicine and published groundbreaking research studies on healthy aging, cardiovascular health, stress management and corporate disease management programs.

Pelletier feels that genes certainly play some role in how long we live, but he stresses that the genes we inherit are far less important than the *way* we choose to live our lives. "Even if some people have the genetic predisposition to live a long time, they may die young because of an unhealthy lifestyle. By contrast, people who may not have the 'longevity' genes can live very long lives despite their genetic predisposition," he says. "The transfer of DNA takes place in that infinitesimal moment when the egg and sperm unite and engender genetic expression. But everything that you do for the rest of your life actually determines whether or not that genetic predisposition is realized."

In one of his books, Pelletier cites research to support this position. For example, he summarizes one study of longevity based on life insurance records that compared two groups of people of a similar age, one group with parents who were long-lived and one group with short-lived parents. The people with long-lived parents had a life expectancy at age twenty that "probably did not exceed by three years" the life expectancy of the second group. Statistically, at least, having parents who lived a long time did not necessarily confer a longevity advantage.

Pelletier's interest in aging began more than twenty years ago when he was researching preventive medicine—particularly in the area of heart disease. "I had written a book in the early eighties (*Holistic Medicine: From Stress to Optimum Health*) looking at conventional and alternative methods to prevent disease," he recalls. "But I quickly realized that the same factors that promote the *quality* of life, by promoting good health, also contribute to the *quantity* of life.

In his research at Stanford and now at the University of Maryland and University of Arizona Schools of Medicine, Pelletier and his colleagues continue to investigate the best ways to ensure a healthy, long life. "We are seeing a phenomenon that has been termed 'squaring the curve,'" he says. "People who live longer seem to have more years of health and vigor before they die. And when they finally do die, they do not seem to linger and suffer with long-term disease. Their ultimate death is fairly quick and involves relatively brief periods of suffering, disability and pain, by comparison with people who die in their sixties and seventies. It would seem that if you can stay healthy until your sixties, you have a good chance of staying healthy well into your eighties, if not beyond." (Please see boxes for Pelletier's evidence-based suggestions of lifestyle choices that help to achieve a healthy old age.)

One of the problems older people face, says Pelletier, is Western society's attitudes toward aging. "The idea of retirement at age sixty-five is based on a completely arbitrary decision made about a hundred years ago in the German Weimar Republic in order to save money on social security," he says. "As a result, sixty-five is now considered the age at which people outlive their usefulness—at least in Western cultures. There is no biological reason for retirement, yet people are made to feel useless and less intelligent, and these feelings can contribute to depression and health problems. By contrast, many Asian cultures revere and respect the wisdom that comes with age."

✓ TAKE ACTION ✓

Best lifestyle changes to make now—to improve both the quality of life and the quantity of years
(from Kenneth R. Pelletier, Ph.D., M.D., (hc)

"There is an enormous difference in the way people age," says Pelletier. "There's the eighty-year-old in the nursing home and the eighty-year-old who hikes to the base of Mount Everest to celebrate his birthday." By making healthy lifestyle choices now, you may be able to influence your aging process.

1. **Examine your physical environment:** Bright lights and access to natural light help to avoid injuries due to falls as well as SAD (seasonal affective disorder): Sadness and depression are often associated with the lack of natural light in winter. Access to nature is also important for general buoyancy of spirit. Even if you don't live near a park or green space, a small window garden might suffice. (Remember eighty-six-year-old Jinny Chapin: Both she and her vegetable garden continue to flourish.)

2. **Social support and connection with other people of** *all* **ages** help to mitigate the depression that is often associated with aging. Maintaining friendships and connections with people of all ages, whether through family, or through community or religious groups has been associated with good health. (See the research conclusions of the New England Centenarian Study in this chapter.) If you are in a long-term care facility, inquire into joint programs with local schools or daycare centers. (See "The Joy of Creating" for an example of one such facility that hosts regular "tea and art" afternoons with a nearby daycare program.)

3. **Open yourself up to the possibility of forgiveness,** both of yourself and others who may have harmed you in the past. In his book, *Forgive for Good* (Harper Collins), Frederick Luskin, Ph.D., describes the health benefits of forgiveness. His research demonstrates that people who went through a structured program of learning how to forgive had measurable improvements in their health. This effect is even more important for older people, who may have accumulated years of resentment and anger. (See chapter 8 for details about Dr. Luskin's research.)

4. **Appreciate the assets of growing older,** including the accumulation of wisdom, the opportunity to reflect and to convey that wisdom to others. Writing journals or memoirs, or expressing yourself in the creative arts is one way to do this. (Please see "The Joy of Creating.")

(continued)

5. **Continued physical intimacy and sexuality** appear to be a common denominator among long-lived people. Although the relationship between sexuality and longevity may not be clear, says Pelletier, what is clear is that people who hug, kiss and remain sexually active seem to lead longer and happier lives.

6. **Nutrition after sixty** (some say after forty) should be less rich, lighter, simpler and more focused on whole grains, beans, cooked (but not overcooked) vegetables and fruit. Pelletier recommends a multivitamin every day because "foods are often depleted of nutrients, either in growing or in preparation." Two recent research studies demonstrate the importance of nutrition in preventing the mental and physical deterioration that comes with age:

   —One study at the University of Iowa found that most people over seventy-nine living independently were not getting enough nutrients, including folate (a B vitamin that helps to prevent heart disease and stroke), vitamin D and calcium (which help to prevent osteoporosis and fractures).

   —While the best way to improve nutrition is an adequate diet, supplements were found to be helpful as well. A study found that people over sixty-five who were given a supplement of vitamins and trace minerals showed improvements in short-term memory, problem-solving, abstract thinking and attention. The author recommended a supplement containing the recommended doses or less of most vitamins and minerals and somewhat larger amounts of beta-carotene and vitamin E. In a previous study, the author found that a similar supplement helped to boost immunity to infectious disease.

Successful Aging with Complementary Methods: What's the Evidence?

Keep your balance with tai chi

Major fractures due to falls are frequently fatal in the elderly. Studies have shown that the regular practice of tai chi, a series of slow, flowing exercise movements originating from traditional Chinese medicine improves balance, coordination and strength in the elderly and helps to prevent falls. (See Appendix I and chapter 6 for details about Chinese medical practices.)

A 1996 study found that elderly people who took a tai chi course reduced their risk of falling by 47.5 percent, compared with a control group that took a training course in balance. Another study compared tai chi to balance training, strength training, and combined balance and strength training in people with an average age of eighty. Those who learned tai chi gained significantly more balance and strength than the other groups.

In addition to describing the studies above in his book, Pelletier conducted his own research into tai chi: "A study I was involved in with my colleagues at Stanford indicated that loss of balance with age is not inevitable," he says. "Our preliminary findings show that even people of advanced age with balance problems can restore their equilibrium by using tai chi. Anecdotal evidence also suggests that the practice can enhance mood."

(Please also see "A Closer Look at Yoga" for the benefits of yoga—another mind/body method—in improving balance, posture and flexibility.)

Ginkgo biloba for clear thinking

A supplement made from the leaves of the world's oldest living deciduous tree is used with some success to treat the symptoms of dementia-related memory deficits, concentration problems, depression and vascular-related problems in the elderly according to Kenneth R. Pelletier,[8] who also points to what he refers to as an important 1997 study of Alzheimer's patients by LeBars and associates, published in the *Journal of the American Medical Association*. "[G]inkgo induced modest improvement in, or a delay in the decline of, cognitive function, living skills, and social behavior." In addition, says Pelletier, the extract may be capable of producing noticeable increases in intellectual performance in normal, healthy subjects.[9] *(NOTE: It is important to check with your doctor before taking any supplement or medication.)*

While the final word about ginkgo biloba is still not established, many herbs are useful antioxidants. (Antioxidants remove free radicals which can cause cell damage.) A few examples of other herbs with health benefits include green tea, as well as other teas made of nettle leaf, peppermint, chamomile, rooibos or raspberry leaves. (These herbs are suggested by Alexa Fleckenstein, M.D., whom you met in chapter 3.)

Ease those aching joints

"As we age," says Pelletier, "inflammation is a problem. This might include inflammation in the joints, causing the pain of osteoarthritis, as well as inflammation in the vascular system and in the bowel." Chemical anti-inflammatories may have major side

---

[8] K. R. Pelletier, *The Best Alternative Medicine: What Works? What Does Not?* (New York: Simon & Schuster, 2000), 163.
[9] Ibid.

effects, but Pelletier has identified several herbal and nutritional supplements that seem to work just as well to reduce the pain of osteoarthritis, with fewer side effects. These include glucosamine sulfate, which was found to be as effective as ibuprofen, with fewer adverse reactions. "Glucosamine is currently being investigated in a large NCCAM-funded multicenter randomized controlled trial as an effective nutritional supplement (for arthritis). Considerable animal research indicates that glucosamine alone may arrest arthritic deterioration."[10]

Several other complementary treatments have been shown in research trials to be effective for alleviating the pain of arthritis and joint inflammation. These include SAMe, a nutritional supplement that was as effective and better tolerated than a nonsteroidal anti-inflammatory drug; the herb capsaicin, which reduced pain in arthritis patients; and pulsed electromagnetic field stimulation, which is a method of physical medicine. (For more research about pain relief, please see chapter 7.)

In March 2000, the *Journal of the American Medical Association* published a review of glucosamine and chondroitin for the treatment of arthritis. The authors concluded that trials of both supplements demonstrated that these preparations were "probably" effective. The authors were concerned about "quality issues" and "likely publication bias " causing "exaggerated" claims.

[10] Ibid., 186, 325.

SUCCESSFUL AGING: RESEARCH IN PROGRESS

Several ongoing research projects will soon provide more evidence about what contributes to healthy aging. (No final results yet.)

A three-year demonstration project at the Stanford Medical School is showing that 100 people between 55 and 85 can learn to combine conventional and complementary medicine to create healthy lifestyles, reduce disability and disease and enhance optimum health. The SAGE (Successful Aging Growth Experience) project, founded by Kenneth R. Pelletier, Ph.D., M.D., (hc), began in April 2000 and is training three small groups of about thirty older adults in optimal nutrition, mindfulness meditation (See "A Closer Look at Meditation"), guided practice in tai chi and moderate exercise. Leaders also help group members share their experiences of the training as well as their feelings about aging.

"We hope to demonstrate that older adults can learn to take an active responsibility for improving their health and that this flexible approach will develop sustained positive change in lifestyle," says Pelletier, who was the former project director as well as founder. "Once SAGE has demonstrated its effectiveness, it is our intention to use the success of this program to influence health plans, HMOs, and Medicare to offer comprehensive lifestyle modifications programs in their health plans for older adults to achieve and sustain 'successful aging' for us all."

In other research at Stanford, Pelletier and his colleagues have been involved in ongoing studies of:

Ginkgo biloba and its effect on memory, blood clotting factors and quality of life in men and women between sixty-five and eighty-five;

A "Round the Clock" Wellness Program for people over fifty-five, to evaluate strategies for improving daytime and nighttime quality of life, focusing on such topics as aging, nutrition, use of supplements, exercise, sleep and disease prevention;

The "Community Health Advice by Telephone" (CHAT) study to compare the effectiveness of different telephone-based counseling strategies to motivate participants to start and maintain a regular exercise program;

The "Wellness Interventions for Self Enrichment" (WISE) study to evaluate a one-year program of tai chi exercise, a standard program of Western exercise and a health education class that will include the latest information on wellness and disease prevention.

✦ ✦ ✦ ✦

The Joy of Creating

A delightful surprise awaits you in the Laurelmead retirement residence. If you walk down the long passageway from the independent living apartment complex toward the attached building that contains the Assisted Living, Skilled Nursing and Alzheimer's units, you will see four large windows displaying colorful and whimsical scenes. The four form part of a row of sun-filled windows lining the passageway.

Each of the stained glass windows beautifully illustrates a folktale from a different cultural tradition: "The Magic Brocade" is a story of courage from ancient China. "The King With the Dirty Feet," from India, is about creativity and the invention of shoes. From Africa comes the story of "Kimwaki and the Weaver Birds," teaching a lesson about cooperation and friendliness. "Meshka the Kvetch (complainer)" comes from Russia, and tells the story of a woman who learned to see the beauty in life rather than her own miseries. A fifth window, about Native Americans and Rhode Island's first settlers, will be installed soon.

All of the windows are low enough to be seen from a wheelchair, and each window has a comfortable chair next to it, along with a frame holding the text of the folktale (in easy-to-read large print.) "It feels good to see people from the nursing home being wheeled along the hallway, looking at the windows, and either reading the stories or having the attendants read to them," says Lillian Weisz in her melodious voice. She is a petite woman of seventy-nine with a light step, deft hands and bright hazel eyes that seem permanently crinkled into a smile.

It is the artistry and imagination of Lillian Weisz that has transformed this hallway into a place of joy, hope and optimism. Lillian lives with Paul, her husband of almost sixty years, in one of Laurelmead's independent living apartments. Almost as soon as they moved into the complex just a few years ago, she began her stained glass project, teaching a group of residents to work with her. "We are excited that we have almost completed our fifth window," she says.

Before they begin work on each window, Lillian and the group of residents select the folktale, discuss it and begin to draw illustrations. When they agree on the images to include, Lillian incorporates the ideas into designs that are feasible for cut glass shapes. "Some people cut the glass, others wrap the edges of each piece in copper foil, and then we solder the pieces together," says Lillian. "It is truly a group effort."

Lillian did not discover her creative abilities until she was sixty-five years old. "Both my father and grandfather were talented amateur artists," she says. "But I was too busy raising three children and volunteering to think about art!" Her life in stained glass began fifteen years ago with a snowstorm and a broken window. "We were shoveling a huge mound of snow in front of our house when a handle flew off a shovel and cracked one of the leaded glass panes at our front door," she remembers. "I was wondering how we were going to get it fixed when I happened to see an advertisement in the newspaper for a stained glass course at a nearby senior center."

Lillian signed up for the class. "I had never thought of working with stained glass before this," she says. She soon realized that the course at the senior center was not technical enough to teach her how to repair the thick leaded glass at their house, but by then she was hooked. She had become so fascinated by what she was learning that she stayed in the class and has been working with stained glass ever since. In the years that followed, she continued to create her own fanciful designs, began to teach classes in the technique, and built windows of ever-increasing beauty and complexity. Several "Weisz windows" now decorate her neighborhood: They can be seen in the children's hospital, the library and a nearby synagogue. When she and Paul, a former professor of biology and a scientific textbook author, moved into the Laurelmead residence, it seemed only natural for her to use her growing skill to create stained glass windows to brighten up the facility.

"That first class unleashed a flood of creativity in me that I never suspected," she says. "For me, working in stained glass is all about connections. There are so many interweaving links in life, and if we remain alert and receptive, even as we grow older, we can make connections with others and with our own accumulated thoughts and experiences. Working with other people to create meaningful designs has helped me realize that we do not have to be alone. Enthusiasm is catching!"

Perhaps inspired by his wife, Paul Weisz worked with Lillian to design and create a "Window of Hope." Paul is the only member of his immediate family in Vienna to survive the Holocaust. Today, at eighty, he moves with an inner strength and possesses a dignity that is reminiscent of his European heritage. His white hair and the penetrating, inquisitive expression in his dark eyes make it easy to understand the powerful impact he had on hundreds of biology students during his tenure at Brown University. (He still has a large notebook filled with the letters they continue to write to him.) The window he designed shows a golden Star of David rising from a dark, stormy sea into a rainbow of light. In 1994, this window was installed during a special dedication ceremony at the Jewish Community Center. During the ceremony, the Weisz's three children and seven grandchildren read excerpts from Paul's only nonscientific book, *Family in War*, which chronicles the story of his family during the Holocaust. "Both this window and the book honor the memory of my parents, sister and other family members who were murdered," says Paul.

The folktale windows in the retirement home passageway have created another unexpected benefit: an intergenerational connection between the senior residents and a local daycare center. "When the teachers at the center heard about our first windows, they asked if they could bring the children to see them," says Lillian. "Now, whenever we install a new window, we invite the children and the senior residents to a special tea party and window-viewing. We read the folktale and talk about its meaning as we look at the window." When "The Magic Brocade" was first unveiled, Laurelmead residents put on a puppet show and acted out the story for the children. The puppets (designed and made by the seniors) are now arranged on a trellis that decorates the wall opposite The Magic Brocade window, along with photographs of the children enjoying the show.

As they enter their eighties, Lillian and Paul have developed a lifestyle that seems to promote health, creativity and vigor. In addition to working on her windows, Lillian swims and takes an aerobic class several times a week. Paul walks every day; a few years ago, he founded "Laurelmead College," to allow residents with particular expertise to teach classes in the building. He taught biology and Lillian is currently taking classes in origami (Japanese paper art), American history and French.

"So many older people are angry and depressed because they are focusing on what they can no longer do, making themselves and others miserable, just like 'Meshka the Kvetch' in the Russian folktale," says Lillian. "I believe that it is okay to be angry and sad, as long as you are creative and patient as well: Channel that anger and sadness and create something—anything!"

WHAT IF AGING HAS ALREADY TAKEN ITS TOLL? IT'S NOT TOO LATE!

Not everyone is fortunate enough to reach old age in good health. Some people are mentally or physically impaired and cannot follow most of the suggestions in this chapter. The "Knitting With a Purpose" story tells about the experiences of some of these elders, and Enza Stabilé, a special care geriatric counselor, has some professional advice to add. Enza is Social Activities Coordinator at Place Kensington in Montreal, which has independent-living apartments as well as several assisted-living units for residents who need more nursing care.

"The assisted-living residents have short and long-term memory problems and are not able to take care of their own daily needs without nursing assistance," says Enza. "But these residents can still participate in activities, as long as they are at a slower pace with more direction. We help them to exercise while they are sitting down, using light weights and stretching their muscles. They also enjoy games such as mini-putt, beanbag toss and a modified game of bowling. We use a point system to make it more interesting and competitive." The residents also enjoy Bingo, which is played slowly and with the numbers being repeated.

(continued)

Music is a popular activity. "We have tea and music two afternoons a week," says Enza. "We invite musicians to play accordion, guitar and piano and we sing songs from the good old days. We also encourage the residents to play along on musical instruments and the staff helps people to get up and dance. People love this, and by the end everyone is smiling and singing."

The knitting program (See "Knitting with a Purpose," below) has been especially successful at encouraging both manual dexterity and social interaction among residents who had previously been more socially isolated. "We started a similar group program called the Cooking Club," says Enza. "Like knitting, cooking is a skill that they remember from the past, and with staff supervision, they can work in the kitchen together. They share their recipes and talk about how they used to cook for their families."

Residents also participate in "reminiscence therapy," a discussion group led by staff members that encourages people to talk about their life experiences. "The residents have better memories of their childhood and early years and really enjoy talking about them," says Enza. "The staff also helps people focus on the present by encouraging discussions about general knowledge, geography and current events.

One of the most successful programs is the Women's Nail Club. "Every two weeks the staff gives manicures to any woman who wants one," says Enza. "We have four people to a table and they talk and joke together, remembering when they used to go to a salon. We use bright colors, and they choose the nail polish they want. Even women who are almost always sleepy wake up when we tell them it is manicure time. They feel cared for and their hands look beautiful! At the end, some who think this is a real salon, will ask, 'How do I pay for this?' and we always say, 'Just give us a smile.' And they always do, usually with a big laugh as well."

Knitting with a Purpose *or* Never Too Old to Care

When Elinor Cohen had a stroke at seventy-three that incapacitated her right arm and leg, she was sure that she would never do anything useful again. From the time she was a child, her mother had taught her knitting, crocheting, sewing and other crafts and she had become proficient in each. "I was really down and depressed after the stroke," she says. "After spending time in a rehabilitation hospital and having occupational and physical therapy, I could take care of myself and walk with a cane, but I was awkward and clumsy. My writing was terrible, and I had given up hope of ever doing the handicraft work I loved."

Then she and her husband, Seymour, moved into an independent living apartment in Place Kensington, a senior residence in Montreal. "Shortly after we arrived, some of the women asked if I would join their knitting club," remembers Elinor. The group had been started about a year before by resident Miriam "Mimi" Berger, who came up with the idea of making blankets for the young teens in a homeless shelter. "Our mottos were 'Knitting With a Purpose' and 'Never Too Old to Care,' says Mimi. An energetic woman of eighty-three, Mimi is a former social worker known both for her creative ideas and her ability to make things happen.

The shelter chosen by the knitters—called *Dans la rue* ("In the street")— sends two vans out almost every night to find homeless adolescents and teenagers, including young single mothers, on the streets of Montreal. The staff invites them back to the shelter for a hot meal, clothing and a place to sleep. In a separate building, the program offers daycare for the children of teen mothers, high school classes, health services, and educational and vocational counseling. (For more information, see their Web site: *www.danslarue.com.*)

Elinor was initially reluctant to join the knitting group but decided to try one meeting. "I went that first time with a 'ho-hum' attitude," she remembers. "I wanted to please my new friends, but expected nothing for myself. I was sure that my knitting days were over. They gave me some needles and yarn, and I fiddled around for about ten minutes. Then my hand got tired, so I had a cup of tea and went home. That was all I felt good for."

Her friends encouraged her to try again, and she soon found herself there every week, sitting in a circle with the others, knitting as best she could, and chatting. "Everyone was sweet and encouraging, tea time was fun, and I enjoyed being with them, so I kept it up," she says. The women were knitting large squares of yarn, in bright colors. When they had enough for a blanket, they would spread the squares on the floor and decide together on the arrangement.

"Simplicity is key," says Mimi, the group's founder. "We all use the same size needles, the same number of stitches, and knit the same size squares. Then we all have a say in how the squares are put together. We insist that each blanket be beautiful and in good taste, the best we can turn out. Creating something for children who are homeless and poor means that we try harder!"

Within a few weeks, Elinor's knitting speed and stamina had improved, and she began taking needles and yarn back to her apartment to keep working. "Somewhere along the line, I realized that I was producing as many squares as anyone else," she says. "I wasn't even aware of it happening, but with their encouragement, I went from feeling helpless and useless to saying, 'Hey, I can do this!' I began to notice that my right hand was growing stronger and more agile in other ways as well. I could write and do small motor tasks more easily."

Elinor had joined the group at an exciting time. Over the previous year, the women had already created more than thirty blankets. By November 2001, forty blankets were ready to go. The knitters invited the shelter founder, Father Emmett "Pops" Johns, and one of his staff members to a "fashion show and blanket donation" tea party, complete with a guest pianist. "They even pinned a blanket around my shoulders, so I could model it while walking with my cane," says Elinor. "That made me feel just great."

Soon after the fashion show, stories about the Kensington Knitters and their blankets began to appear in several Canadian newspapers as well as in local and national television news. As word spread, skeins of donated yarn began to arrive and several knitters who had no connection to Place Kensington called to volunteer their services. "One woman sent us fifteen squares, more than enough for a whole blanket, that she made while her husband drove their car to Florida and back for the winter," says Elinor.

Later in the year, after the knitting club donated a second group of blankets, *Dans la rue* executive director Toni Cochand visited Place Kensington to meet the knitters and tell them how much their gifts were appreciated. "Our kids need to feel that someone cares about them," says Toni. "Having a homemade blanket reminds them that a senior took the time to make every stitch, just for them. We put them on the beds at our shelter for twelve- to eighteen-year-olds to make the rooms feel cozy and bright." At Christmastime, the shelter gave blankets to the teenage single mothers to take home. "Some took two or three to brighten up their apartments, cover up worn furniture, as well as to put on the beds," says Toni.

Under Mimi Berger's leadership, the knitting club has grown from three to more than twenty committed women. "The group gives us the chance to social-ize while contributing to our community," says Mimi. "Knitting is excellent physical therapy for old hands, and helping others with purposeful activity alle-viates or even prevents the depression that is common to older people." (Knitting has, in fact, been called "the new yoga," and is being touted as an excellent stress-reduction method. See, for example *Zen and the Art of Knitting*, by Bernadette Murphy.)

Within just a few months, Elinor had regained all of her former knitting prowess. "I became one of the knitting consultants and 'blanket finishers,' cro-cheting together the completed squares," she says. But she didn't stop there. "The shelter staff told us that they also needed scarves for the kids as well as slip-pers for them to wear in the centers after they leave their snowy or muddy shoes in the hallway. And the teenage moms needed sweaters and baby clothes for their children." Working with Mimi, Elinor designed a simple way to make slip-pers out of leftover yarn. They also designed a child-sized sweater made out of extra blanket squares. "Nothing goes to waste," says Elinor.

The new slippers were a big hit, according to Toni: "After dinner, the street kids go upstairs and have a shower. Then they put on clean nighties and paja-mas and the handmade slippers. It's a wonderful way to make them feel special again. If they want, they can keep the slippers."

The knitting program has spilled into the second floor of Place Kensington, the assisted-living unit for semi-autonomous residents. Once a week, Elinor and a few of the "downstairs knitters" go up to the second floor to provide knitting guidance to anyone who seems interested. "They don't talk very much, but we do sit and knit quietly together, and they seem to enjoy it," says Elinor. "One woman, who will do nothing else, has become a furious knitter. She kept call-ing downstairs every day, asking us to come up and start her on a new square.

Finally, we brought up a whole lot of yarn and told her to make sixty-inch scarves for the kids at the shelter. Each scarf takes her a week to do. We get a break, and she feels great about what she is doing!"

Doreen Friedman, one of the recreation and social activities coordinators of Place Kensington, is impressed by the therapeutic value of knitting, especially for the people in the assisted-living unit. "It seems to be like riding a bicycle," she says. "Once people have learned to knit, even if it was fifty years ago, they seem to always be able to do it. We have residents in the assisted-living unit who have difficulty with speech, but put some knitting in their hands and they just whirl away at it. And for the autonomous residents, the knitting group encourages active, healthy communication and a sense of purpose. It is certainly better than having them sit alone in their apartments watching television."

Working with Place Kensington, Mimi Berger and the Kensington Knitters are already planning another blanket fashion show and presentation. "We've got some absolutely gorgeous designs coming up," she says. "Being in our eighties and nineties (with a few seventies) doesn't faze us. In fact, we hope we will encourage other groups in the community to get involved in keeping our children warm and letting them know we care."

RESOURCES FOR ELDERS

www.longevityworld.com. This site provides timely discussion of age-related issues.
www.ThirdAge.com publishes a weekly health newsletter, *The Long Life Letter,* which provides updates on the latest research into health, longevity, diet and exercise.
AARP Andrus Foundation, *www.andrus.org*
Alliance for Aging Research, *www.agingresearch.com*
American Federation for Aging Research, *www.afar.org*
National Institute on Aging, *www.nih.gov/nia/*
American Association of Retired Persons, *www.aarp.org*
American Society on Aging, *www.asaging.org*
International Federation on Aging, *www.ifa-fiv.org*
International Year of Older Persons, *www.un.org/esa/socdev/iyop.htm.*

References

Caruso, I., et al. "Italian Double-Blind and Multicenter Study Comparing S-adenosylmethionine, Naproxen, and Placebo in the Treatment of Degenerative Joint Disease." *American Journal of Medicine* 83, no. 5A (1987): 66–71.

Chandra, R. K. "Effect of Vitamin and Trace Mineral Supplementation on Cognitive Function in Elderly Subjects." *Nutrition* 17, no. 9 (September 2001): 709–712.

Cousins, N. *Anatomy of an Illness.* New York: Bantam, 1981.

Deal, C. L., et al. "Treatment of Arthritis with Topical Capsaicin: A Double-Blind Trial." *Clinical Therapy* 13, no. 3 (1991): 383–395

Leaf, A. "Unusual Longevity: The Common Denominators." *Hospital Practice* (October 1973): 75–86. In K. R. Pelletier, *Longevity: Fulfilling Our Biological Potential*, New York: Dell, 1981.

Le Bars, P. L., et al. "A Placebo-Controlled, Double-Blind, Randomized Trial of an Extract of Ginkgo Biloba for Dementia." *Journal of the American Medical Association* 278, no. 16 (1987): 3127–3132.

Marshall, T. A., et al. "Inadequate Nutrient Intakes Are Common and Are Associated with Low Diet Variety in Rural, Community-Dwelling Elderly." *Journal of Nutrition* 131 (2001): 2192–2196.

McAlinson, T. E., et al. "Glucosamine and Chondroitin for Treatment of Osteoarthritis: A Systematic Quality Assessment and Meta-Analysis." *Journal of the American Medical Association* 283, no. 11 (2000).

Pelletier, K. R. *The Best Alternative Medicine: What Works? What Does Not?* New York: Simon & Schuster, 2000.

Pelletier, K. R. *Longevity: Fulfilling Our Biological Potential.* New York: Dell, 1981.

Murphy, B. *Zen and the Art of Knitting* (in press).

Perls, T. T. and M. H. Silver. *Living to 100: Lessons in Living to Your Maximum Potential at Any Age.* New York: Basic Books, 1999.

Trock, D., et al. "A Double-Blind Trial of the Clinical Effects of Pulsed Electromagnetic Fields in Osteoarthritis." *Journal of Rheumatology* 20, no. 3 (1993): 456–460.

Wolf, S., et al. "Reducing Frailty and Falls in Older Persons: An Investigation of Tai Chi and Computerized Balance Training." *Journal of the American Geriatrics Society* 44 (1996): 489–497.

Wolfson, L., et al. "Balance and Strength Training in Older Adults: Intervention Gains and Tai Chi Maintenance." *Journal of the American Geriatrics Society* 44 (1996): 498–506.

A Closer Look at Pilates Exercise:
Like a Butterfly in the Sky

Julie Gleason still likes to tease her brothers about the time they kicked her off their pickup baseball teams. "I hit too many homers, so they decided that girls weren't allowed to play," she remembers. "I went home crying because I loved sports and didn't like dolls. Now, I beat them on the golf course." She has also become something of a fitness mentor for about two hundred clients, presiding over the Pilates exercise studio that she founded in 1992. Those who make the three-story climb up to the top floor of the converted Mansard home of Cambridge Health Associates ("The stairs are our *warm-up*," says Julie.) step into a large, sunlit room filled with the melodies of Mozart or Bach and several machines that look like they belong in a medieval torture chamber.

But no one looks tortured. Using their arms, legs and the "core" muscles deep in their trunks, the women and men using the machines look peaceful, graceful, even happy as they stretch and strengthen their bodies. Teachers (who look like dancers, athletes or both) watch them closely, giving friendly but firm instructions: "Reach *long* with those legs; *squeeze* those thighs; *relax* those shoulders; *hollow* out those abs—navel to the spine; *tighten* that butt." The slow, dancelike movements are done while lying, sitting or standing on movable wooden platforms, working against the resistance created by several complex arrangements of straps, springs, bars and pulleys. Those who stick to the regime of one-hour workouts two or three times a week are rewarded with long, lean muscles in their arms and legs, flatter abdomens, flexibility, better balance, straighter posture and a strength that comes from the deep inner muscles of the trunk.

"And there is no stress on the joints," points out Julie. "So anyone can do this. My clients range in age from fourteen to eighty-six, and include people with polio, hip and knee replacements and many other physical problems." They also include dancers, athletes and stage performers—people who are paid to look good and whose bodies must perform every day and recover quickly from injury. "The beauty of this system is that you can work around your disability or injury. Even if you can't use a limb, you can strengthen any other part of the body that can function," says Julie.

In the early 1900s, German athlete Joseph Pilates began experimenting with an exercise system to help himself recover from severe asthma. He designed a series of mat exercises to balance the body, improve ease of motion and promote mental and physical harmony. Later, during World War I, while working as a nurse, he tried to help hospital patients recover from their injuries by attaching springs to their beds, enabling them to start exercising their arms and legs even before they could walk. The "Reformer" and other types of apparatus used in modern Pilates studios are all based on the principles of exercise that he developed. In the 1920s, Pilates came to the United States and started his own studio, with machines he designed. He taught his system to dancers and also used it to rehabilitate people with injuries and disabilities.

"I didn't understand the full power of the system until I had a badly injured ballet dancer as a client," says Julie. "She had had surgery on her foot and was wearing a heavy cast almost up to the knee. But she came to exercise three times a week anyway, and we focused on the muscles of her inner thighs, deep abdominals and muscles supporting her back, pelvis and hips. When the cast came off three months later, she was almost immediately back on stage, in her *"pointe"* shoes, jumping high in the air and landing just fine—like a butterfly in the sky. I believe that maintaining her core strength helped her recover so quickly."

❖ ❖ ❖ ❖

Once the "secret" of dancers and athletes, the Pilates method is now gaining rapid popularity among the fitness-seeking public. Julie Gleason herself discovered it by a circuitous path. She grew up one of thirteen children in an Irish-French family in Boston. Her father worked for the telephone company. "We knew that we couldn't afford college," she says. "My oldest sister joined a convent and one brother joined the army, so their educations were paid for. The youngest one got to go to college because there were no more after her. But for the rest of us, higher education was not an option." After high school, Julie took business courses and learned to type, supporting herself by working as a secretary for local colleges. "That was the only way to be around other kids my age," she said.

But she wasn't happy. "I was bursting with energy and always needed to be doing *something*—whether running, basketball, field hockey, bicycling, whatever," she says. "I hated sitting behind a desk all day." Her solution? Work for the post office: "I liked the idea of being paid to take a walk every day." Julie became, in fact, one of the first women mail carriers in Massachusetts. "They even wrote a story about me in the *Boston Globe, 'Neither dogs, hills nor ugly black shoes will stop her from her appointed rounds,'* something like that." She carried thirty-five-pound bags of mail for nearly eight years, eventually straining her back.

"I was in pain and decided to go for a massage," says Julie. "I had never had one before, but once I was on the table, I remembered that I used to love giving massages to my football player brothers and cheerleader sisters when I was a kid! They used to say they would pay me fifty cents a massage, but they always fell asleep in the middle and never paid up." Julie enrolled in the Muscular Therapy Institute in Cambridge, studied massage, and began to hear about the Pilates method. "I realized I was finally on track," she says. "I wanted to work with people's bodies, help them feel better, get well and function. Delivering mail was a way of making money so I could eat, but in the end I didn't care if I starved. This is what I loved to do!"

She stopped delivering mail and began a full-time therapeutic massage practice. At the same time, she began traveling to New York City once a week to study Pilates with long-time expert Fran Lehan, as well as with Mary Bowen in Northhampton, Massachusetts. "Both of these women helped me get started," she says. In 1992, she gave up the massage practice (much to the dismay of her clients) and opened her own Pilates studio with four machines and one other teacher. Today, she has six machines and a rotating staff of six teachers. (Each workout is closely supervised. The teacher/student ratio is rarely greater than 1:2, even for advanced students.)

"The best thing about having this studio is that people come to me because they want to get well or stronger, not because someone is dragging them in," says Julie. "I felt like I was good at something, which I had never felt before. Growing up with twelve brothers and sisters, it's easy to get lost and feel unnoticed."

One of the most important benefits of Pilates exercise is the effect on the mind/body connection says Julie, and this can help with emotional as well as physical problems. "The exercises are gentle and peaceful, although they can be made more difficult by increasing the weight resistance of the springs. But even at their most difficult, the movements slow down the mind. You have to focus on your mind within your body, understand where your weaknesses are and learn how to use your mind to work with your body in a supportive way. It requires full concentration. We work from the 'inside out,' to develop deep core strength, flexibility and balance."

Pilates has been helpful to people with chronic back pain ("We strengthen the muscles that support the spine," says Julie), fibromyalgia, arthritis, neurodegenerative diseases like multiple sclerosis and osteoporosis ("This is weight-bearing, so it builds up bone mass," she says.) And the clients, many of whom have been with Julie since she opened the studio, can attest to the benefits: Jinny Chapin, whom you met in chapter 11, is eighty-six years old and started Pilates when she was seventy-nine. She still comes twice a week, had her knee replaced and regained full range of motion in eight months. She says it helps her balance and keeps her spirits up. (She climbs the two flights of stairs to the studio slowly, with a cane and a smile on her face.) Another client, eighty years old, had a plate put in her hip forty years ago and says nothing has helped reduce pain and increase mobility like Pilates. She's been with Julie since the studio opened and won't do any other form of exercise. And a sixty-four-year-old woman has been diagnosed with severe osteoporosis. "She has an eighty-five-year-old spine," says Julie. "And she hasn't broken a bone. In fact, none of my clients with osteoporosis has ever had a broken bone!"

Julie herself is a good advertisement for the Pilates method. With blond hair pulled back in her trademark ponytail and her lean, powerful form, she bounces around the studio like a teenager, instead of the forty-something woman she is. She seems to have an unending storehouse of energy. When she is not working, she walks, jogs, bicycles or plays golf (sometimes all in the same day). No "restful" vacations for her, either. She likes to go skiing, hiking, on bike trips, and she's even done hang-gliding in the Colorado mountains. "Hey, if it's out there, I'll try it!" she says.

Author's note: I have been going to Julie's Pilates studio twice a week for about four years, after I had a stroke. When I started, I could barely move the platforms, especially with my left arm. Now, both sides of my body are equally strong, and while I don't do any of the really advanced, spine-bending exercises, my teachers have helped me develop my own personal routine. I now notice muscles in my arms and legs that I never knew I had and have improved the strength of my abdominal area and trunk—considered to be the source of all strength in the Pilates system. An added benefit: Pilates has even helped me stay connected to my teenager. My daughter Elizabeth, now fifteen, goes with me every week and loves how it makes her feel about her body.

WHAT DO I DO NOW?
PUTTING IT ALL TOGETHER

By now, you have read the stories, perused the research data, learned the opinions of experts and "met" some doctors and practitioners. You may be deciding that you want to begin to integrate complementary and alternative practices into your conventional health care, but at the same time you are wondering, "How do I go about this myself? Where do I begin?" In this chapter, several experts in the field answer your questions and give you practical next steps.

Combining the best of both worlds
to create your personal prescription for health.

First, we hear from Brian Berman, M.D., founder and director of the Complementary Medicine Program at the University of Maryland, the first university-based center of its kind in the United States focusing on research. "Just making the decision to stand up for yourself, to feel you have the right to be involved in your own individual plan for health and well-being, and to not just accept the 'norm', is a critical step in the process of recovery and of health," says Berman, "So feel good that you are already on this path!" In addition to being professor of family medicine at the University of Maryland School of Medicine and principal investigator of a number of multicenter research studies in complementary medicine, Berman has trained extensively in complementary therapies such as acupuncture and homeopathy. He sees patients in the clinical program of the Complementary Medicine Center, including two whose stories appear in this book. (Please see chapters 5 and 7.)

As you embark on your exploration of integrative care and finding practitioners who are respectful of your desire to be in charge of your life, says Berman, there are several important points to consider:

"You are at the center of your own healing; it is your self-healing process that the therapies you use and the practitioners you consult should be trying to facilitate. There is no one "right" approach for everyone, just as there is no one "right" system of medicine. Both conventional and alternative medicine have their weaknesses and strengths; both have their share of wisdom and of foolishness. The challenge is to look around objectively and take those elements that make sense to you for your condition, and then to work with knowledgeable, experienced practitioners who will help guide and assist you. Remember that medicine is an art—an art that uses the tools of science and the information gleaned from scientific research—but that draws on human qualities such as compassion and trust and works with the beliefs, preferences, and needs of each individual person to make its practice truly effective. You, therefore, are an integral and vital part, an active participant in the process."

✓ TAKE ACTION ✓

Best ways to become your own integrator: combining conventional care and complementary and alternative medicine

Following is a synthesis of suggestions from Brian Berman, M.D., Wayne Jonas, M.D., and Alexa Fleckenstein, M.D. (We met Dr. Fleckenstein in chapter 4. Dr. Jonas, whose textbook is quoted in research sections throughout this book, was the second director of the Office of Alternative Medicine of the National Institutes of Health (NIH). He led the Office through its transformation into the National Center for Complementary and Alternative Medicine (NCCAM), staying on as the first director.[1]

Picking a doctor or practitioner

1. One source for finding an integrative physician is The American Board of Holistic Medicine, which is beginning to certify doctors for holistic care (the same as integrative medicine). The Web site lists the names and contact information of certified holistic doctors by state.[2]

2. Whether you choose an integrative physician or conventional physician, make sure your doctor is well-trained and competent. It is important that you get the best that modern medicine has to offer.

3. The same should be expected of any CAM practitioners with whom you work. How many years of training and experience have they had? Are they licensed or are they members of professional organizations? (Appendix II lists some licensing organizations.) Be aware, however, that some CAM approaches are further along than others in establishing standard licensing and credentialing and in monitoring the behavior of those in practice.

4. *Always let everyone involved with your health care know about everyone else!* The CAM practitioner should be willing to communicate with the doctor you are seeing and not advise you to change your conventional treatment without consulting your doctor. Likewise, make sure your doctor is willing to communicate with your CAM practitioner.

(continued)

---

[1] As noted in chapter 1, NCCAM has expanded rapidly, evidence of the country's interest in CAM therapies. The agency's budget grew from $2 million in 1992 to $92 million in 2001. As of this writing, NCCAM provides funding to twelve medical research centers around the country that are evaluating alternative treatments for many specialty areas or chronic health conditions including: aging, arthritis, cancer, cardiovascular disease, neurological disorders, neurodegenerative diseases and pediatrics.

[2] American Board of Holistic Medicine. Address: 614 Daniels Drive NE, Wenatchee, WA 98802; telephone: (509) 884-1062; fax: (509) 886-3708; Web site: *www.amerboardholisticmed.org.*

5. Make sure you feel valued, respected and listened to, whether by your doctor or CAM practitioner. Are they interested in your family, work, diet and lifestyle? Are you at ease talking about both personal and financial aspects of your care with them? Is your doctor open to discussing all your treatment options? If you feel good about all of these questions you are on your way to co-creating a meaningful healing partnership.

6. You should feel comfortable that the treatment is provided in an appropriate and safe environment. (For instance, does the acupuncturist use disposable needles?) Ask what could go wrong with the treatment, as well as the potential side effects. Is there a process for reporting adverse reactions to the treatments?

7. Has the practitioner treated anyone else with your problem? Is the treatment appropriate for your problem?

8. Does the practitioner treat all information and data in a confidential manner? Do you feel comfortable with the practitioner and does he or she respect your personal boundaries? The latter is obviously especially important in the case of therapies that involve a lot of physical contact such as massage or manipulation. Do not tolerate anything that makes you feel physically or sexually uncomfortable. Trust your instincts! What do friends or other professionals have to say about this person?

Getting going on your own integrative care

1. First off, you obviously need to try and get a clear diagnosis of your problem. If such a diagnosis cannot be made, have common problems been excluded?

2. Have you determined whether there is a conventional treatment for your condition that is proven to be effective? For example, most conventional and complementary cancer experts strongly advise patients *NOT* to reject conventional cancer treatments such as chemotherapy, surgery or radiation; people should *supplement* conventional treatment with CAM therapies.

3. Use your physician and those you consult as sources of information in addition to your own research. Make sure your doctor works in *partnership* with you. Give your doctor the information you have collected about CAM therapies, ask how it seems to fit in with your illness, health history and medical history, and ask your doctor to review the medical literature before coming back to you with advice. Take this as an opportunity to educate your doctor as well as yourself! Your doctor may also appreciate knowing about the National Center for Complementary and Alternative Medicine (*www.nccam.nih.gov/*) and the centers it has funded focusing on specific diseases at different academic centers and also about the Cochrane Collaboration Complementary Medicine

(continued)

Field (*www.compmed.umm.edu/Cochrane/index.html*)—all good sources of high-quality information.

4. With any treatment that is suggested to you, you will want to be very aware of how invasive it is and how likely to cause harm. If either is the case, there should be very good evidence for its immediate use. Be cautious of invasive procedures such as intravenous therapies, colonics, and putting chemicals into your body orally or by injection. Check to make sure that your practitioners are licensed and that your conventional doctor is aware of what you are doing.

5. Expect that a practitioner should be able to set guidelines at the first appointment for how the treatment should progress. Should you expect a response after two or three sessions of acupuncture, for example, or are you more likely to need eight or ten? If you are being told to sign up for indefinite treatment or for this treatment exclusively, alarm bells should be ringing in your head! Also, ask about the projected cost of treatment.

6. What is the evidence for or against a therapy? At this point there is a lot of research still to be done to find out how most alternative therapies work, if they work, or if they are safe. In this book we discuss some of the best research that currently exists for the approaches we have focused on. The evidence is stronger for some, for instance a variety of mind/body approaches, and practically nonexistent for others, for example Ayurvedic palmistry diagnosis. Throughout the book and in the Appendices are further resources for you to use in your own investigations.

7. A lot of what you can do for yourself is good self-care. Whether you are seeking treatment from professionals or not, part of owning your health is doing things like eating well, exercising, looking at the stresses in your life and finding ways to deal with them even if you can't change them (there are many easy mind/body ways to start with, such as meditation). Don't be hard on yourself! Above all, taking control of your health should not add more stress to your life, nor should you feel any sense of guilt, either about your condition or your reaction to it. Laugh, take time for yourself and the things you love to do, appreciate and spend time with those you care about.

Notes of caution

1. It is important not to embrace all alternative approaches just because they are touted as "natural" or "holistic." Knowledge is power, and the more you inform yourself from reputable resources, the more able you will be to tell the fraudulent from the worthwhile. (Two organizations that focus on this topic are The National Center Against Health Fraud (*NCAHF.org.*) and *Quackwatch.com.*

(continued)

2. Be alert to potential toxic effects: Some alternative therapies are relatively non-toxic, including homeopathy, massage, mind/body practices, spinal manipulation (although if done improperly, this could have negative bone, muscle or joint effects), biofeedback, regular doses of vitamins and minerals and properly delivered acupuncture. Be aware that herbs, for instance, although natural, can have powerful ingredients that do not mix well with certain pharmaceutical drugs. *Make sure you understand any potential negative interaction between herbs and prescription medicines.*

3. On the subject of herbs, if you buy them, do so from a reputable company. Herbs are not regulated by the FDA so their quality can be highly variable; also, there have been cases where herbs have been doctored with other products, such as pharmaceutical drugs. There is no national certification for herbalists (except for doctors of traditional Chinese medicine and doctors of naturopathy), so, even though some may be excellent sources of information, you need to do your own research. You could start with the Center for Science in the Public Interest,[3] the American Botanical Council in Austin, TX[4] and the Herb Research Foundation in Boulder, CO.[5] See also "A Closer Look at Healing Herbs." *With any treatment, find out if it will interact negatively with something you are already doing or taking.*

4. Beyond a simple fee-for-service arrangement, do not get involved in any business-related transaction with your practitioner (e.g., selling products or investing).

5. If you are seriously ill, do not avoid conventional treatments that are known to be effective, in favor of CAM treatments. In cancer treatment, for example, it is unethical for anyone to recommend that you not use the best of conventional medicine. At the same time, however, you can integrate CAM treatments into your therapy to support your quality of life and deal with side effects.

---

[3] Center for Science in the Public Interest. This nonprofit organization publishes the *Nutrition Action Healthletter*, a small but information-packed newsletter that provides objective, evidence-based nutrition and supplement information (they accept no advertising) in an entertaining, easy-to-read format. Always interesting and up-to-date. My teenage daughter especially likes their "Food Porn" column, which trashes (by name) unhealthy food products with details of their ingredients. Address: 1875 Connecticut Avenue, NW, Suite 300, Washington, DC 20009-5728; fax: (202)-265-4594; E-mail: *circ@cspinet.org;* Web site: *www.cspinet.org.*

[4] American Botanical Council. Web site: *www.herbalgram.org/browse.php/defaulthome.*

[5] Herb Research Foundation: *www.herbs.org/index.html.*

Why "meaning" and "context" are important in medicine

"Patients are interested in results," says physician, researcher and writer Wayne B. Jonas, M.D. "Patients are usually satisfied to know their chances of getting better. For example, if you can tell them that they have an 80 percent chance of getting rid of their complaint with a treatment, they usually don't care how the treatment compares to placebo. They want to know if there are side effects and if they will feel better."

By contrast, says Jonas, scientists want to know what the mechanism is, and whether one treatment works better than no treatment. They find this out through "randomized controlled trials," (using matched experimental and control groups) and "placebo" (something that looks identical to the treatment being investigated but is designed to have no medical effect, like a sugar pill.) "Scientists ask different questions, and they are looking for different kinds of information," says Jonas. "The scientific investigation is essential for the development of a body of knowledge, but often overlooks using what I call the 'context' or 'meaning' response to treatment."

As you face your own health challenges and try to make decisions about which treatments to choose, this "context" or "meaning" becomes essential. Are you a risk taker or more cautious? Do you have confidence in your doctors? How would you deal with the necessity of choosing between a treatment with severe side effects and the material risk of a life-threatening disease? (In this book, B.J. Goodwin and Julie Arredondo in chapter 5, Charlotte Harrington in chapter 4, and Sarena Morello in chapter 7 all handled these choices differently, each according to her own values about health, healing and the meaning of illness in her life.) Above all, remember that not everything can be decided by evidence, but you and your partners in health can together weigh risks and benefits and arrive at a thoughtful, reasonable decision that is right for you. And remember, as cardiologist Eugene Lindsey, M.D., says in chapter 4, "As long as you are alive, there are very few decisions in life that cannot be reversed!"

❖ ❖ ❖ ❖

Wayne Jonas has a story to illustrate the importance of the mind/body connection in health and illness. He describes a recent research study that was trying to determine whether St. John's wort works better for depression than either a drug or a placebo. "The study found that, surprisingly, the placebo actually worked better than the other two; and statistically, there was no difference among all three," says Jonas. "The problem with this study was the context of the research. Researchers invited all three groups of patients into the medical center, spending time interviewing and talking with them about their feelings; perhaps no one had done that before for them. The study created a caring context that was itself healing, and the effect of this context was so large that it obscured the additional effects of the various treatments. The results suggest that the context in which a therapy is delivered may have greater effects than the specific chemical interactions of the therapy itself."

In other words, the mind/body connection works in mysterious ways. Science, says Jonas, is one of the most powerful tools for exposing the "spurious claims of truth" that many people seem to make about alternative medicine. Yet when it comes to understanding how and why people heal, science has its limitations. "The complexity of disease and the powerful healing capacity of the body often make it difficult to apply science to clinical medicine, especially when evaluating chronic disease," he writes in one of his textbooks.[6]

One study demonstrated that nearly 80 percent of those who seek out medical care get better "no matter what hand-waving or pill-popping is provided.[7] This is called the '80 percent rule,' meaning that data collected on novel therapies delivered in an enthusiastic, clinical environment typically yield positive outcomes in 70 to 80 percent of patients."[8] In homeopathy treatments, for example, "even taking the health history is a contextually rich, elaborate event," explains Jonas. "Regardless of your opinion of the science of homeopathy, paying attention to the patient, being warm and delivering the service with confidence all have been shown to enhance healing—or, if you wish to call it that, the placebo effect."

---

6 W. B. Jonas and J. S. Levin, *Essentials of Complementary and Alternative Medicine* (Baltimore, MD: Lippincott, Williams & Wilkins 1999), 6.

7 K. B. Thomas, "The Placebo in General Practice," *Lancet* 344 (1994): 1066–1067.

8 W. B. Jonas, *Essentials of Complementary and Alternative Medicine*, 6 and W. B. Jonas, "Therapeutic Labeling and the 80% Rule," *Bridges* 5, no. 1 (1994): 4–6.

But what happens all too often, says Jonas, is "a communication gap between science and the public. In our research and our practice, we need to better combine the fundamental differences between science—which seeks to eliminate the symptoms of disease; and healing—which seeks to stimulate the natural ability of our minds, bodies and spirits to overcome illness and maintain health."

A SCIENTIST WHO IS ALSO A HEALER

Wayne Jones, M.D., is a good example of the kind of doctor that many people are looking for. He became interested in alternative medicine when he was a military physician stationed in Germany in the early 1980s. "I was surprised to find out that many of the German physicians used alternative practices—such as herbal medicine, acupuncture and homeopathy—which were disparaged when I went to medical school," says Jonas. "They told me that these methods worked well. I could see that they were rational people, not quacks, and this intrigued me." Jonas started observing these colleagues as they treated their patients and he began to learn about herbs, homeopathy and acupuncture.

"After I saw the success of these methods, I obtained permission from the military to use them in my practice as well," says Jonas. "I was pleasantly surprised at the effectiveness. I treated one child, for example, who had been getting chronic ear infections for years, including breakthrough infections even while he was on antibiotics. Tubes did not help much. But homeopathy cleared up these infections in several months."

During twenty-four years as a military doctor, Jonas directed a medical research training program at the Walter Reed Army Institute of Research, focusing his work, in part, on the role of complementary medicine in bioterrorism response. Jonas has been researching and writing about complementary, alternative and integrative medicine for nearly a quarter of a century and is considered an international authority in the field. He teaches medical students and cares for patients; and is trained not only in conventional medicine, but also in a variety of complementary practices, including diet and nutritional therapy, homeopathy, mind/body methods and electro-acupuncture. Among his more than 140 publications are some of the first medical textbooks on integrative medicine. In addition to directing the National Center for Complementary and Alternative Medicine, he also served on the White House

(continued)

Commission for Complementary and Alternative Medicine Policy, made hundreds of presentations on the subject around the world and is on the editorial boards of seven peer-reviewed journals.

Jonas is now director of the Samueli Institute for Informational Biology and an associate professor in the Department of Family Medicine at the Uniformed Services University of Health Sciences in Bethesda, Maryland. He continues his research, writing and teaching while maintaining a family medicine practice in Maryland. "I still love being a family physician and incorporating integrative medicine into my practice," he says. "To see patients from birth to death you need a very large medicine bag, with many tools."

Where to Find It and Who Pays?

The medical insurance landscape is constantly changing, so that a definitive list of insurers, health maintenance organizations and hospitals that are offering or covering CAM is not available, according to Kenneth R. Pelletier, M.D., Ph.D., (hc), author of *The Best Alternative Medicine: What Works? What Does Not?* However, while he was director of the Complementary and Alternative Medicine Program at Stanford University School of Medicine, he and his colleagues completed research that produced some answers. The research identified hospitals that have CAM programs, or that collaborated with centers that offered CAM.

The most common types of CAM therapies offered through these hospitals include chiropractic, acupuncture, massage, guided imagery and tai chi. However, reports Pelletier, "few, if any, of these services are covered by insurance. For virtually all providers, the individual patient must pay out of pocket for these services."[9] Some health maintenance organizations (HMOs), seem to be more amenable to covering CAM: A 1995 survey found that 86 percent of HMOs covered chiropractic, 69 percent covered weight-loss programs,

---

[9] K. R. Pelletier, *The Best Alternative Medicine: What Works? What Does Not?* (New York: Simon & Schuster, 2000), 280.

31 percent acupuncture, 28 percent relaxation therapy, 17 percent mental imagery therapy, and 14 percent massage therapy and hypnosis. However, the survey also found that some 46 percent of HMOs actively discouraged patients from using one or more alternative therapies.[10]

At a recent seminar for the Integrative Medicine Alliance in Massachusetts, Robert Scholten of Harvard Medical School's Division for Research and Education in Complementary and Alternative Medical Therapies provided information about currently available coverage for CAM:

Health plans that provide varied reimbursement for CAM services do so through full or partial coverage for these therapies via some third-party payers through standard plans, discount programs or rider clauses and through some employers who have "defined contribution plans" as part of their employee health package. A number of insurance companies nationally that are participating to some extent in CAM coverage, according to Scholten, include Aetna U.S. Healthcare, United Health Group, CIGNA Healthplan, Kaiser Permanente (Northern California Kaiser is very innovative in CAM coverage), Humana Health Care and Blue Cross of California. Some businesses with CAM coverage in their defined contribution health plans include Textron of Rhode Island, Medtronics of Minnesota, and Raytheon of Massachusetts.[11]

Unfortunately, the changing insurance landscape makes access to CAM therapies both difficult and confusing for patients. There are, however, several resources where you can find updated information. These include:

- The Collaboration for Healthcare Renewal. *www.thecollaboration.org*. "The Collaboration" has ongoing working committees publish white papers to its Web site and is a source of information on CAM coverage.
- The Integrative Medical Alliance. *www.integrativemedalliance.org*.

---

[10] N. Goodwin, "A Health Insurance Revolution," *New Age Journal* (March/April 1997): 95–99.
[11] For additional information, see the article by Linda Kenney on the Web site of the Integrative Medical Alliance: *www.integrativemedalliance.org*.

AFTERWORD
A Call to Action: Comments from an Allopathic Physician

"It is time for us to own our profession."

by H. Eugene Lindsey, Jr., M.D.,
cardiologist and primary physician;
Chairman of the Board, Harvard Vanguard Medical Associates[1]

This book is both a call to action and a challenge for allopathic Western physicians to think more broadly about better ways to help our patients. There is much to be proud of in the achievements of allopathic medicine, a system to which I have devoted my entire medical career. The system is a wonderful tool and can usually provide accurate diagnoses and treatment. For example, when a patient comes into my office with swollen ankles and shortness of breath, I know just what to do. A medical exam and such diagnostic tools as an EKG and a chest X ray might reveal that the patient has congestive heart failure. An echocardiogram and a cardiac catheterization might explain the reasons. With

---

[1] H. Eugene Lindsey, Jr., M.D., specializes in cardiology and internal medicine. He is a graduate and on the faculty of the Harvard Medical School and has been practicing for more than 25 years. He is chairman of the board of Harvard Vanguard Medical Associates (HVMA), a large, multispecialty group practice with a staff of 1,000 medical professionals serving 300,000 patients in 15 sites. Recently, HVMA has created an Alternative Medicine Program, offering such services as acupuncture, massage and yoga to its patients. Robert Ebert, M.D., former dean of the Harvard Medical School, founded HVMA in 1969 as the Harvard Community Health Plan. Dr. Ebert's vision was to create a prepaid group practice offering innovative, effective medical care to patients while training future physicians and providing leadership in medical research and the effective delivery of care. Today, the Harvard Medical School Department of Ambulatory and Preventative Care (DACP) still uses HVMA outpatient offices as clinical sites.

medicines and advice about lifestyle and dietary changes I can usually reduce both his symptoms and his risk of future heart damage. Even if a patient comes to me with a problem beyond my expertise, in gastroenterology or neurology, for example, I can refer her to a colleague who specializes in that field. In either scenario, I am on familiar, allopathic turf.

While appreciating the strengths of allopathic medicine, however, we physicians must also be honest with ourselves about its limitations. Perhaps more than half of the patients who come to my office do so with complaints that have no obvious organic cause. They may be having pain, fatigue, or a sense that something "just isn't right." These patients are part of a much larger and growing population who feel there is something missing from their allopathic treatment, that our approach to human suffering and illness is not helping them. This book presents the possibility—along with some compelling evidence—that the answer for some of these patients may lie in the field of integrative medicine, which combines alternative/complementary treatments with conventional medicine.

Who can benefit from integrative medicine?

Although the terms "integrative" or "complementary" medicine did not exist at the time, I realize that I have been recommending at least one complementary technique to my patients since the 1970s. This is the "Respiratory One Method," a form of meditation (based on Transcendental Meditation) that was developed and researched by Herbert Benson, M.D., founder and president of the Mind/Body Institute at Beth Israel Deaconess Medical Center and faculty member of the Harvard Medical School. One of the most important pioneers in the field of complementary medicine, Benson researched this form of meditation, which resulted in what he termed "The Relaxation Response." He found in clinical trials that meditating patients were able to enter a state of deep relaxation that resulted in lower blood pressure, slower heartbeat and respiration rates and other physiological and biochemical changes and were beneficial to health, including reduced anxiety.

For the past thirty years, I have been recommending Benson's book, *The Relaxation Response*, to hundreds of my patients with hypertension, heart disease, asthma, obesity and gastrointestinal problems. Many of these patients "took the bait," and began to practice the meditation, improving their symptoms to such an extent that we were often able either to reduce medications or eliminate them altogether. As a result, many patients became further motivated to introduce changes in their diet, add exercise and create healthier lifestyles.

The successful outcome for the patients who practice Benson's meditation method has prompted me to think about different kinds of patients who might benefit from other forms of integrative medicine:

- Patients whose diagnostic tests are negative or inconclusive, but whose symptoms are real and disabling and for whom psychiatric referral is not helpful (Barbara Kivowitz, one of my patients whose story is described in chapter 7, is one example);
- Patients with chronic diseases such as stroke, congestive heart failure, arthritis and cancer, for whom our best treatments are inadequate or fail to help them maximize their health.

We allopathic physicians have little to offer in these situations, aside from empathy and palliative medication, and it is in the treatment of these two broad groups of patients that integrative medicine holds the most promise. My own enthusiasm for the integrative approach has grown out of my failure to help patients like these with allopathic medicine alone.

Consider just one example: A forty-eight-year-old corporate attorney whose only previous health problems were a slightly elevated blood pressure, borderline cholesterol and a slight tendency to be overweight is now complaining of a rather sudden onset of fatigue so extreme that she can "no longer function." She has to take a disability leave from a job she loves and stay home, too exhausted to do much more than occasionally buy groceries or go for a walk. She also complains of slight gastrointestinal problems. A myriad of tests, including blood analysis and magnetic resonance imaging reveal only minor abnormalities that do not add up to a diagnosis.

The frustration for both of us is that we can neither identify a cause nor find anything that seems to give her the energy she needs to live a normal life. As her doctor, I am left with a lingering sense of uncertainty that I have somehow missed something important by not ordering the right test or discovering the right approach. At this point, most doctors will respond to this uncertainty by either ordering more tests, referring the patient to still more specialists, or by simply sending the patient on her way with the assurance that there is nothing seriously wrong.

Overcoming uncertainty, our near-constant companion

This book offers another course of action for doctors in this kind of ambiguous medical situation: We can look outside of allopathic medicine for answers. But as we begin to explore this unfamiliar world, we are immediately confronted with barriers that include lack of knowledge, unreceptive patients and those elusive commodities: time and resources.

- *Knowledge:* There is no systematic way for most allopathic physicians to consult with someone who is an expert in a wide range of complementary fields. Would it help to use Chinese medicine to remove blockages to the qi energy of this attorney? Would Ayurvedic medicine build up her prana (life force)? What about Reiki or therapeutic massage? Might there be herbs or special foods that could give her a nutritional boost? Does she need cold showers? (See chapter 3.) There are many choices, but what is the best choice for this particular patient?

Despite the recent advances in complementary and alternative medicine research and practice, our knowledge is still rudimentary. I can generally imagine, from anecdotal evidence and from the research studies both in this book and elsewhere, that complementary modalities can indeed help certain patients and conditions. But when I am faced with a patient who has profound constitutional problems, including fatigue, pain or a sense of "malaise," I am not sure what to offer after I have exhausted the allopathic treatments. It seems that each of the complementary or alternative treatments bills itself as "the be-all and end-all," while discounting the benefits of other modalities. We need more objective, evidence-based comparative information and advice on which to base the process of diagnosis and management. References referred to in this book are helpful, and *Own Your Health* is itself an important breakthrough: Not only is it a resource for patients, but it also can become a tool for discussion between patient and doctor. More resources like this need to be available, as well as more consulting physicians who can objectively advise on the best complementary treatments for each patient.

The knowledge and tools exist to serve our patients more holistically, humanely and effectively than we are now doing, but this knowledge must be proven with clear, evidence-based medicine before insurers will recognize the benefits of integrative medicine. Such research has already begun through the Cochrane Collaboration and through the integrative studies being carried out at such forward-thinking academic medical centers as the University of Maryland, the University of Arizona, the Harvard and Stanford Schools of Medicine and the University of Illinois at Chicago. But, for this knowledge to be available to all patients, it must also be readily available to allopathic physicians who have little time for extensive research. I envision, for example, a consultation system where I might have regular access to an integrative medical practice for diagnostic and treatment advice for particular patients.

- *Unreceptive patients.* We doctors also need to help patients be more receptive to integrative medicine, especially when allopathic approaches have failed to meet their needs. While many patients are looking for alternatives to conventional medicine, there also seem to be those who are opposed to the very idea. Sometimes, conventional solutions are not the answer, however. It may well be that our enchantment with the physical sciences—on the part of doctors and patients alike—has prevented us from recognizing and using some complementary tools that may promote health and treat disease.

In fact, I have found that unless suggestions for complementary treatments come from the patient, there is little likelihood that they will be accepted. Both as a result of this book, and from my own explorations, I have begun to suggest such treatments as massage, meditation, acupuncture or the Alexander

Technique to patients who I think might benefit from them. More often than not, the response is, "I don't believe in that stuff;" or "I tried that once and it didn't work." These patients believe that their health problems are organic and fixable, either by surgery or by a pill, and that is the solution they want. It almost seems as if they view their bodies as automobiles: When it is broken, leave it with a mechanic until it is fixed, then pick it up and drive it home. The philosophy of integrative medicine takes the opposite approach: The message to patients is: "When there is something wrong with your body, both you and your doctor need to make a commitment of time and energy to find the solution." This sense of personal responsibility is the meaning of "owning your health," and too often, this sense is missing from conventional medical treatment. As a physician, I would appreciate being able to consult with integrative medical experts about how to help introduce the potential benefits of complementary treatments to patients who are not receptive to the idea.

- *Time and resources.* Another problem facing the allopathic physician, especially within a managed care setting, is finding both the time and the resources to provide more in-depth care. On any given afternoon, I might have sixteen patients on my schedule. If I am wondering whether the legitimate but unexplained physical symptoms of some of these patients might be coming from some intangible emotional or spiritual source, I need to have a real conversation with my patient. This kind of conversation would need to fully explore her symptoms, lifestyle, work, family situation and cultural perspective, in order to begin to determine which complementary modalities would be both acceptable and helpful. But in the fifteen minutes that is allotted for each appointment, such a conversation is impossible. Physicians who do engage in these kinds of important conversations do so at their own expense because they are often not reimbursable, and even when they are, the doctors' schedules are full.

As chairman of a medical group practice that serves 300,000 patients in 15 sites, I understand only too well the budgetary constraints that are putting pressure on doctors to serve more patients in less time and with fewer expenses. But the very nature of allopathic medicine actually encourages the ordering of expensive tests, procedures and medication—often because there is no time to use the doctor-patient relationship to more fully explore the problem. Managed care has, in fact, evolved as the allopathic reaction to this tendency towards expensive practice. Patients want answers and doctors, in response, order tests. The results of these tests might be inconclusive, so doctors order more tests. Eventually, a medicine might be indicated, which may or may not help, and which might point to the need for further tests, which may or may not reveal anything of value. This redundant testing is often ineffective, but testing—and then testing again—is how we in allopathic medicine often deal with the uncertainty that is our near-constant companion.

Integrative medicine seems to offer an additional way to help our patients. If complementary methods reduce the costs of health care, so much the better, but it should be efficacy rather than cost that is the predominant consideration in the practice of medicine. I find it interesting, however, that at least one research study in this book has compared the costs of allopathic and complementary treatments, finding significant savings with equally good results for the complementary methods.

Own Your Health is an impressive combination of the inspirational, the factual and the potential for integrative medicine. By telling the stories of patients who became "medical pioneers," determined to discover how to choose the best treatments from both worlds of medicine, this book is both a welcome breakthrough and valuable tool for all patients and their doctors. *Own Your Health* and similar resources will arm allopathic physicians with the solid evidence we need to become advocates with our patients for better health care. Together, we will demand from the government, employers and the insurance payers sufficient resources to take advantage of proven treatments from the full range of conventional and complementary medicine, drawing on new knowledge as well as the traditions of thousands of years of ancient healers. Just as this book helps patients to "own their health," it may also help those of us who are physicians to "own our profession."

APPENDIX I
ALTERNATIVE AND
COMPLEMENTARY MEDICINE:
EXPANDED GLOSSARY

The list below is by no means complete. However, most experts say that these practices are worth considering as complements to conventional medicine. Anecdotal evidence or research studies suggest that they have been effective in the treatment of particular conditions for certain patients.

(Note: The definitions below are adapted from interviews with practitioners as well as the reference books *Natural Health Complete Guide to Integrative Medicine*, by Dr. David Peters & Anne Woodham, Dorling Kindersley, London. 2000) and *The Desktop Guide to Complementary and Alternative Medicine: An Evidence-Based Approach*, Edzard Enrst, ed. (Edinburgh, Mosby, 2001).

IMPORTANT: Please make sure to keep your doctor as well as any alternative practitioners fully informed of all of your treatment choices, and consult with your conventional doctor *before* using these or any other complementary practices.

Alternative Medical Practices

- *Traditional Chinese Medicine* (TCM): A three thousand-year-old system that includes acupuncture, acupressure, herbalism and diet; qigong and tai chi (special movements); and *tui na* and shiatsu (forms of massage). TCM views the human body as a whole and as a part of nature. Disease occurs when the balance or harmony within the body—or between the body and nature—is disrupted. TCM focuses on both preventing and treating disease by restoring harmony and the balanced flow of qi (pronounced "chee")—universal energy—within the body.

- *Homeopathy:* A system of diagnosis and treatment that uses highly diluted remedies made from natural substances. Based on the theory that "like cures like," homeopathic medicines are given to boost the body's own "vital force" and promote its self-healing powers to fight disease and infection.

- *European Natural Medicine:* Based on principles developed by Sebastian Kneipp, a Bavarian Catholic priest, in the mid-nineteenth century: This system posits that the body has innate healing powers that are supported by "five pillars of health:" cold water (to boost the immune system and mood); movement (it's never too little or too late); proper nutrition; herbs; and an ordered life (balancing work, relationships, art, beauty and living in harmony with nature).

- *Naturopathy:* A healing system that emphasizes nutritional and herbal treatment, which grew out of European Natural Medicine (see above), naturopathy is based on the belief that an unhealthy lifestyle can disturb organ function and contribute to disease. Practitioners use whole foods, medicinal herbs and exercise to stimulate the body's self-healing.

- *Ayurvedic Medicine:* Originating in India more than five thousand years ago, Ayurveda uses meditation, yoga, breathing exercises and nutritional guidance to create a balanced mind and body, in order to free the body from illness. Ayurvedic doctors prescribe specific diets, medicinal herbs and physical activities—especially yoga (see below) carefully tailored to individual patients based on their particular body types (*doshas*). The system is based on the belief that no two individuals react in the same way to particular foods, exercise or medication.

Mind/Body Interventions

- *Alexander Technique:* Improves ease and freedom of movement, balance, support, flexibility and coordination. Teachers help their students develop "conscious awareness" of habitual patterns of movement that cause muscle tension and pain. Once students are aware of their tension-creating movement habits, they can "inhibit" them, freeing their bodies to move with ease. (The Feldenkreis Technique is a similar therapy.)

- *Meditation:* This practice strives for "relaxed awareness in the present moment," using various techniques to free the mind from the constant barrage of thoughts of the past (which is gone) or the future (which is not yet here). Meditation practices are found in all major religious traditions, but the techniques are often practiced outside of religion as well. Perhaps the best known proponent of secular meditation is Herbert Benson, M.D., of the Harvard Medical School, who has spent many years researching the physiological and therapeutic effects of what he has termed the "relaxation response."

- *Yoga:* This regime of mental and physical training is part of the Indian Ayurvedic health system (see above). Yoga is now taught throughout the world according to several different methods, ranging from strenuous aerobic workouts ("power yoga") to slow, deeply meditative movements, breathing and deep relaxation techniques. Students of all ages report increased flexibility, balance, ease of movement, calmness, increased mental acuity and ability to focus the mind.

- *Hypnotherapy, visualization and guided imagery:* These practices use a state of profound relaxation or hypnosis, when the mind is more open to suggestion, to plant positive ideas of healing. They can be done either by a practitioner or by the individual patient, using pre-recorded taped messages. (See "What Is Guided Imagery?")

- *Biofeedback:* This system teaches patients to control involuntary bodily functions, such as heart rate, skin temperature or muscle tension, by using breathing, visualization or other relaxation techniques. It is done through the use of sensors that signal when the desired result is achieved. (See chapter 7.)

- *Spiritual healing:* With a practice that can be traced back to the Bible, spiritual healers believe that the therapeutic effect results from the channeling of "energy" from an assumed source via the healer to the patient, thereby promoting self-healing in the patient. Types of spiritual healing include distant healing, faith healing, intercessory prayer, paranormal healing and psychic healing.

- *Reiki, therapeutic touch and other forms of energy healing:* An increasingly popular form of energy healing, Reiki was "founded in the late ninteenth century by Dr. Mikao Usui, a Japanese theologian, and allegedly based on ancient Buddhist healing rituals. Practitioners claim to channel 'reiki energy' to areas of need, both in their patients and in themselves. Reiki is said to work at an atomic level, making the body's molecules vibrate so intensely that energy blockages are dissolved" (Peters & Woodham).

  Practitioners of therapeutic touch, developed by Dr. Dolores Kuieger, professor of nursing at New York University, also balance energy flow in the body to promote self-healing. The technique, involving the use of sweeping hand motions, was designed to introduce healing techniques into the patient-nurse relationship, and is now widely practiced by nurses in hospitals in the United States and the United Kingdom.

- *Shamanic healing:* Based on ancient cultural traditions in which the "shaman" served as the primary spiritual and physical healer in the community, this practice is being increasingly used to treat the mental and physical effects of trauma as well as other psychological and physical ailments. The belief is that parts of the patient's "soul" become dissociated or "lost," especially as the result of trauma. Shamanic healers—some of whom been trained in Western psychotherapy as well—practice "soul retrieval" and energy balancing to help the patient become spiritually and psychologically whole again.

Herbal Therapies

Many of the practices discussed above, including traditional Chinese medicine, homeopathy, Ayurvedic medicine, European Natural Medicine and naturopathy make extensive use of diet, supplements and herbs. Many herbs and supplements can now be bought over the counter to treat a variety of conditions, and while some research is underway to determine both safety and efficacy, there are no definitive answers yet. This book discusses what is currently known about some herbal treatments. (See, for example, "A Closer Look at Healing Herbs.")

NOTE: It is very important, if you do take herbal remedies or vitamin supplements, to discuss it with both your conventional doctor and your practitioner, especially if you are also taking prescription medications or have heart disease, high blood pressure or glaucoma. There can be dangerous interactions between herbal medicines and prescription drugs.

Diet and Nutrition

Many complementary and alternative therapies, including traditional Chinese medicine, Ayurvedic healing, European Natural Medicine and naturopathy use diet and nutrition as a mainstay of the treatment. Conventional medicine, thanks to the research of Dean Ornish, M.D., and others, recognizes that cardiovascular disease and other illnesses can be prevented and even reversed by changes in diet. Also in conventional medicine, nutrition has long been a standard part of diabetic treatment—both type 1 and type 2 diabetes; and in early stages of type 2, nutrition is considered a cure for the disease. In type 1 diabetes it is an important, although not sufficient, part of the treatment.

Body-Based and Manipulative Systems

- *Osteopathy:* This system was developed in the late 1800s by an American physician, Andrew Taylor Still. In the United States, osteopathic physicians (D.O.) have the same licensure as medical doctors (M.D.) and practice the full range of medical specialities, use all conventional diagnostic tools and perform surgery. In addition, they use osteopathic manipulation, including cranial osteopathy to treat a wide variety of conditions, including pain, ear infections in children and menstrual problems. Osteopaths use hands-on treatment in order to restore the body's ability to heal itself. It is believed that healing occurs when the natural circulation, nerve impulses and body rhythm are restored. The system is based on several principles including:

—The body is a unit; the person is a unit of body, mind and spirit. The body is capable of self-regulation, self-healing and health maintenance.

—Structure and function in the whole body are related.

• *Chiropractic:* This practice is based on the premise that the body can heal itself if the musculoskeletal system is properly aligned. "The spinal cord carries nerves to the whole body. Chiropractors think that . . . (A)ny strain, damage, or distortion of the spine is said to promote problems in the internal organs, glands, and blood vessels and undermines the body's self-regulating and healing processes. . . . Chiropractors have tended to concentrate on joint manipulation" (Peters & Woodham). Treatment usually involves detailed medical history, X rays and other diagnostic tools, and the use of precise, controlled techniques to realign the spine and joints and release muscle tension.

• *Craniosacral therapy:* This is an extremely gentle technique aimed at removing restrictions in the flow of cerebrospinal fluid (which cushions and bathes the spinal cord.) The technique was founded in the 1970s by J. E. Upledger, an osteopathic physician, based on the work of osteopathic physician W. G. Sutherland in the 1930s. Restoring the regular "pulse" of cerebrospinal fluid is thought to treat conditions that include chronic pain, migraines, depression and trauma. Young children seem to respond particularly well, especially in the treatment of chronic ear infections. Health professionals who practice craniosacral therapy include chiropractors, osteopaths, naturopaths, physiotherapists, dentists and medical doctors.

• *Massage therapy:* The touch of another human's hand is perhaps the oldest form of medical care. Massage of many kinds "has been used for thousands of years around the world to promote well-being, ease pain of all kinds, and relieve anxiety" (Peters & Woodham). Massage techniques include relaxing "Swedish" methods, involving long, stroking motions; more intense, (sometimes uncomfortable) deep tissue, "trigger point" or "Rolfing" massage; shiatsu or acupressure massage, which uses the meridians and acupuncture points of Oriental medical systems; and "Trager" bodywork therapy, a mind/body approach. But no matter what the technique, the goal is to increase circulation, along with the supply of oxygen and nutrients to the skin and body tissues. Less tangible benefits include stress reduction and relaxation.

- *Pilates exercise:* Developed at the turn of the last century by Joseph Pilates to help people recover from injury, Pilates exercise has become increasingly popular as a way to strengthen the whole body (from the "inside out") while reducing stress on joints and ligaments. A typical Pilates routine, using moving platforms and springs to create resistance, focuses on the core muscles of the trunk, strengthens limbs and stretches the whole body. The effect is long, lean strength, rather than bulk, and while the system is popular among dancers and athletes, people of nearly any condition and age can benefit.

- *Aromatherapy:* Inhaling deeply when walking past a fragrant flower or tree gives a good idea of the practice of aromatherapy. Essential oils, extracted from plant roots, stalks and flowers, have been used for centuries for healing and relaxation. As they are inhaled, chemicals in the oils are "thought to act on the hypothalamus, the part of the brain influencing mood and the hormonal system" (Peters & Woodham). Certain oils, such as tea tree, for example, can be used directly on the skin. Depending on the needs of the client, practitioners select oils that have calming, uplifting, stimulating, antiseptic or decongestant properties. Essential oils (along with self-help instruction books) are also available in health food or "New Age" stores.

APPENDIX II
WHERE TO FIND IT; WHAT TO READ

This Appendix contains organizations, Web sites and books that provide information on complementary and alternative medicine (CAM) and research. Much of the information in this Appendix is excerpted from *Complementary Therapies on the Internet: Guide for Health Care Professionals*, by William M. Beckner and Brian M. Berman, M.D. (London: Churchill Livingston, 2002). Used with permission of the authors.

Government Resources

The National Center for Complementary and Alternative Medicine (NCCAM), *www.nccam.nih.gov/*

The NCCAM is dedicated to exploring complementary and alternative healing practices in the context of rigorous science; training CAM researchers; and disseminating authoritative information to Health care consumers and patients.

Research Resources in CAM:

NCCAM funds and monitors more CAM research than any other institution in the United States. The level of appropriation for NCCAM has been increased twice, to a budget of $113 million for the year 2003. As a result of partnering with other National Institutes of Health (NIH) institutes, NCCAM has achieved aggregate funding totaling roughly $200 million for 2002.

ClinicalTrials.Gov

ClinicalTrials.Gov provides a complete listing of all CAM trials sponsored by the NIH. For a complete listing of clinical studies in CAM search under the keyword "Alternative Medicine." As of April 2002, there were 147 clinical trials listed. (*www.clinicaltrials.gov/*)

In addition to funding individual clinical trials, NCCAM has funded or provided cofunding to fifteen research centers across the U.S. Each program concentrates on prevention and treatment of at least one major disease condition or on the health issue of a particular population. These centers in turn have the ability to fund pilot studies called "development-of-feasibility projects." Given the focus of each of these centers, they are in a position to conduct, assess and stimulate research within their field. There are now quite a few research organizations focused on complementary medicine; most often these are academic medical schools that are involved in performing research and teaching medical students. A number of them have also developed integrative clinics where patients are treated. Some institutions such as the University of Maryland include a focus on information, research, education and clinical care.

NCCAM Public Information Clearinghouse

As one of its mandates from Congress, NCCAM is charged with "the dissemination of health information . . . in respect to identifying, investigating, and validating complementary and alternative treatment, diagnostic, and prevention modalities, disciplines, and systems." (Public Law 105-277) The NCCAM Clearinghouse serves this mission. It is the public's point of contact for scientifically based information on complementary and alternative medicine (CAM) and for information about NCCAM. Contact the Clearinghouse at:

P.O. Box 7923
Gaithersburg, Maryland 20898
Tel: 1-888-644-6226; outside U.S.: (301) 519-3153
Fax: 1-866-464-3616 (Toll-Free)
TTY: 1-866-464-3615 (Toll-Free)
E-mail: *info@nccam.nih.gov*
www.nccam.nih.gov/nccam/fcp/clearinghouse/

NCCAM Newsletter

www.nccam.nih.gov/nccam/ne/newsletter/

NCCAM Fact Sheets

Considering Complementary and Alternative Medicine Therapies?
www.nccam.nih.gov/fcp/faq/considercam.html

Frequently Asked Questions about CAM and the NCCAM

www.nccam.nih.gov/fcp/faq/index.html

General Information about the NCCAM

www.nccam.nih.gov/an/general/

NCCAM Clearinghouse

www.nccam.nih.gov/fcp/clearinghouse/index.html

CAM on Pub Med

This collection of more than 220,000 citations is accessed through the Pub Med database, which also includes Medline. Sponsored by the National Center for Pub Med can be accessed at:

www.nlm.nih.gov/nccam/camonpubmed.html

Combined Health Information Database (CHID)

The federally supported Combined Health Information Database (CHID) is another service in which NCCAM participates, which includes a variety of materials not available in other government databases. CHID aggregates health information for the public on numerous topical areas related to health and disease.

www.chid.nih.gov/

National Cancer Institute (NCI)

The National Cancer Institute has funded a number of CAM clinical trials, many in conjunction with NCCAM, including evaluation of the value of vitamins and minerals in cancer prevention and treatment, Gonzales nutritional therapy, angiogeneisis effects of shark and bovine cartilage, the effects of caratinoid nutrients on human papilloma viral lesions, the effect of natural inhibitors of carcinogenesis, and other types of natural products research.

www.nci.nih.gov/

NCI Office of Cancer and Complementary and Alternative Medicine

The Office of Cancer Complementary and Alternative Medicine (OCCAM) was established in October 1998 to coordinate and enhance the activities of NCI in the arena of complementary and alternative medicine (CAM). The goal of OCCAM is to increase the amount of high-quality cancer research and information about the use of complementary and alternative modalities

www3.cancer.gov/occam/

NCI Cancer Trials Database

www.nci.nih.gov/clinical_trials/

Quality and Safety Issues:
The Food and Drug Administration (FDA)

The FDA regulates dietary supplements under a different set of regulations than those covering "conventional" foods and drug products (prescription and over-the-counter). Under the Dietary Supplement Health and Education Act of 1994 (DSHEA), the dietary supplement manufacturer is responsible for ensuring that a dietary supplement is safe before it is marketed. FDA is responsible for taking action against any unsafe dietary supplement product after it reaches the market. Generally, manufacturers do not need to register with FDA nor get FDA approval before producing or selling dietary supplements. Manufacturers must make sure that product label information is truthful and not misleading. FDA's postmarketing responsibilities include monitoring safety, e.g., voluntary dietary supplement adverse event reporting, and product information, such as labeling, claims, package inserts and accompanying literature.

www.fda.gov/

FDA Food Safety Site

www.cfsan.fda.gov/

Dietary Supplements/Food Labeling Electronic Newsletter

www.cfsan.fda.gov/~dms/infonet.html - fda-dsfl

The Centers for Disease Control (CDC)

In the area of CAM, the CDC has taken a role in monitoring herbal supplements and has also analyzed data on nutritional supplements. Although their Web site does not post an area dedicated specifically to alternative medicine, a subject search yielded 40 documents, primarily reports in pdf files. All entries are relevance ranked to the topic. Of the first 20, 19 were published within the past 15 months. The CDC site also provides excellent up-to-date information regarding infectious disease, outbreaks, and epidemiology.

www.cdc.gov/

The Federal Trade Commission (FTC)

The FTC protects consumers by pursuing organizations that fraudulently market products and services on the Web. Recent enforcement actions have been taken and are currently underway.

www.ftc.gov/opa/2001/06/cureall.htm

Canadian Natural Health Products Directorate

This new office will have the authority to approve natural health products for the Canadian market, ensuring Canadian consumers safe, natural health products.

www.hc-sc.gc.ca/hpb/onhp/welcome_e.html

Health Protection Branch, Canada

Regulation and control of medical devices, product safety, drugs, etc.
www.hc-sc.gc.ca/hpb/

MedlinePlus

Designed for both health professionals and consumers MEDLINEplus has extensive information from the NIH and other trusted sources on about 500 diseases and conditions including CAM. There are also lists of hospitals and physicians, a medical encyclopedia and dictionaries, health information in Spanish, extensive information on prescription and nonprescription drugs, health information from the media, and links to thousands of clinical trials.

www.nlm.nih.gov/medlineplus/alternativemedicine.html

Healthfinder.gov

The Government Healthfinder is a massive directory that provides links to Web sites. It is essentially a searchable health portal linked to pre-selected quality government and private health-related sites, including those on complementary therapies. The Healthfinder can be searched by broad topic, by diagnosis and by therapy, linked primarily to Web resources and organizations.

A search on the keywords "alternative medicine" produced 149 Web resources and 66 organizations.

www.healthfinder.gov/

White House Commission on Complementary and Alternative Medicine Policy

President Clinton formed this commission to make recommendations on public policy and legislation pertaining to complementary and alternative medicine. Web site contains the Full White house Commission Report and transcripts of Town Hall meetings.

www.whccamp.hhs.gov/

CAM Directories:

The Rosenthal Center

A comprehensive and authoritative listing from Columbia University, NYC, of complementary and alternative medicine resources.

www.cpmcnet.columbia.edu/dept/rosenthal/

University of Pittsburgh

Alternative Medicine Home Page
www.pitt.edu/~cbw/internet.html

McMaster University Alternative Medicine Resources

A comprehensive Canadian directory of Web sites on the Internet.
www-hsl.mcmaster.ca./tomflem/altmed.html

New York Online Access to Health (NOAH)

Complementary and Alternative Medicine
www.noah-health.org/english/alternative/alternative.html

Yahoo Alternative Medicine

Contains a listing of over 500 CAM sites.
www.dir.yahoo.com/Health/Alternative_Medicine/

HealthWell

Features comprehensive information regarding alternative health and integrative medicine
www.healthwell.com

Popular Health Sites with Good CAM Information:

Ask Dr. Weil

DrWeil.com is a leading provider of online information and products for optimum health and wellness.
www.drweil.com/app/cda/drw_cda.php

InteliHealth

A comprehensive CAM site with a broad range of timely information.
www.intelihealth.com/IH/ihtIH/WSIHW000/8513/8513.html.

MedWeb Plus—Alternative Medicine

Extensive directory of CAM sites organized using the same "Alternative Medicine" Medical Subject Headings used by the National Library of Medicine.
www.medwebplus.com/subject/Alternative_Medicine.html

WebMD/Medscape

WebMD/Medscape—is quite a comprehensive site offering Internet-based medical information for consumers and professionals. Site includes extensive content on alternative and complementary medicine resources for patients. Registration is required.
www.medscape.com/

WholeHealthMD

WholeHealthMD.com is a partnership between leading companies in the health-care field: American WholeHealth and Rebus.
www.wholehealthmd.com/

Topical Sites and News:

HealthWell Natural News

www.healthwell.com/news/index.cfm

Natural Health Line

www.naturalhealthvillage.com/

Alternative Health News Online

www.altmedicine.com/FrameSet.asp

USA Today Health

www.usatoday.com/life/health/health.htm

Science Daily News

www.sciencedaily.com/index.htm

Health Watch Web Site

www.trufax.org/menu/health1.html

Medscape Medical Research News

www.medscape.com/medscapetodayhome

CNN Daily Updates on Health Topics

www.medscape.com/Home/Topics/multispecialty/multispecialty.html

Reuters Health Information Services, Inc.

www.reutershealth.com/

ABC NEWS.com: Health & Living News Index

www.abcnews.com/sections/Living/

New York Times Daily Health News: Your Health Daily

www.yourhealthdaily.com/

Laser Acupuncture:

www.Acupuncture.com/Acup/Naeser.htm
www.Acupuncture.com/Acup/laser.htm

Selected CAM Associations:

Complementary Medicine Association	Complementary Medicine	UK	www.the-cma.org.uk/
American Academy of Medical Acupuncture	Acupuncture	US	www.medicalacupuncture.org/
British Medical Acupuncture Society	Acupuncture	UK	www.medical-acupuncture.co.uk/
American Association of Naturopathic Physicians	Naturopathic	US	www.naturopathic.org/
American Chiropractic Association	Chiropractic	US	www.amerchiro.org/
The Canadian Chiropractic Association	Chiropractic	Canada	www.ccachiro.org/
British Chiropractic Association	Chiropractic	UK	www.chiropractic-uk.co.uk/
The American Herbalists Guild	Herbal Medicine	US	www.healthy.net/herbalists/
American Herbal Products Association	Herbal Medicine	US	www.ahpa.org/
British Herbal Medicine Association (BHMA)	Herbal Medicine	UK	www.info.ex.ac.uk/phytonet/bhma.html
American Holistic Medical Association	Holistic Medicine	US	www.holisticmedicine.org/
American Massage Therapy Association	Massage	US	www.amtamassage.org/
The Association of Physical and Natural Therapists	Herbal and Manual Therapies		www.apnt.org.uk/

British Homeopathic Association	Homeopathy	UK	www.trusthomeopathy.org/trust/tru_over.html
National Center for Homeopathy	Homeopathy	US	www.healthy.net/nch/
Touch For Health Association	Therapeutic Touch	US	www.tfh.org/

Academic Research Organizations and Institutions:

Bastyr University

A leading research center in natural health sciences.
www.bastyr.edu/

Beth Israel Medical Center, NY

Continuum Center for Health and Healing
The facility provides fully integrative care, employing safe and effective conventional and complementary therapies.
www.healthandhealingny.org/

Palmer Center for Chiropractic Research

Consortial Center for Chiropractic Research
www.palmer.edu

Harvard University

Osher Center for Alternative Medicine Research and Education
A leading research organization in CAM research programs, research, education information and clinical treatment. The center sponsors annual conferences:
www.bidmc.harvard.edu/medicine/camr

Minneapolis Medical Research Foundation

Center for Addiction and Alternative Medicine Research (CAAMR)
www.mmrfweb.org/caamrpages/caamrcover.html

Stanford University

Center for research in Disease Prevention

The Complementary and Alternative Medicine Program at Stanford (CAMPS) is researching the topic of successful aging.

www.camps.stanford.edu/

Tzu Chi Foundation

This Canadian organization's activities include clinical treatment programs, research, education and information.

www.tzuchi.org/

University of California Irvine

Susan Samueli Center for Complementary and Alternative Medicine

www.ucihs.uci.edu/com/samueli/

University of California San Francisco

Osher Center for Integrative Medicine

www.ucsf.edu/ocim/

University of Texas

M. D. Anderson Cancer Center Complementary Therapy Reviews

Extensive list of evidence-based summaries conducted on complementary therapies used in the treatment of cancer.

www.mdanderson.org/departments/cimer/dIndex.cfm?pn=6EB86A59-EBD9-11D4-810100508B603A14

Research Council for Complementary Medicine (RCCM)

A UK-based research organization and originators of CISCOM database.

www.gn.apc.org/rccm

Münchener Modell

Leading German CAM research organization dedicated to research education and patient care.

www.lrz-muenchen.de/~ZentrumfuerNaturheilkunde/

Exeter University

Research organization and publisher of FACT—Focus on Alternative and Complementary Therapies. A review journal that aims to present the evidence on complementary medicine in an analytical and impartial manner.

www.ex.ac.uk/

Some Evidence-Based Databases:

The Cochrane Library is an electronic publication produced by the Cochrane Collboration to supply high quality evidence to inform people providing and receiving care, and those responsible for research, teaching, funding and administration at all levels. It is published quarterly on CD-ROM and the Internet, and is distributed on a subscription basis. Contains over 5,700 reports of randomized controlled trials, and over 80 systematic reviews in complementary medicine.

www.cochranelibrary.com/clibhome/clib.htm

Cochrane Complementary Medicine Field Registry

To meet the growing need for evidence-based complementary medicine the Complementary Medicine Field promotes and facilitates the production and collection of systematic reviews in Complementary Medicine and continually maintains and updates a registry of randomized controlled trials. Registry contains over 6,000 trials. Located at the University of Maryland, Complementary Medicine Program (CMP).

Complementary Medicine Program Databases

This program facilitates systematic literature reviews and evaluation. Other databases include: The Arthritis and Complementary and Alternative Medicine

Database (ARCAM) and the Complementary and Alternative Medicine and Pain Database (CAMPAIN).

www.compmed.umm.edu/

CAM on PubMed:

National Center for Complementary and Alternative Medicine bibliographic citations obtained from the National Library of Medicine's PubMed (Medline) database that uses a feature to locate citations with a predetermined CAM search criteria.

www.nlm.nih.gov/nccam/camonpubmed.html

Selected Bibliography:

(Additional books on chapter topics can be found in footnotes and references throughout the text.)

Health and Aging:

Ornish, D. *Love & Survival: 8 Pathways to Intimacy and Health.* New York: Harper Collins, 1998.

Pelletier, K. R. *Longevity: Fulfilling Our Biological Potential at Any Age.* New York: Delta/Seymour Lawrence, 1981.

Perls, T. T and M. H. Silver. *Living to 100: Lessons in Living to Your Maximum Potential at Any Age.* New York: Basic Books, 1998.

Shealy, C. N. *Sacred Healing: The Curing Power of Energy and Spirituality.* London: Element Books, 1999.

Weil, A. *Spontaneous Healing.* New York: Knopf, 1995.

Ayurvedic Medicine

Frawley, D. *Ayurvedic Healing.* Salt Lake City: Morson Publishing, 1989.

Frawley, D. and V. Lad. *The Yoga of Herbs.* Santa Fe: Lotus Press, 1986.

Lad, V. *Ayurveda: The Science of Self-Healing.* Santa Fe: Lotus Press, 1986.

Lad, V. *Ayurvedic Cooking for Self-Healing.* Albuquerque: The Ayurvedic Press, 1994.

Morrison, J. J. H. *The Book of Ayurveda: A Holistic Approach to Health and Longevity*. New York: Simon & Schuster, 1995.

Singh Birla, G. *Destiny in the Palm of Your Hand: Creating Your Future through Vedic Palmistry*. Rochester, VT: Inner Traditions International, Limited/Destiny Books, 2000.

Svoboda, R. E. *Ayurveda: Life, Health and Longevity*. London: Penguin, 1992.

Svoboda, R. E. *Prakruti: Your Ayurvedic Constitution*. Albuquerque: Geocom Limited, 1989.

Cancer—General

Gearin-Tosh, M. *Living Proof: A Medical Mutiny*. New York: Scribner, 2002. An eloquent account of how one man grappled with cancer treatment decisions.

Gordon, J. S. *Comprehensive Cancer Care: Integrating Alternative, Complementary, and Conventional Therapies*. Cambridge, MA: Perseus: 2000. Dr. Gordon is the former Chair of the White House Commission on Complementary and Alternative Medicine and the founder/director of the Center for Mind/Body Medicine in Washington, DC. Please see Chapter Nine for a profile of Dr. Gordon and his work.

Lerner, M. *Choices in Healing: Integrating the Best of Conventional and Complementary Approaches to Cancer*. Cambridge, MA: MIT Press, 1994. This book provides information with compassion and humanity. In the Foreword, Jon Kabat-Zinn, Ph.D., writes:

"None of the alternatives presented here, as Lerner emphasizes, provides in any sense a definitive cure. But at the very least, the reader can gain a new vantage point from which to look at cancer and at possible ways to approach treatment decisions and the question of alternative therapies. At the same time, the reader can take comfort in Michael's assuring tone and the wisdom of his own deeply personal as well as professional inquiry into what is 'out there' in the way of treatment approaches and what is 'in here' in the way of different attitudes and disciplines one might explore for facing questions of health and illness, mind and body, diet, pain, death and dying."

Michael Lerner is founder and director of Commonweal Cancer Help

Program, a residential non-medical, educational program for people with cancer. Address: P. O. Box 316, Salinas, CA 94924; Phone: (415)-868-0970.

Cancer and Fruits and Vegetables

The Alpha-Tocopherol, Beta Carotene Cancer Prevention Study Group. "The Effect of Vitamin E and Beta Carotene on the Incidence of Lung Cancer and Other Cancers in Male Smokers." *New England Journal of Medicine* 330 (1994): 1029–1035.

Block, G., B. Patterson, and A. Subar. "Fruit, Vegetables, and Cancer Prevention: A Review of the Epidemiological Evidence." *Nutrition And Cancer* 18 (1992): 1–29.

Fariss, M. W., et al. "The Selective Antiproliferative Effects of Alpha-Tocopheryl Hemisuccinate and Cholesteryl Hemisuccinate on Murine Leukemia Cells Result from the Action of the Intact Compounds." *Cancer Research* 54 (1994): 3346–3351.

Omenn, G. S., et al. "Effects of a Combination of Beta Carotene and Vitamin A on Lung Cancer and Cardiovascular Disease." *New England Journal of Medicine* 334 (1996): 1150–1155.

Prasad, K. N. "Induction of Differentiated Phenotypes in Melanoma Cells by a Combination of an Adenosine 3',5'-Cyclic Monophosphate Stimulating Agent and D-Alpha Tocopheryl Succinate." *Cancer Letters* 44 (1989): 17–22.

Prasad, K. N. and J. Edwards-Prasad. "Effects of Tocopheryl (Vitamin E) Acid Succinate on Morphological Alterations and Growth Inhibition in Melanoma Cells in Culture." *Cancer Research* 42 (1982): 550–555.

Prasad, K. N., et al. "Vitamin E Increases the Growth Inhibitory and Differentiating Effects of Tumor Therapeutic Agents on Neuroblastoma and Glioma Cells in Culture." *Proceedings of the Society for Experimental Biology and Medicine* 164 (1980): 158–163.

Rama, B. N. and K. N. Prasad. "Effect of Hyperthermia in Combination with Vitamin E and Cyclic AMP on Neuroblastoma Cells in Culture." *Life Sciences* 34 (1984): 2089–2097.

Sahu, S. N. and K. N. Prasad. "Combined Effect of Adenosine 3',5'-Cyclic

Monophosphate Stimulating Agents, Vitamin E Succinate, and Heat on the Survival of Murine B-16 Melanoma Cells in Culture." *Cancer* 62 (1988): 949–953.

Sporn, M. B. and A. B. Roberts. "Role of Retinoids in Differentiation and Carcinogenesis." *Cancer Research* 43 (1983): 3034–3040

Steinmetz, K. A. and J. D. Potter. "Vegetables, Fruit, and Cancer II: Mechanisms." *Cancer Causes and Control* 2 (1991): 427–442.

Steinmetz, K. A. and J. D. Potter. "Vegetables, Fruit, and Cancer Prevention: A Review." *Journal of the American Dietetic Association* 96 (1996): 1027–1039.

Turley, J. M., et al. "Vitamin E Succinate Inhibits Proliferation of BT-20 Human Breast Cancer Cells: Increased Binding of Cyclin A Negatively Regulates E2F Transactivation Activity." *Cancer Research* 57 (1997): 2668–2675.

World Cancer Research Fund. *Food, Nutrition, and the Prevention of Cancer: A Global Perspective*. Washington, DC: American Institute for Cancer Research, 1997.

Cancer and Guided Imagery

Gruber, B. L., et al. "Immunological Responses of Breast Cancer Patients to Behavioral Interventions." *Biofeedback & Self-Regulation* 18, no. 1 (March 1993): 1–22.

Mastenbroek, I. and L. McGovern. "The Effectiveness of Relaxation Techniques in Controlling Chemotherapy Induced Nausea: A Literature Review." *Australian Occupational Therapy Journal* 38, no. 3 (September 1991): 137–142.

Rossman, M. L. *Healing Yourself: A Step-by-Step Program for Better Health Through Imagery*. New York: Pocket Books, 1989.

Simonton, O. C., S. Matthews-Simonton, and J. L. Creighton. *Getting Well Again*. New York: Bantam Books, 1992.

Watson, M. and C. Marvell. "Anticipatory Nausea and Vomiting Among Cancer Patients: A Review." *Psychology & Health* 6, no. 1–2 (January 1992): 97–106.

Yan, L., et al. "The Effect of Psycho-Behavioral Intervention on the Emotional Reaction and Immune Function in Breast Cancer Patients Undergoing Radiotherapy." *Acta Psychologica* (China: Science Press) 33, no. 5 (2001): 437–441.

Cancer and Medicinal Mushrooms

Franz, G. "Polysaccharides in Pharmacy: Current Applications and Future Concepts." *Planta Medica* 55 (1989): 493–497.

Ghoneum, M. "Immunomodulatory and Anticancer Properties of (MGN-3): A Modified Xylose from Rice Bran in 5 Patients with Breast Cancer." Abstract, 87th Meeting of the American Association of Cancer Research (AACR) Special Conference: "The Interference between Basic and Applied Research." November 5–8, 1995, Baltimore, MD.

Ghoneum, M. "Enhancement of Human Killer Cell Activity by Modified Arabinoxlane from Rice Bran (MGM-3)." *International Journal of Immunotherapy* 14, no. 2 (1998): 89–99.

Jong, S. C., J. M. Birmingham, and S. H. Pai. "Immunomodulatory Substances of Fungal Origin." *Journal of Immunology and Immunopharmacology* 11 (1991): 115–122.

Cochrane Collaboration

Berman, B. M. "The Cochrane Collaboration and Evidence-Based Complementary Medicine." *Journal of Alternative and Complementary Medicine* 3, no. 2 (1997): 191–194.

Chalmers, I., K. Dickersin, and T. C. Chalmers. "Getting to Grips with Archie Cochrane's Agenda." *British Medical Journal* 305, no. 6857 (1992): 786–788.

Dickersin, K. and E. Manheimer. "The Cochrane Collaboration: Evaluation of Health Care and Services Using Systematic Reviews of the Results of Randomized Controlled Trials." *Clinical Obstetrics and Gynecology* 41, no. 2 (1998): 315–331.

Ezzo, J., et al. "Complementary Medicine and the Cochrane Collaboration." *Journal of the American Medical Association* 280, no. 18 (1998): 1628–1630.

General Research and Reference

Cassileth, B. R. *The Alternative Medicine Handbook*. New York: W. W. Norton & Company, 1998.

Ernst, E., ed. *The Desktop Guide to Complementary and Alternative Medicine: An Evidence-Based Approach*. London: Harcourt Publishers Limited, 2001.

Freeman, L. W. *Best Practices in Complementary and Alternative Medicine: An Evidence-Based Approach with Nursing CE/CME*. Gaithersburg, MD: Aspen Publications, 2001

Fugh-Berman, A. *Alternative Medicine: What Works*. Philadelphia: William & Wilkins, 1997.

Goldstein, M. S. *Alternative Health Care: Medicine, Miracle, or Mirage?* Philadelphia: Temple University Press, 1999.

Gordon, J. S. *Manifesto for a New Medicine: Your Guide to Healing Partnerships and the Wise Use of Alternative Therapies*. Cambridge, MA: Perseus, 1996.

Horstman, J. and W. J. Arnold. *The Arthritis Foundation's Guide to Alternative Therapies*. Atlanta: Arthritis Foundation, 1999.

Jonas, W. B. and J. S. Levin, eds. *Essentials of Complementary and Alternative Medicine*. Baltimore: Lippincott, Williams & Wilkins, 1999.

Murray, M. and J. Pizzorno. *Encyclopedia of Natural Medicine*. Roseville, CA: Prima Publishing, 1998.

Pelletier, K. R. *The Best Alternative Medicine: What Works? What Does Not?* New York: Simon & Schuster, 2000.

Peters, D. and A. Woodham. *Natural Health® Complete Guide to Integrative Medicine: Combining the Best of Natural and Conventional Care*. New York: DK Publishing, 2000.

Pressman, A. and D. Shelley. *Integrative Medicine: The Patient's Essential Guide to Conventional and Complementary Treatments for More Than 300 Common Disorders*. New York: St. Martin's Press, 2000.

Healing

Dossey, L. *Meaning and Medicine: A Doctor's Tales of Breakthrough and Healing*. New York: Bantam Books, 1991.

Moyers, B. *Healing and the Mind*. New York: Doubleday, 1993.

Herbal Medicine

Duke, J. *The Green Pharmacy*. Emmaus, PA: Rodale Press, 1997.

Meditation and Health

Benson, H. *The Relaxation Response*. New York: William Morrow & Co., 1976.

_____. *Timeless Healing: The Power and Biology of Belief*. New York: Scribner, 1996.

Hanh, Thich Nhat. *Peace is Every Step: The Path of Mindfulness in Everyday Life*. New York: Bantam, 1991.

Kabat-Zinn, J. *Full Catastrophe Living: Using the Wisdom of Your Body and Mind to Face Stress, Pain, and Illness*. New York: Delacorte, 1990.

_____. *Wherever You Go, There You Are: Mindfulness Meditation in Everyday Life*. New York: Hyperion, 1994.

Traditional Chinese Medicine

Eisenberg, D. and T. L. Wright. *Encounters With Qi*. New York: W. W. Norton, 1995; 1985.

Kaptchuk, T. *The Web That Has No Weaver*. Chicago: Contemporary Books, 2000.

Reid, D. *The Complete Book of Chinese Health and Healing: Guarding the Treasures*. Boston: Shambhala, 1995.

Rothfeld, G. and S. Levert. *The Acupuncture Response: Balance Energy and Restore Health*. Chicago: Contemporary Books, 2002.

Tse, M. *Qigong for Health and Vitality*. New York: St. Martin's Griffin, 1995.

Women's Health

Balch, J. F. and P. A. Balch. *Prescription for Nutritional Healing*, 3rd edition. New York: Avery-Penguin Putnam, 2000.

Colbin, A. *Food and Our Bones: The Natural Way to Prevent Osteoporosis*. New York: Penguin Group, 1998.

Gaby, A. *Preventing and Reversing Osteoporosis*. Roseville, CA: Prima Publishing, 1995.

Northrup, C. *Women's Bodies, Women's Wisdom: Creating Physical and Emotional Health and Well-Being*. New York: Bantam, 1998.

INDEX

Own These Great
Principles of Health

Never Be Sick Again

One Disease • Two Causes • Six Pathways

Health Is a Choice
Learn How to Choose It

Raymond Francis, M.Sc.
with Kester Cotton

Foreword by
Harvey Diamond
Coauthor of the
#1 *New York Times*
Bestseller *Fit for Life*

Code #9543 • Paperback • $12.95

Never Be Sick Again is health in one lesson. Through provocative case studies and cutting-edge scientific research you will learn an entirely new way to look at health and disease. It is an approach that is easy to understand, yet so powerful that you may, indeed, never be sick again.

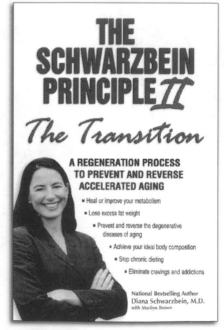

THE SCHWARZBEIN PRINCIPLE II

The Transition

A REGENERATION PROCESS TO PREVENT AND REVERSE ACCELERATED AGING

- Heal or improve your metabolism
- Lose excess fat weight
- Prevent and reverse the degenerative diseases of aging
- Achieve your ideal body composition
- Stop chronic dieting
- Eliminate cravings and addictions

National Bestselling Author
Diana Schwarzbein, M.D.
with Marilyn Brown

Since the release of her best-selling book, *The Schwarzbein Principle*, people have discovered a revolutionary way to lose weight, be healthy and feel younger. Now, in this groundbreaking follow-up Dr. Schwarzbein helps you live a more healthful lifestyle through a regeneration process to prevent and reverse accelerated aging.

Code #9640 • Paperback • $14.95

Available wherever books are sold.
To order direct: Phone 800.441.5569 • Online www.hcibooks.com
Prices do not include shipping and handling. Your response code is BKS.